THE SELF-HEALTH HANDBOOK

Brent Q. Hafen, Ph.D.
with Molly J. Brog, MA, and
Kathryn J. Frandsen,
Research Associates

PRENTICE-HALL, INC., Englewood Cliffs, New Jersey 07632 A SPECTRUM BOOK

Library of Congress Cataloging in Publication Data

HAFEN, BRENT Q
   The self-health handbook.

   (A Spectrum Book)
   Includes bibliographical references and index.
     1. Drugs—Popular works. 2. Therapeutics—Popular
works. I. Brog, Molly J., joint author. II. Frand-
sen, Kathryn J., joint author. III. Title. [DNLM:
1. Drugs—Popular works. 2. Drugs, Non-prescription—
Popular works. 3. Self medication—Popular works.
4. Cosmetics—Popular works. WB120 H138s]
RM301.15.H33 1980   615.5′8   80-17911
ISBN 0-13-803304-8
ISBN 0-13-803296-3 (pbk.)

Editorial/production supervision and
interior design by Carol Smith
Cover design by Judith Kazdym Leeds
Manufacturing buyer: Barbara A. Frick

© 1980 by Prentice-Hall, Inc.
Englewood Cliffs, New Jersey 07632

A SPECTRUM BOOK

10 9 8 7 6 5 4 3 2 1

Printed in the United States of America

PRENTICE-HALL INTERNATIONAL, INC., *London*

PRENTICE-HALL OF AUSTRALIA PTY. LIMITED, *Sydney*

PRENTICE-HALL OF CANADA, LTD., *Toronto*

PRENTICE-HALL OF INDIA PRIVATE LIMITED, *New Delhi*

PRENTICE-HALL OF JAPAN, INC., *Tokyo*

PRENTICE-HALL OF SOUTHEAST ASIA PTE. LTD., *Singapore*

WHITEHALL BOOKS LIMITED, *Wellington, New Zealand*

contents

iii

preface

For too many of us, medicine is shrouded in mystery. We wake up one morning with vague and mysterious symptoms. When that happens, we can either call a doctor or treat ourselves.

If we decide to see a doctor, we often find that from the time we enter the office until we leave with a prescription and have it filled by a pharmacist, we never understand fully exactly what we have, what caused it, or what we're taking to cure it. If we decide to treat ourselves with the ointments, pills, and capsules in our medicine cabinets, we might take something that cures us—but we could also harm or even kill ourselves.

This book has been written to take some of that mystery out of medicine, to help you understand drugs and how they work, how safe they are, which medicines can be taken under which conditions, and how to save money on prescriptions. It will also familiarize you with things you use every day—both medications and nonmedicinal items such as soap, shampoo, cosmetics, mouthwashes, and so on—and what you should have on hand.

Once you become acquainted with over-the-counter and prescription drugs, you'll know when it's safe to treat yourself and when you should consult a physician. Once the mystery is gone, you'll be able to take an active part in the care and well-being of your own body.

Acknowledgments

Special thanks to the following for their permission to reprint material:

- illustration of a prescription form on page 121 reprinted with permission from *Drug Therapy*, July 1979.

- herbs for specific areas of the body on pages 220–222 excerpted from *The Way of Herbs* by Michael Tierra. Published by Unity Press, Santa Cruz, CA (1980).

- "Medicinal Uses for Culinary Herbs" on pages 222–225 from *Well-Being* by Barbara Salat and David Copperfield. Copyright © 1975, 1976, 1977, 1978, 1979 by Well-Being Productions. Reprinted by permission of Doubleday & Company, Inc.

- herbal preparations and glossary on pages 225–227 from *Nutrition Almanac* by John D. Kirschmann. Copyright © 1979 by John D. Kirschmann. Used by permission of McGraw-Hill Book Company.

- "Toxic Reactions to Plant Products Sold in Health Food Stores" on pages 227–229 from *The Medical Letter*.

- chart on inorganic minerals on pages 252–257 from *The Vitamin Book* by the Editors of Consumer Guide®. Published by Simon & Schuster, Inc., 1979.

- chart on fiber content on certain foods on page 260 from *Journal of Human Nutrition* courtesy of John Libbey Co.

part one

OVER-THE-COUNTER DRUGS

1

using otc drugs

Over-the-counter (OTC) drugs—drugs that can be purchased without a prescription—are the most widely used in the country today. In fact, in 1977, $4 billion was spent on over-the-counter remedies.[1] The table that follows shows the breakdown of how much money was spent for which type of remedy.[2] Even those who do not visit a doctor regularly or who never have a prescription filled are likely to purchase and use over-the-counter drugs (the most common of which is aspirin) to get relief from headache, indigestion, constipation, mild aches and pain, skin irritations, or sleeplessness.

HOW MUCH AMERICANS SPENT ON OTC MEDICATIONS IN 1977

ITEM	DOLLARS SPENT
Cough and cold remedies	$ 843,520,000
Pain killers (internal)	832,490,000
Vitamins	519,580,000
Antacids	459,290,000
Laxatives	273,090,000
Pain killers (external)	147,700,000
Antiseptics (external)	83,880,000
Contraceptives	66,820,000
All others (burn remedies, eye washes, hemorrhoidal preparations, sleeping aids, etc.)	1,132,600,000
Total	$4,358,970,000

Currently, thousands of over-the-counter drugs are on the market.[3] But just because you can get them without a prescription is no reason to believe that they are harmless or that they should be used any time or all the time. The reason is that nonprescription drugs generally treat *symptoms*, that is, the changes from your normal healthy state that indicate something is wrong with your health. If you hide symptoms too long, you may think your health is restored. Actually, all you are doing is preventing your body from warning you of a possibly serious problem. Some OTC drugs are safe and beneficial in relieving minor symptoms, but none can ever "cure" disease—they only relieve the *symptoms*. The continuation of those symptoms is a sign that you should seek medical attention and that you will probably need a prescription medication. The improper or prolonged use of over-the-counter drugs may only aggravate your symptoms or even hide a condition that needs to be brought to the attention of your doctor.

PRECAUTIONS

Before we consider specific over-the-counter drugs and their effects, you should know several ways to protect yourself when dealing with OTC drugs in general.

1. *Get into the habit of reading labels.* The label tells you all you need to know. Read the drug's label carefully, and make sure the drug is the right one for your symptoms. You could avoid a serious complication or reaction by simply studying the ingredient listing; be especially careful if you know you have allergies. By law, labels on over-the-counter drugs must list the complete ingredients. To be a wise consumer, you should also be aware that federal law requires the following information on all OTC drug labels:

- *The name of the product*, along with the name and address of the manufacturer, distributor, or packer.

- *The active ingredients.* Some ingredients in medication are *inactive*; that is, they serve only to make the product a liquid or gel, to color it, to flavor it, or to do something that has no direct effect on healing or relieving symptoms. *Active* ingredients are the ones that actually help you—or harm you, if used improperly. This information is valuable for those with allergies. Also, by checking the active ingredients, you may be able to buy an identical product for less.

- *Directions for safe use.*

• *Cautions or warnings.* These caution you about such things as driving or operating machinery while taking the drug. They also warn about how long you should take the drug before seeing your doctor. A typical warning might read, "If symptoms persist for more than 24 hours, see your doctor."

2. *Follow directions.* The label on the bottle or tube contains important information regarding who can take the drug, the conditions under which the drug can be taken, whether it is safe to drive your car when you are taking the drug, and whether the drug is safe for children. If a leaflet is tucked inside the drug's box, read and study the leaflet also. Then make sure you follow the directions *exactly*—including, of course, dosage information.

Driving is a particular problem. We all know that we shouldn't drink and drive, but it's just as important that we do not "drug and drive," expecially on nonprescription drugs. Most of the pills, tablets, and capsules in your medicine chest—including aspirin, cold tablets, and allergy medication—can have definite adverse effects on your vision, your ability to concentrate, your coordination, and your judgment.[4] Whenever your doctor prescribes a drug, you have the opportunity to ask if it's safe to drive while you're using it. Whenever you buy and use a nonprescription drug, it's up to you to find out about its safety. Read the label—it usually tells you. And follow *all* directions on the label; it's foolish to take too many pills at once, to take them more often than you should, or to combine several drugs unless you know they are safe. If you can't figure out a label, call your doctor or pharmacist; they are happy to advise you.

Even after you have discerned that a drug is safe to use while driving, it's smart to find out how you react to the drug before you hit the road. Observe your own reaction. Each person reacts differently to a given drug, and your own reaction is based on a lot of things: your general health, your state of mind, your own chemical makeup, and the foods you have eaten today. If you start feeling lightheaded, dizzy, shaky, sleepy, or if your vision blurs while you are driving, pull over to the side of the road or take the nearest exit. Rest until you feel better. If you have to, call home and arrange for someone to come and get you. If you manifest any such symptoms before you set out, take a taxi or bus instead, or find a ride with someone else.

Finally, there's no substitute for sleep. Too many people try to drive long distances on too little sleep, using the various stay-awake pills that are available on the market. The major ingredient in those pills is caffeine, which won't kill you but which can give you a severely upset stomach if you get too much of it—making it hard for you to concentrate on your driving. And if you get motion sickness, the medication you need for that makes you drowsy too. Pull off the road and sleep, or let someone else drive. Driving takes acute concentration and the ability to make split-second decisions—which often spell the difference between life and death.

3. *Keep advertising in the proper perspective.* Before you buy an OTC drug, ask yourself whether you really need it. Or have you been convinced that you "need" it by a TV commercial, a friendly neighbor, or a magazine or newspaper? We've all seen commercials on television for products that promise instant relief from stomach gas, constipation, or headache. Use your common sense: Don't buy a drug to treat a problem you don't really have, don't expect instant cures, and don't require more from the drug than you can reasonably expect it to deliver. Remember: No drug can make you look younger, make you lose weight, or relieve a headache in two minutes.

4. *Ask questions.* If you are confused or unsure about which product to buy, ask a pharmacist for a recommendation. Pharmacists cannot legally diagnose disease or prescribe prescription medication, but they can (and will) advise you about over-the-counter drugs. If they tell you to see a doctor, take the advice. If you are unable to consult a pharmacist, call your doctor; he or she will be happy to advise you concerning the effectiveness of over-the-counter medications.

5. *Be extremely wary about mixing medications.* Before you take more than one drug at a time, ask your doctor about the consequences of mixing the medications. Some drugs just don't mix; others can create serious—even fatal—reactions. For instance, a man with a heart disease who regularly takes blood-thinning medication can die of hemorrhage shortly after taking two aspirin for a headache: The aspirin can further the blood-thinning action of the heart medication. More commonly, you might need to treat a combination of symptoms—typical among flu victims—and you might consider taking several over-the-counter drugs at the same time to relieve the symptoms. Ask your doctor or pharmacist first to make sure the drugs are compatible.

6. *Don't drink alcohol and use other drugs simultaneously.* Alcohol is a drug. Sleeping pills and antihistamines are only two of the drugs that result in extreme drowsiness when combined with alcohol; in some cases, coma results.

7. *Protect children from drugs.* If you have children, keep medications out of their reach—either in a high, inaccessible cabinet or in a locked cupboard or drawer. Also, check for safety packaging whenever you buy medications of any kind. Ask pharmacists to package the drugs that they dispense in child-proof packaging; when buying over-the-counter drugs, choose the ones with child-proof caps.

8. *Don't change packaging without consulting your pharmacist.* Some drugs are packaged in a certain way to preserve their potency and freshness. If you transfer the drug to a different bottle or container, you might destroy its potency. Your pharmacist can tell you whether you can safely switch containers.

9. *Stop taking the drug immediately if you suffer from adverse reactions.* Most labels can help you determine what the possible adverse reactions might be. So read the label, and pay attention to what your body is trying to tell you. If the reaction is particularly serious, you should consult your doctor.

10. *Be careful that you don't overdose.* Over-the-counter drugs that are completely safe in normal doses may cause kidney disease, enzyme imbalance, or even accidental poisoning and death if taken in large doses. Follow the directions carefully.

11. *Report your suspicions about a possible problem drug.* If you have a bad experience with an OTC drug, call the local office of the Food and Drug Administration. (The offices are listed in the telephone directory under "United States Government, Department of Health, Education, and Welfare.") Drugs that don't seem right or that cause unexpected or bizarre reactions may have been manufactured improperly, and federal law provides for the inspection and regulation of over-the-counter drugs.

12. *Learn how to take medication, that is, how to "deliver" it.* Know the most common forms of delivery for OTC drugs, as well as the correct way to use an OTC product. These guidelines may help you:[5]

- *Tablets and capsules:* Swallow a mouthful of water or wet the inside of the mouth with water before taking the medication. Place the capsule on the back of the tongue, and then drink water.

- *Liquids:* The problem with liquids is that some people do not read the labels to be sure they are getting the proper dosage. Also, they do not use a uniform measuring implement to take the medication. How many different-sized spoons do you have at your house? Pharmacists can help you solve this problem. Ask them to give you a special measuring spoon so that you are taking the same dosage of the product at all times. Also remember to shake the medication thoroughly. Some liquids have a tendency to separate; in other words, the doses that come off the top of the bottle may be less potent than those at the bottom.

• *Powders:* Sprinkle the product evenly on the affected area making sure that you do not inhale any of the powder.

• *Ointments and creams:* Apply these products as thinly as possible, and massage them into the skin until there is no trace. If you have especially dry skin, moisten or immerse the skin before applying the ointment or cream.

• *Aerosol sprays:* Shake the product thoroughly. Hold the container upright about 4 to 6 inches from the area. Press the nozzle for several seconds, and then release. Do not use the spray near your face or eyes.

• *Eye drops:* Wash your hands before applying drops. Lie or sit down, and tilt your head back. Pull the lower lid down to form a pouch. Hold the dropper close to your eye, but do not touch it. Drop the liquid into the pouch (not directly onto the eyeball—the medicine will be blinked out). Close your eyes, and keep them closed for a few minutes.

• *Eardrops:* Tilt the head to the side, with the affected ear up. Grasp the ear lobe, and pull it back. Do not touch the ear canal with the dropper. The drops should be neither too cool nor too warm. A good way to bring them to a comfortable temperature is to roll the bottle back and forth between your hands. Never warm them in boiling water; they should not be too warm.

• *Nose drops and sprays:* Before applying either product, gently blow your nose. To apply drops, tilt your head back and put the drops into the nose without touching the nasal linings with the applicator. Keep your head tilted back, and sniff gently. For nasal sprays, keep your head in an upright position. Insert the applicator into your nose, trying not to touch the linings. Squeeze the container and sniff the medication into the nose at the same time. Keep squeezing the bottle until you withdraw it from your nose so that mucous and bacteria are not sucked into the sprayer. The problem with sprays and drops is that bacteria can build up and multiply in the container, causing more serious effects than the original problems. So do not use someone else's nasal spray or drops. Do not use any nasal drops or spray longer than one week from one bottle.

13. *Make sure all OTC drugs in your possession are fresh and potent.* On a regular basis, clean out your medicine cabinet and throw away the drugs that you have had on hand for more than a year. (A good method of disposal is flushing the drugs down the toilet—children may find a handful of attractive tablets in a trash can and mistake them for candy.)

14. *Just as foods can interfere with the results of clinical laboratory tests, so can certain common prescription and over-the-counter drugs.* Tests results have been upset by antibiotics, tranquilizers, aspirin, laxatives, cough and cold remedies, oral contraceptives, and vitamins. These medications can give a "false positive" or "false negative" reading in tests. Certain changes can also occur such as physical changes (such as a change in the color of urine) and biological changes (changes in the electrolyte concentration of blood and urine for example).[6]

Finally, you will be able to use over-the-counter drugs intelligently if you learn the symptoms and illnesses they treat, the symptoms of common illnesses, how the drugs work, and which brands are most effective.

SUPPLYING YOUR MEDICINE CABINET

Before going into detail throughout the other chapters in *part one,* we recommend taking a close look at the contents of your medicine cabinet. Is it ready for an emergency? You might check the contents of your cabinet with the OTC medications listed below.[7] Be sure to come back to this table to reevaluate the list after you have read the section on OTC drugs.

- Aspirin, used to reduce fever, reduce swelling, and relieve pain; should not be used by those with gastrointestinal disease or allergy.
- Band-Aids.
- Caladryl Lotion, used for skin irritations.
- Bandages and compresses.
- Di-Gel liquid, used to combat gas and acid indigestion.
- Fleet Enema, for severe constipation.
- Neosporin ointment, on minor skin abrasions that could lead to infection.

- Robitussin CF Syrup or some other cough syrup you have found effective and safe in treating your own cough.

- Tylenol, or some other nonaspirin pain reliever.

- Vaseline.

- Nose drops or spray.

- Cold medication you have found safe and effective.

- Milk of Magnesia, for constipation.

- Kaopectate, for diarrhea.

- Eye drops, if you suffer from frequent eye irritations due to pollutants in the air or glare from sun or snow.

- Syrup of Ipecac, used to induce vomiting in cases of accidental poisoning.

- Sunscreen lotion.

- An antacid you have found safe and effective.

- Adhesive tape.

- Elastic bandages.

- Iodine, hydrogen peroxide, or rubbing alcohol, to use as an antiseptic for mild abrasions or cuts.

- Some type of gargle or mouthwash for relief of throat symptoms.

- An antihistamine compound for allergies.

- Moisturizing creams and lotions for dry skin.

- Hemorrhoid preparations.

- Baking soda.

BEING YOUR OWN DOCTOR

When you take nonprescription drugs, you are responsible for what happens because you are the one in control. You decide occasionally—with the help of your doctor—that you need to take the medication to begin with. You stand in the aisle at the pharmacy or drugstore, surrounded by neat little rows of brightly colored boxes, tubes, and bottles. You choose what to buy. And you take the medicine for yourself.

When you do so, you join a large segment of this country's population. For every American who sees a doctor, three treat themselves, usually with over-the-counter drugs. In any two-day period, 40 percent of the population in the United States take some kind of over-the-counter product. Women are the greatest users of nonprescription drugs; they report more muscle and joint pains, sleeplessness, backache, nervousness, weight problems, faintness, constipation, and headaches than men do. Men report more coughing.[8] All ages use nonprescription drugs. People from higher social and economic classes use more, because they tend to be more aware of symptoms and more apt to do something for relief. Whites spend much more than blacks.

Well over half of the symptoms that these Americans are trying to relieve are gastrointestinal disorders, symptoms of the common cold, or headache. So despite the almost limitless numbers of medicines available over the counter, only a very narrow product category is represented: Most OTC drugs are designed to relieve the symptoms of the common cold, digestive distress (including constipation), skin problems (most notably acne), and simple pain (predominantly headache).

These over-the-counter drugs are generally a good buy—*if* you use them as intended, of course. Nonprescription drugs account for only 3 cents of the American health dollar: We spend 42 cents for hospital care, 20 cents for doctors, 7 cents for prescription drugs, and 7 cents for dental care. Nonprescription drugs haven't soared very high on the inflation spiral, either. In a ten-year period, while the average price of consumer goods rose 64.6 percent and the cost of hospital care soared 73.5 percent, the cost of over-the-counter remedies went up only 32.5 percent.

From a consumer's point of view, you have the right and the opportunity to complain about dissatisfaction. You should be satisfied with the products you buy over the counter. If you're not, contact the local chapter of the Food and Drug Administration; they are an agency specifically created to make sure that Americans get a fair shake on the remedies they buy over the counter.

You have the ability to become an intelligent and safe user of over-the-counter drugs. Use your common sense and any knowledge you can gain from reading books like this one. When you're bothered with a symptom, try to determine what is causing it; you might be able to alleviate the cause and do without the medicine. For instance, when you realize you are constipated because you haven't been drinking enough water, you need a tall, cool glass of water, not a laxative. Try to gauge the severity of your symptoms; at times, it's wise and safe to treat yourself, and other times it is critical that you see a doctor. Don't try to mask your symptoms with over-the-counter remedies when you know you should seek medical attention. Use over-the-counter drugs as a temporary way to gain relief while you are waiting to see the doctor.

Again, you are responsible for yourself when it comes to self-treatment, and you're worth taking the time to do it right.

2

colds, coughs, and the flu

The most widespread human illness is the common cold.[1] It is also the most expensive illness in the United States. Over $500 million is spent each year on OTC drugs in an attempt to relieve cold symptoms. Almost $5 billion is lost each year through lost wages and medical expenses, making the common cold a condition that causes more time lost from work and school than all other diseases combined.[2] In terms of productivity, that $5 billion figure means about one million person-years of work is lost each year—all from the common cold.[3]

SYMPTOMS

Besides the cold's most common characteristic, a runny and stuffy nose, the signs of a common cold include a sore or dry throat, headache, cough, hoarseness, and sneezing; sometimes a cold is accompanied by burning eyes, muscle aches, or chilling. Colds are generally not characterized by a fever over 100°, chest pains, diarrhea, or vomiting. Generally lasting from one to two weeks, by the time a cold has run its course, it usually affects the linings of the nose, throat, bronchial tubes, and lungs.

Other infectious diseases, however, may at first have the very same symptoms. The runny or stuffy nose might indicate just a cold or the onset of several other common illnesses, such as:[4]

1. The *flu*, also caused by a combination of viruses, usually lasts from three to seven days (in some rare cases, up to ten days). It is characterized by fever (usually over 101°), headache, a "blah" feeling, loss of appetite, vomiting, diarrhea, coughing, muscle aches (including backache), burning and redness of the eyes, and some nasal discharge. Less frequent symptoms of the flu include hoarseness, a sore throat, sneezing, and chest discomfort.

2. *Strep throat*, which lasts up to five days in adults and up to ten days in children, is occasionally accompanied by nasal discharge or obstruction. Other symptoms include a severe sore throat, fever (usually over 102°), swollen glands (especially in the neck), headache, loss of appetite, pus on the tonsils, and occasional cough, ear ache, and nausea and vomiting. Strep throat can be a very dangerous condition in children; if not treated, it can turn into rheumatic fever which can cause permanent heart damage.

3. *Sinusitis*, a bacterial infection of the sinuses, can be determined where there is a pain and tenderness over the sinuses in the head and face, a headache that gets worse at night and better during the day, or a fever.

4. *Allergy*—especially hay fever—is among the ailments most commonly confused with a cold. The most obvious way to distinguish between the two is to determine the regularity and pattern of the symptoms' occurrence: The average American adult gets two to three colds a year. Although catching colds may seem to be fairly unpredictable, more people tend to have colds during three peak seasons: in the autumn (a few weeks after school opens), in mid-winter, and in the spring.

On the other hand, allergy symptoms can occur regularly as the seasons change, or only when you are around cats, or whenever you pick certain flowers, or whenever you are in a particularly dusty room. Besides a running or stuffy nose, an allergy is marked by sneezing (especially in the morning), severe itching of the nose, eyes and throat, and redness and tearing of the eyes. The air passages are frequently blocked; less often, victims suffer from coughing, wheezing, and asthma.

CAUSES

A virus causes the common cold. In fact, any one of 125 different viruses can cause a cold, and over 60 are directly responsible for the telltale runny or stuffy nose.[5] Despite the popularity of many myths, colds are not caused by walking in the rain, getting your feet wet and cold, going outdoors after a shower or bath, washing your hair and going outside, exposure to a north wind, or standing in a draft. In fact, you are less likely to catch a cold while walking in the rain barefooted by yourself than you are while sitting in a warm room, enjoying the company of friendly snifflers and sneezers. And you don't have to kiss persons to catch their colds, or even be close to them while they sneeze and cough. You are more likely to catch a cold by shaking hands or by handling a contaminated object—a pencil sharpener at the office, a bus railing, a bathroom doorknob, or a drinking glass that has been handled by someone with a cold.[6]

TREATMENT
Because the cold is caused by a virus, you can do only so much to combat it:

1. There is no cure for the cold. Drugs and home remedies simply serve to relieve the cold's symptoms, making the cold more bearable. They bring only temporary relief while the body builds its own defenses. If $5 billion are lost in wages and medical expenses each year due to the common cold, you might ask how much would be lost if we didn't use any cold medication at all? Or if we used *twice* as much? The answer is $5 billion—the same amount! Increased drug dosing for colds does not shorten a cold, nor does it increase a worker's productivity.

2. A cold must therefore run its course, but you should take whatever measures you can to make yourself more comfortable while you have the cold.

3. Be wary if a fever develops. It's a sign of a secondary infection. Call your doctor if your fever lasts more than two days or if it climbs over 101° in adults and 102° in children.

4. Be careful of a sore throat, which can also be a sign of secondary infection—especially a strep throat. Untreated, a strep infection can result in kidney inflammation or rheumatic fever. Call your doctor if your throat is sore for longer than two days.

5. Antibiotics are not effective in fighting viruses. So do *not* take an antibiotic that was prescribed for someone else or an antibiotic delivered by a well-meaning friend. Not only is an antibiotic ineffective, it can hurt you: If you take an antibiotic needlessly, your body can build up a resistance to the drug. Then, when you really need it to fight off a bacterial infection, you will be immune to its healing action.

6. Stay in bed (if you can) and drink lots of fluids. We aren't sure why, but these old home remedies really seem to work in lessening the cold's severity and in shortening its stay.

7. Take whichever drugs you choose for as long as the cold lasts—*but no longer*. A cold should never last longer than ten days; if it does or if the symptoms get worse instead of better, call your doctor.

8. Change medications during a cold as your symptoms ease up. In other words, "let the punishment fit the crime." Treat only the symptoms you have—not the ones you anticipate. Also, treat each symptom individually by an active ingredient and by the amount of the ingredient that you need. For example, suppose you have been using a decongestant (to break up stuffiness and to dry up a runny nose) that also contains aspirin (to cool a slight fever)—such as Alka-Seltzer Plus Cold Medicine. Once your fever is gone, you should switch to a drug that contains only a decongestant, such as Dristan time capsules or Neo-Synephrine drops.[7]

As a general rule, avoid products that combine two of these active ingredients for the treatment of a single symptom, such as fever or stuffiness. Also avoid products that do not indicate the amounts of the active ingredients on the label.

CLASSES OF DRUGS
To select the right drug for treatment of a given set of symptoms, you have to know which *class* of drug is best suited for what ails you. Tailoring your drug-therapy program therefore means you have to determine, first, which symptoms you have to treat and, second, which drugs will do what you want them to do. There's a lot to know. So let's examine the major classes of drugs commonly used to combat cold symptoms.

Analgesics
Analgesics act to relieve pain and to reduce fever.[8] The most common one, of course, is aspirin. A number of cold medications (capsules, tablets, drops, and sprays) contain analgesics (including aspirin):[9] Alka-Seltzer Plus Cold Medicine, Bayer Decongestant Cold Tablet, Cenagesic, Chexit, Colrex, Coricidin "D," Coryban-D, Co-Tylenol, Dristan, Duadacin, Duradyne-Forte, Flavihist, Ginsocap, Kiddisan, Neo-Synephrine compound cold tablet, Pyrroxate, Romilar, Super Anahist, Triaminicin, Sinarest, Sine-Off, Sinulin, Sinustat, Sinutab, Ursinus, Bayer Children's Cold Tablet, Bromo Quinine, Congespirin, Ornex,

4-Way Cold Tablet, Sine-Aid, Sinutab II, Coricidin, Coricidin medilet, and Toloxidyne.

Take drugs containing an analgesic only as long as you suffer from a headache or a low-grade fever; they are also helpful in minimizing any muscle aches or pains that may accompany a cold. As soon as these symptoms disappear, switch to a cold medication that does not contain aspirin or some other analgesic. Because aspirin and other analgesics can have some bad side effects, you should not continue to use a product containing aspirin if you no longer need it. (You can also choose, of course, to take *only* aspirin when you have a cold; we will discuss aspirin and its effects later in this chapter.) Many cold remedies have aspirin or acetaminophen in them as secondary ingredients. Read the labels so you know whether the medication you are taking contains an analgesic. If you don't check and are already taking aspirin or acetaminophen, you may be doubling up on analgesics and experience an adverse effect.

People who have an allergy to aspirin, asthma, a heart condition for which they are taking medication, a stomach ulcer, gastritis, or frequent stomach upsets should *not* take any cold medications containing aspirin. Instead, they should read labels and find a medication that contains acetaminophen or salicylamide, not aspirin. Co-Tylenol, Neo-Synephrine cold tablet, and Sinutab are examples.

Several analgesics (especially phenacetin) can damage the kidneys if the drug is taken for a long period of time—another good reason to switch to a different drug once you no longer need an analgesic. Phenacetin is listed on the label of any medication that contains it; in addition, most of the labels warn that kidney damage may result from prolonged use.

Decongestants

Decongestants work on the victim of most of the cold's ill effects, the nose.[10] They unplug a stuffy nose and dry up a runny nose, making them a valuable medication in the relief of cold symptoms. Decongestants work by constricting the small arteries in the lining of the ears, nose, sinuses, and bronchial tubes. This constriction reduces inflammation. As the inflammation disappears, the linings shrink in size, drainage takes place, pain decreases, and stuffiness is relieved. Thus the person can "breathe easy" once more.

Decongestants generally come in two forms: tablet or capsule and spray or drops. Tablets and sprays contain the same medicine; it is just applied differently. Sprays and drops, applied directly to the nasal lining, reach greater areas of congestion and give quick relief. Sprays tend to be more convenient than drops. A tablet or capsule releases drugs into the blood stream, where they eventually work their way to the nasal lining. At that point, they work in much the same way as a spray or drops. Oral decongestants tend to work for a longer period of time, but they don't produce as much constriction of the arteries as sprays or drops do.

You should note some dangers with these drugs. Oral decongestants can change your blood pressure, so persons having high blood pressure should ask their doctors before using them. Tablets or capsules also increase blood sugar, which may be a danger for diabetics. Because the action of sprays or drops is spontaneous, you can easily get too much, and too much can inflame the nasal lining even more on the "rebound" up to several days after you begin using the medication. It has been found that those nasal sprays or drops that cause the least "rebound" effect are Afrin, Duration, and Sinex, L.A.

Several cautions should be exercised when using decongestant drugs:[11]

• *Don't take decongestants at night.* A common side effect is difficulty falling asleep. Take your evening dosage of decongestant two to three hours before bedtime; that way, the drug will still be working on your nasal passages—so you can breathe—but it will not be potent enough to keep you awake.

• *If the mucus in your nose is thick or viscid, don't use drops or spray.* The mucus will form a barrier, and the medicine won't be able to touch the swollen membranes.

• *Don't take an oral decongestant at the same time you are using a spray or drops.* Overdosing is easy.

• *Don't use nose drops that have an oil base.* First of all, a water-based drop makes more efficient contact with the membrane. Second, inhalation of droplets of oil can cause irritation in the lungs, leading to lipid pneumonia.

• *Jellies are not as effective as drops or sprays.* They often merely coat the debris in the nose. Most are washed out with the discharge or with blowing the nose.

• *Use decongestants for congestion or pain in your ears.* The medicine also acts to shrink membranes in the ear passages, which swell and put painful pressure on the middle ear. In some cases of eustachian tube swelling, you might feel no pain, but you become dizzy; decongestants are also recommended in this case.

• *Decongestants make some people slightly nervous.* (since they stimulate the central nervous system). If the nervousness becomes a problem, you should discontinue use.[12]

• *Don't use any kind of decongestant, if* you are under treatment for diabetes, thyroid disease, high blood pressure, or heart disease, unless it is prescribed by a doctor. Decongestants directly oppose the effects of insulin.[13]

• *Decongestants might make urinating difficult.* So it might be wise to urinate just before taking them.

On labels, decongestants appear as: phenylephrine hydrochloride (HCl), phenylpropanolamine HCl, ephedrine, naphazoline HCl, tetrahydrozoline, I-desoxyephedrine, methoxyphenamine, pseudoephedrine HCl, and oxymetazoline HCl.

Nose sprays, nose drops, and inhalers that contain *only* a decongestant include: Afrin (spray), Alconefrin (drops, spray), Anit-B (spray), Benzedrex (inhaler, also contains aromatics), Coryban-D (spray), Duration (spray), Forthane (inhaler), Gluco-Fedrin (drops), Isophrin (drops, spray), Neo-synephrine (drops, spray, jelly), Privine (drops, spray), Rhinall (drops, spray), Sine-Off Once-A-Day (spray), Vicks (inhaler), and Vicks Sinex (spray).[14] Two liquids—Novafed and Sudafed—contain only a decongestant.

Tablets, capsules, and sprays that contain a decongestant combined with an analgesic or other auxiliary drug include: Bayer Children's Cold Tablets, Bromo Quinine, Congespirin, Ornacol, Ornex, 4-Way Cold Tablet, Sine-Aid, and Sinutab II.

All the decongestant tablets currently on the market—except Sudafed tablets—are combinations of decongestants and antihistamines; they will be listed in the next section with the antihistamine drugs.

Antihistamines

Antihistamines[15] stop sneezing and clear stuffy noses. They do so by blocking the action of *histamines*, which are released in excessive amounts in both allergies and colds. They represent a kind of allergic reaction on the part of the body either to the virus that causes the cold or to the agent that causes the allergy. The result for the victim is sneezing and a stuffy nose. Antihistamines, then, keep the histamines from doing their job—and presumably stop your sneezing and clear your stuffy nose. Antihistamines are found in almost all cold remedies, because serious toxicities are seldom noticed in adults and they are safe for children to take.

Despite their relative safety, exercise two cautions if you decide to take an antihistamine. First of all, because they cause drowsiness, don't operate machinery or drive a car after taking medicine containing an antihistamine. Second, antihistamines increase the effects of alcohol;

so don't drink beer, wine, or hard liquor while you're taking the medicine.

Antihistamines also have other side effects with high doses. In adults, the side effects may be a dry mouth, blurred vision, inability to urinate, and constipation. In children, an accidental overdose may cause excitement, lack of coordination, muscular twitching, convulsions, and flushed skin.

Antihistamines appear on the medicine label as: chlorpheniramine maleate, methapyrilene fumarate, pyrilamine maleate, pheniramine maleate, phenindamine tartrate, phenyltoloxamine dihydrogen citrate, thonzylamine HCl, thenyldiamine HCl, and chlorcyclizine HCl.

Only a few cold remedies on the market contain *only* antihistamines. Chlor-Trimeton liquid and tablets contain only antihistamines. Several contain an antihistamine and an analgesic;[16] these are Coricidin tablets, Coricidin medilet chewable children's tablets, and Toloxidyne tablets.

Because decongestants and antihistamines work together well and because they help cancel out each other's bad effects, it is recommended that you take an antihistamine/decongestant if you do not need the pain-relieving benefits of an analgesic. Cold remedies that contain both antihistamines and decongestants include:[17] Allergesic, Allerest, A.R.M., Axon, Chlor-Trimeton decongestant tablet, Demazin, Dristan, Fedrazil, Ginsopan, Novafed A, Novahistine, Novahistine Fortis, Novahistine LP, Novahistine Melet, Tetramine T. R., Triaminic syrup, Triaminicin children's chewable tablet, Vasominic, Allerest spray, Contac spray, Coridicin spray, Dristan spray, Dristan vapor spray, Mistol Mist spray, Naso-Mist spray, NTZ drops and spray, Soltice spray, Vicks Va-tro-nol drops, and 4-Way spray.

When you have all of the common cold's symptoms, however, you may need the effects of antihistamines, decongestants, and analgesics. *For as long as you need all these medicinal effects,* you might try one of the following:[18] Alka-Seltzer Plus Cold Medicine, Bayer Decongestant Cold Tablet, Cenagesic, Chexit, Colrex, Contac tablets, Coricidin "D" tablets, Coricidin demilet, Coryban-D, Co-Tylenol, C3, Dristan tablets, Duadacin, Duradyne-Forte, Flavihist, Ginsocap, Kiddisan, Neo-Synephrine compound cold tablet, Pyrroxate, Romilar, St. Joseph's children's decongestant cold relief tablet, Super Anahist, Triaminicin, Sinarest, Sine-Off, Sinulin, Sinustat, Sinutab, and Ursinus.

Home Remedies

Besides the over-the-counter tablets, capsules, drops, or sprays, you can find nonmedicinal remedies in the kitchen cupboards that help you relieve some of the miseries of the common cold.[19]

Sore Throat. The most popular home remedy for a sore throat, of course, is to gargle with hot salt water. A sore throat can also be soothed if you take a spoonful of sugar, suck on a piece of hard candy, or use a vaporizer to moisturize the air. (A pot of boiling water works too.) Antibacterial mouthwashes, gargles, and cough drops do not work against a common cold, because a cold is caused by a virus, not by bacteria.

Hoarseness. Gargles, washes, or drops are all ineffective against hoarseness, because they can't reach your vocal chords, which are located at the top of the windpipe. The best remedy for hoarseness is to rest your voice; you can also try humidifying the air, along with avoiding dust, smoke, and fumes of any kind.

Coughing. If your chest is congested but your cough isn't expelling any mucus, the mucus is probably too thick. Drink plenty of water and other fluids, and try humidifying the room.

What About Vitamin C?
In 1970, Nobel Prize winner Dr. Linus Pauling recommended vitamin C as useful both for preventing colds and for reducing the severity of the cold's symptoms. Since Dr. Pauling's announcement, chemists and physicians have been testing the vitamin to see if it does indeed reduce the severity of the cold or prevent its occurrence in the first place. No one can argue that sound nutrition is important in the body's ability to fight off any infection, but Dr. Pauling recommended a dosage of vitamin C that was 300 times the recommended daily allowance. Such a high dosage can actually be harmful to the body in the following ways:[20]

• High doses of vitamin C cause diarrhea, which can lead to dehydration in severe or prolonged cases.

• Vitamin C increases the amount of uric acid in the urine and may lead to kidney stone formation.

• Vitamin C affects the amount of insulin manufactured by and needed by the body, and it can be extremely hazardous in large amounts to diabetics. In addition, vitamin C affects the "testape" reading, affecting a diabetic's ability to determine the insulin level of his blood.

• High doses of vitamin C interfere with the actions and benefits of other drugs.

• High doses of vitamin C may prompt spontaneous abortion.

• High doses of vitamin C may wash calcium from the bones, causing severe problems in elderly people who may have osteoarthritis.

A cough—basically just an explosive release of air from the lungs—is generally caused by some kind of irritation, either of the lungs themselves or of the linings of the air passages within the lungs. Over-the-counter medications can suppress certain kinds of coughs. You've got a wide variety to choose from when you go to the drugstore for a cough medicine: There are over 800 cough remedies on the druggists' shelves.[21]

There are three general types of coughs:[22]

1. A *productive cough* produces phlegm or mucus, which is raised with the coughing. A productive cough is the body's way of cleansing the lungs; it gets rid of debris lodged in the lungs as a result of infection or disease.

2. A *nonproductive cough* (dry cough) is just that—nonproductive. This kind of a cough does *not* raise sputum or mucus; the typical dry cough is the "smoker's hack." A dry cough usually accompanies the late stages of a cold, but it can also come in the early stages of serious diseases such as lung cancer and tuberculosis. You should be concerned with a nonproductive cough that accompanies severe chest congestion: The body wants to cleanse the debris out of the lungs, but for some reason it is unable to do so—probably because the mucus or phlegm is too thick.

3. A *croupy cough* results from a great deal of phlegm. Someone with the "croup" has a hard time breathing and experiences spasms of the voice box.

CAUSES
You must determine specifically what is *causing* the cough so you can treat the cause, not just the symptom. Coughs can be caused by:[23]

• infections of the upper respiratory tract (including flu and the common cold),

• infections of the lungs or air passages (either bacterial or viral, such as pneumonia or bronchitis),

- infections in the lungs caused by yeasts or tuberculosis,

- tumors (in the lungs or the lung passages),

- blood clots in the lungs or air passages,

- irritations of the lungs and air passages (from cigarette smoking, coal dust, aerosol sprays, paint fumes, or other chemical toxins),

- allergies,

- heart failure and heart disease,

- diseases of the lung (such as emphysema),

- nervousness, or dryness of the mouth and throat.

TREATMENT

As you can see, some causes of a cough are actually serious diseases or conditions that require prompt medical attention. Coughing is also the first symptom of lung cancer. You should see a doctor immediately if any of the following happens:[24]

- You cough up blood. It can be either rusty-colored or bright red, and it can be either in clots or mixed with the sputum.

- You notice a fever, weight loss, or shortness of breath accompanying the cough.

- The coughing is extremely painful.

- The sputum that accompanies the cough is foul-smelling or foul-tasting.

- You experience a change in the pattern of coughing.

- Your cough lasts for more than ten days.

- Your cough does not respond to over-the-counter cough medicines. Coughs that respond are usually only a symptom of a cold or the flu; coughs that do not respond are usually indicative of a more serious problem.

- You faint during or after a coughing spell.

Even if a cough is not a symptom of serious illness, certain kinds should still not be treated with drugs and should not be suppressed. A cough can sometimes be literally a lifesaver: A woman who is choking on a piece of roast beef should be encouraged to cough with vigor so that she can dislodge the obstruction in her throat. A man with a lot of debris in his lungs needs to cough to get rid of it. Certain people who are unable to cough (victims of stroke, polio, or muscle disease or persons under the influence of barbiturates, opium, or anesthesia following surgery) can drown in their own bronchial secretions. And, of course, people who cough because they are nervous or because they are trying to get attention should not be treated with drugs. We are concerned only with the kinds of coughs that should be treated with drugs.

Before you look for a drug, try a few nonmedicinal remedies. If one of them provides relief, you do not have to take a drug needlessly.[25] For example, sucking hard candy sometimes does the trick by soothing a scratchy throat, one of the leading causes of a dry cough. Of the more than 43 billion cough drops sold each year in this country, most have a soothing effect and a pleasant taste, yet none of them is more effective than simple hard candy, and most of them are much more expensive than candy, too. In addition, most cough drops contain two ingredients that are not effective in treating a cough: antibiotics and anesthetics. Try using a vaporizer of some kind—the cool mist and heated mist types are equally effective. If you don't have a vaporizer, you can moisturize the air with a tea kettle or a pan of boiling water.

If neither remedy works, you are in the market for an over-the-counter drug medication. Cough medication in tablet form is just as effective as cough medication in syrup form—as long as it contains the same chemicals. Cough medication has to enter the bloodstream before it can work, and tablets do so as well as liquids and syrups. Several different kinds are on the market.[26]

Suppressants
Suppressants work directly on the "cough center" located in the brain to depress the cough reflex. Generally, suppressants should be used with either an uncontrollable cough or a dry nonproductive cough.

Two major cough suppressants are used in cough medicines. *Dextromethorphan*, the more common, is safe in proper dosages and generally quiets a cough for eight to twelve hours. The second type, *codeine*, is a narcotic. Pharmacists who sell over-the-counter medicines containing it must register the buyer's name in a narcotics registry book; in some states, cough medicines containing codeine are available only by prescription. Only one cough product on the market contains *only* a cough suppressant: Silence Is Golden cough syrup.

Both types sometimes have undesirable side effects. Dextromethorphan causes nausea and drowsiness in some. Codeine may also produce nausea, vomiting, dizziness, heart palpitations, drowsiness, and constipation. Because codeine is a narcotic, however, dextromethorphan is usually tried before codeine mixtures.

Expectorants

Expectorants act to break up and liquify the phlegm produced in the throat and bronchial passages. Expectorants increase the watery secretions produced by the cells in the upper respiratory tract. These watery secretions loosen thick mucus and phlegm. When phlegm is watered down, the cough reflex moves it out of the tract. Once the phlegm is broken up and moved out, the throat and bronchial passages ae no longer irritated, and the cough stops. Expectorants are normally used with nonproductive or heavily productive coughs. A combination expectorant/suppressant may be used with a productive, uncontrollable cough.

Expectorants commonly contain four chemical ingredients:[27]

• *Aluminum chloride* increases fluid in the respiratory tract by irritating the mucosa in the stomach. Caution: Overdoses of medications containing aluminum chloride may cause poisoning; large doses may cause the acid–base balance of the body to be upset.

• *Guaifenesin* has the same action as aluminum chloride. Caution: In rare instances, guaifenesin may cause nausea.

• *Syrup of ipecac* has the same action as aluminum chloride and guaifenesin. Caution: Because the effects and toxicities of small doses of ipecac are not known, it is not recommended for use of over one week's time. It is also not recommended for children under age 6.

• *Terpin hydrate* increases respiratory fluid volume by stimulating the secretory glands of the lower respiratory tract. Caution: Terpin hydrate use may cause gastrointestinal distress (specifically nausea and vomiting). It also has the potential for alcohol abuse. Because of these two factors, cough medications containing terpin hydrate should not be given to children under age 12.

Some cough medications on the market act *only* as expectorants, with no suppressant medication: Creomulsion, Creo-Terpin, G-G Tussin, Ipsatol, Kiddies pediatric, Penetro baby cough syrup, Pinex regular, Rasp, Rem, Robitussin, and 2/G.

Most cough expectorants on the market are combined with suppressants or with suppressants and decongestants/antihistamines (for the relief of cold symptoms that accompany the cough). Those that are combined with suppressants only include: Arrestin, Cheracol D, Creo-Terpin Plus, DeWitt's, Duad, Ipsatol DM, Pertussin wild berry, Pertussin 8-Hour Cough Formula, Robitussin D-M, Romilar children's, Sorbutuss (sugar-free), St. Joseph children's, Vicks cough syrup,

2/G-DM, Cheracol (contains codeine), Coasdein (contains codeine), Sedatole (contains codeine), and Terpin Hydrate with Codeine.

Combination Remedies

If you are suffering from a cough that accompanies a cold, you can choose cough remedies that combine suppressants, expectorants, decongestants, and antihistamines in several ways:

- *Suppressant plus decongestant:* Contac Jr., Cosanyl-DM (improved formula), Orthoxicol, and Vicks Daycare.

- *Expectorant plus decongestant:* Amonidrin (only tablets), Robitussin-PE (sugar-free), Soltice, and Trind.

- *Suppressant plus decongestant/antihistamine:* Naldetuss, Pertussin Plus Night-Time Cold Medicine, and Vicks Nyquil.

- *Expectorant plus decongestant/antihistamine:* Chlor-Trimeton expectorant, Coldene Children's, Coricidin cough formula, Covanamine expectorant, and Ryna-Tussadine expectorant (both liquid and tablet).

- *Suppressant/expectorant plus decongestant:* Dimacol, Dorcol pediatric, Novahistine DMX, Robitussin CF, Romex Jr., Romilar III, and Trind-DM.

- *Suppressant/expectorant plus antihistamine:* Anahist antitussive, Consotuss, Endotussin-NN, Romilar 8-Hour Cough Formula, Supercitin, Vicks Formula 44, Endotussin-C (contains codeine), G-G Tussin C. F. (contains codeine), and Robitussin-AC (contains codeine).

- *Cough suppressant/expectorant plus decongestant/antihistamine:* Axon (contains vitamin C), Codimal DM (sugar-free), Coldene Cough and Cold, Colrex (sugar-free), Coryban-D (contains vitamin C, sugar-free), Dondril anticough, Dristan cough formula, Histabite-D, Penetro, Quelidrine, Romex, Synephricol, Tonecol, Triaminicol (alcohol-free), and Tussagesic. Those that contain codeine are Codimal PH, Efricon, Histadyl E.C., Novahistine-DH, Novahistine expectorant, and Triaminic Expectorant with Codeine.

Drops, Lozenges, Gargles

As mentioned, you can obtain a soothing effect by sucking a piece of hard candy as well as by sucking a cough drop. If the cough is accompanied by a sore throat, however, you may want to find a cough drop, lozenge, or gargle that also contains a local anesthetic that numbs your throat.

Drops, lozenges, and gargles that *only* soothe include Cepacol throat lozenges, Hall's Honey-Lemon cough drops, Hall's Mentho-Lyptus cough drops, Ipsatol troches, Listerine throat lozenges, Luden's cough drops, Parke-Davis throat discs, Robitussin-DM Cough Calmers lozenges, Romilar cough discs, Silence Is Golden lozenges, Sucrets lozenges, Sucrets children's lozenges, Tonsiline liquids, and Vicks cough drops.

Products that contain a local anesthetic include Aspergum, Axon lozenges, Cepacol anesthetic troches, Chloraseptic gargle/lozenge/spray, Hold lozenges, Isodettes, Listerine Cough Control Lozenges, Oracin throat lozenges, Spec-T troches, Sucrets Cough Control Formula lozenges, Sucrets Cold Decongestant Formula lozenges, Thantis Lozenges, Vicks cough silencers, and Vicks Formula 44 cough discs.

CAUTIONS

You should read the labels carefully before selecting a product. Many times, cough medicines contain unnecessary ingredients such as antihistamines, decongestants, alcohol, and aspirin. For instance, many contain a large percentage of sugar, which is added to make the flavor tolerable. This doesn't pose a danger to most of us, but it could be critical for diabetics. Sugar-free cough medications are indicated in the lists throughout this section.[28] As another example, NyQuil contains enough alcohol to make it a 50-proof drink, but it contains only about one-third of the expectorant needed to relieve congestion.[29] Alcohol also constitutes 25 percent (enough for 50-proof) of Creo-Terpin and Pertussin Plus Night-Time Cold Medicine, 20 percent of Cosadein, 15 percent of Coldene Cough Formula Adult and Trind, and 12 percent of Dristan Cough Formula. If you should not use a decongestant (because of high blood pressure, diabetes, or heart or thyroid disease, for example), choose a cough medication that does not contain a decongestant. Unless you are suffering from severe stuffiness and inability to breathe, you might be better off staying away from decongestants: They serve to dry up secretions and remove water from the system—exactly the opposite of what you need, which is to moisten and loosen the membranes.[30] Or if you can't afford to be drowsy—if you'll be operating heavy machinery or driving a car—stay away from cough medications that contain antihistamines. On the other hand, you may wish to choose a medication containing antihistamines only if the cough is caused by an allergy. If you choose a cough medication that also contains an analgesic (they are listed on the label), cut down on or eliminate other analgesics (such as aspirin) that you may be taking for headache, fever, or minor pain. In general, be cognizant of the ingredients before you use a cough medication.

If you decide to use a throat lozenge that contains a numbing agent, you should realize that the lozenge also numbs everything else that it touches—including your tongue and the roof of your mouth. Don't use such a lozenge right before eating if you want to taste your food.

While vaporizers are beneficial when used with plain water, adding an aromatic product (such as Vicks Vaposteam or Vicks VapoRub) does not increase their effectiveness, and it may even pose a hazard. Some evidence shows that exposure to steam vapors from Vicks Vapo-Rub may lower the body's resistance to infection.[31]

INFLUENZA (THE FLU)

Influenza is a viral infection that has many strains. Researchers have been able to identify three major types of virus that cause flu, naming them A, B, and C. Just because you become infected with one does not mean that you are immune to them all. You can be reinfected a number of times with different viruses. In addition, the type A virus seems to be able to mutate itself, making new strains of flu.

There are three distinct forms of flu infection. *Pandemics* spread worldwide, usually occurring when A virus mutates and forms a new strain of flu. These occur about every thirty or forty years. *Epidemics* seem to break out in multiple and widely varied areas of a country simultaneously. Type A virus infections, usually very widespread, occur about every two to three years; type B infections, typically spotty in its distribution, occur every four to six years. *Endemics,* taking place between pandemics and epidemics, are typically confined to small, isolated areas.[32]

SYMPTOMS
In twenty-four to forty-eight hours after the flu bug hits, you start feeling the first of the symptoms—usually a sore throat, slightly stuffy nose, slightly runny nose, mild chest pain, or a moderate unproductive cough. Once the first of the symptoms appears, the flu progresses rapidly and usually affects most of the body.

As the flu is getting started, you experience chills and a fever (usually around 102° in adults, 103° in children). You can develop a headache, loss of appetite, weakness, nausea or vomiting, and general fatigue accompanied by body aches and pains. Your throat usually stays tender until your fever disappears.

In mild cases of the flu, the fever hovers around 102° for two or three days. In more severe cases, it can soar to 104° and continue for as long as four or five days. Once the fever disappears, most of the other symptoms do too. You usually continue to feel weak (and perhaps notice heavy sweating) for a few days after your fever goes away.

If your fever, cough, or respiratory symptoms last for more than five days, you have probably developed a secondary bacterial infection. Some complications often occur from the flu, including ear infections, sinus infections, and lymph infections.

CAUSES

The only way you can catch the flu is by breathing in airborne droplets that contain the virus. In other words, people who sneeze, cough, or breathe the virus into the air are the ones responsible for passing it. Since we all have to breathe, it is difficult to make ourselves incapable of spreading the flu.

What happens when you breathe in the tiny airborne droplets containing the virus? The virus lodges in your nasopharynx—the place where your nasal passages join with the top of your throat. The virus acts to reduce the thickness of the mucous lining in the respiratory passages; they become exposed, and so they are easily penetrated by the spreading and multiplying virus. So the virus sets up house in your respiratory tract—and rarely spreads beyond it. There is only one other chemical change in the body as a result of the flu virus: The white blood count drops to below normal.

TREATMENT
What About Flu Shots?

A general vaccine that contains a mixture that fights some Type A and Type B viruses is available throughout the United States. Flu shots are a bit risky. They have to be administered in just the right amount at just the right time, usually a few weeks to a few months prior to exposure to the virus. Flu shots, of course, are ineffective against new strains caused by the A virus.

Even though they don't always work in preventing the flu, certain people should have yearly injections (usually in two divided doses several weeks apart). *Everyone* over the age of sixty-five should have flu shots. Others who should get vaccinated include pregnant women, diabetics, or any patient who suffers from Addison's disease, chronic rheumatic heart disease, any other heart disease, or chronic broncopulmonary diseases.

Because flu vaccines are produced by culturing the virus on egg proteins, you *should not* get a flu shot if you are allergic to eggs. Your reaction could be so severe that it would kill you. Infants and young children *should not* get flu shots, either. Infants and young children are usually susceptible to convulsions that can lead to death if they develop a very high fever, and flu vaccines often cause symptoms that resemble the flu (including fever).

Treating the Flu
Like a cold, the flu is caused by a virus, and there is no cure for it. Also because the flu is a virus and not a bacterial infection, antibiotics do not help relieve flu symptoms. They are a waste of money, because they are ineffective. Even worse, you could build up a tolerance for the antibiotic, and, if you develop a bacterial infection secondary to the flu (a common problem), the antibiotic would not work against the bacterial infection. Never take an antibiotic that you have left over from some prescription, and never take an antibiotic that a well-meaning friend or family member gives you. Remember: Deaths from the flu are due to the secondary bacterial infections and complications that follow the flu, not to the flu itself. If you take antibiotics when you don't need them, your ability to fight off a secondary infection is seriously compromised.

All you can do with the flu is treat the symptoms: Use a cough syrup to relieve coughing; take aspirin (or some other analgesic) to relieve headache and body aches, as well as to reduce fever; and rest in bed as much as you can.

CAUTIONS
If your fever is not severe, you should probably not take any medications containing aspirin or salicylates; they can cause drenching sweat and severe chills in victims of the flu. You should remember that the same cautions apply to the flu as to the cold: Use good sense in the medications that you take, and keep your limitations in mind. If you are pregnant, check with your doctor before you take any medications aimed at relieving the flu.

3

constipation, diarrhea, and hemorrhoids

CONSTIPATION

Constipation is characterized by infrequent or difficult bowel movements. Approximately 50 million Americans think they are constipated and must do something about it. Over 700 over-the-counter products jump out from the pages of magazines, line up in rows on the pharmacy shelves, and come into our homes via television, all promising to keep us "regular." But what is *regular*? In the minds of some people, regularity has become equated with virtue. Gruberg describes it as an "elusive, highly-touted goal."[1] For some people regularity means two or three bowel movements each day; for others, it is a bowel movement only once every two or three days.[2] In deciding when you need a laxative, then, you must consider the causes of constipation and the times when self-medication is advisable.

CAUSES
Constipation usually results from one of three conditions:

- The waste material may move through the colon at an abnormally slow rate.

- As the waste material moves through the colon, too much water is reabsorbed back into the body making the stool hard, dry, compacted, and difficult to move out of the colon. (When too little water is reabsorbed, diarrhea results.)

• The urge to eliminate when the colon is full is ignored, and, in time, the urge becomes weaker. The urge to defecate is determined by how much stool is present, how sensitive the individual is to the signs, how much and what kind of food has been eaten, and lifelong habits of responding to the urge. Often, natural tendency is to eat to trigger the urge.[3]

Common causes of constipation include the following:[4]

• The "irritable colon" syndrome is a malady that results in intermittent bouts of constipation and the production of hard, small stools. Long-term anxiety and emotional stress is a likely culprit. Ironically, the anxiety is often connected with the victim's inability to void normally.

• The overuse of laxatives produces another irony. People who use too many laxatives often sedate their bowel until they are unable to have a bowel movement *without* the aid of a laxative. In this instance, they're just making things worse.

• A change of diet, commonly encountered during travel, and insufficient liquid intake are two causes.

• Medical conditions (such as tumors of the large bowel, Parkinsons disease, stroke, congestive heart failure, underactive thyroid, and endocrine abnormalities) can cause constipation.

• Certain drugs can cause constipation; these include some sedatives, antacids, tranquilizers, and drugs commonly used to combat high blood pressure. Specific medications that lead to constipation include Codeine, Percodan, Pro-Banthine, Tofranil, Thorazine, Ansolysen, and Inversine.

• Pregnancy may cause constipation because of the pressure of the baby against the colon.

• Bed rest or inactivity may have an effect on the colon.

• Heredity may cause constipation.

• Constipation, as mentioned, may be caused by neglecting the urge to defecate.

• Mental stress may be a causal factor.

• Certain foods harden the stool, such as dairy products and especially cheeses.

• Inactive bowels may be a cause of constipation. The large intestine loses its muscular strength so that the bowel does not hold its normal shape, nor does it contract forcefully enough to expel the feces.

• Constipation may result after a period of diarrhea for two reasons: The bowel empties completely, which means it takes some time for fecal material to accumulate, and the medication taken to control diarrhea may produce constipation.

• Cigarette smoking activates bowel contractions, and, when smoking is stopped, constipation may result.

Before you take a laxative, try to determine specifically what has caused your constipation. You might not need a laxative if you can get to the source of the problem and correct it.[5] Ask yourself:

• Have I become overly dependent on a laxative? (If you have, consult a doctor for help in supplementing your diet with enough fiber and bulk so you can overcome your dependence.)

• Have I been less physically active than usual?

• Have I been taking any medications that might have caused this constipation?

• Have I been under undue stress lately?

• Have I changed my eating habits (maybe because I just started a new diet)?

• Have I traveled lately?

• Are my bowel movements less frequent, or are they also painful because my stools are hard and dry?

• Has something happened lately to make me depressed?

• Have I eaten a lot of foods lately that might have hardened my stools? (Cheese and dairy products are notorious culprits!)

• Have I tried to relieve my constipation by eating better? (You should have daily foods that add roughage and fiber, and you should increase your fluid intake.)

• Do I try to suppress the urge to defecate when it arises? (A great deal of constipation results when people attempt to wait to eliminate their bowel movements; the stool get hard and dry, and the bowel itself becomes numbed.)

TREATMENT
Nonmedicinal Alternatives
Constipation is not generally a serious problem. Normally it corrects itself through a proper diet (combined with eight to ten glasses of water), adequate sleep, and exercise. Do all you can to relieve constipation without laxatives. Normal liquid intake, for instance, keeps stools soft. Exercise tones up muscles, including those of the colon. Also, regular habits help to combat constipation.

An important way to promote regular bowel movements is to insure that you have enough fiber and bulk in your diet.

Fiber is the part of whole grains, vegetables, fruits, and nuts that is not digested. Since fiber holds water, the stools are softer, bulkier, heavier, and pass through the colon more quickly. The following foods are recommended for increasing fiber and promoting healthy elimination:[6]

• Vegetables: artichoke, broccoli, brussels sprouts, carrots, cress, collard, escarole, kale, lima beans, okra, parsley, peas, green peppers, red peppers, potatoes, rutabagas, spinach, squash, string beans, and turnips.

• Fruits: apples, apricots, blackberries, boysenberries, cranberries, figs, black raspberries, red raspberries, and strawberries.

• Cereals and breads: miller's bran, rice bran, pumpernickel bread, rye bread, whole wheat bread, bran cereal, bran flakes, oat flakes, puffed wheat, shredded wheat, wheat germ, buckwheat, kasha, bulgur, oatmeal, brown rice, whole-grain wheat cereal, bran muffins, rye wafers, whole wheat wafers, and popcorn.

• Dried beans, peas, legumes, nuts, and seeds: dried red beans, dried white beans, dried peas, chick-peas, lentils, roasted peanuts, almonds, Brazil nuts, cashews, hazelnuts, pecans, walnuts, pumpkin seeds, soy seeds, and shelled sunflower seeds.

Using Laxatives
You should consider taking a laxative in the following circumstances:[7]

• Before X-ray exams that necessitate an emptying of the bowels (these include gall bladder X-rays, GI studies, barium enemas, or kidney X-rays).

• When the straining during normal elimination might be harmful to or might further damage some medical condition, such as hernia, hemorrhoids, heart disease, and other rectal or anal conditions. (In a case of this kind, your doctor will prescribe a medication that will help to keep your stools soft so that you will not need to strain to eliminate them.)

• You have only a rare or occasional time when it is difficult to release your stools.

• The constipation is only a temporary change in your usual trouble-free bowel habits.

• Your constipation begins only frequently, and you can clearly identify the source: temporary stress, inactivity due to illness or inclement weather, dietary alteration, or traveling.

• Your constipation is not accompanied by nausea, vomiting, or abdominal pain.

• Your constipation clears up within seven days of self-medication.

• The frequency of your bowel movements becomes abnormal (anywhere from three times a day to three times a week is considered normal, and there is not need for a laxative if you fall within this range).

• The frequency of your bowel movements is normal, but your stools have become hard, dry, and/or painful to release.

You should *not* take a laxative of any kind in the following circumstances:[8]

• Your constipation is chronic.

• You have been using laxatives regularly, and think you may have become dependent on them.

• You experience vomiting, nausea, or abdominal pain with the constipation.

• Any change in your bowel habits persists for longer than two weeks.

• Your efforts at self-medication do not produce relief within seven days.

• You have been taking a drug that causes constipation: that is, pain-killers that contain codeine, opium, or morphine; antacids that contain aluminum or calcium; antianxiety drugs such as Equanil, Elavil, or Tofranil; tranquilizers such as Meprobamate or Thorazine; or antispasmodics such as Donnatal or Pro-Banthine.

- You are suffering from some painful anal or rectal irritation (including painful hemorrhoids).

- You experience sudden weight loss.

- You notice blood or tarry material in your stools.

- You notice mucus in your stools.

- Your constipation alternates with diarrhea.

Types of Laxatives

Once you determine that you *do* need a laxative as a temporary measure in relieving constipation, you can pick from several kinds of laxative products.[9] Ideally, you should look for a laxative that is nonirritating, and nontoxic.

Most laxatives work in one of two ways: Either they soften the stool, or they increase peristalsis (the wavelike motion of the colon). The basic types of laxatives follow.

Stimulants. Chemical stimulants act directly on the colon, causing it to contract and eliminate the bowel movement. The waste products are simply pushed along by the increased wavelike movement of the colon. Stimulant laxatives generally work in six to twelve hours; increased doses or certain kinds of stimulants (such as castor oil) may produce results in two to five hours.

Check the labels on stimulant laxatives. The prolonged use of stimulants may excessively irritate the intestinal walls and produce diarrhea, cramping, and fluid depletion. Drugs that are generally good for occasional use include bisacodyl, cascara sagrada, castor oil, frangula, phenolphthalein (both yellow and white; the yellow is more potent), casanthranol, danthron, and senna. Drugs that are potentially damaging due to excessive irritation include aloe, podophyllin, jalap, rhubarb, and oxyphenisatin acetate.

Stimulants should *never* be used if you are experiencing pain in your abdomen, nausea, or vomiting. These symptoms could indicate appendicitis, and use of a stimulant laxative could result in the rupture of the appendix.

Many laxative products combine stimulants with bulk-forming medication or with lubricants and softeners; a few combine stimulants with saline solutions. We will list those under the appropriate categories. Laxative products containing *only* stimulants include: Alophen pills, Caroid and Bile Salts with Phenolphthalein tablets, Casafru liquid and chewable tablets, Cas-Evac liquid, Dorbane tablets, Dulcolax tablets and suppositories, Espotabs tablets, Evac-U-Gen tablets, Ex-Lax pills and chewable tablets, Ex-Lax instant mix, Feen-A-Mint chewing gum and chewable tablets, Fletcher's Castoria liquid, Glysennid tablets, G-W Emulsoil instant mix, Modane liquid and tablets, Modane Mild tablets, Neoloid emulsion, Phenolax wafers, Senokot granules and tablets, Senokot suppositories and syrup, Swiss Kriss mixture, Tonelax tablets, Veracolate tablets, and Zilatone tablets.

Saline. Saline laxatives, containing magnesium and sodium salts, work by retaining water in the intestines, eventually causing a mechanical stimulus that triggers the urge to expel bowel matter.

Some problems are connected with saline laxatives. First, the laxative draws the water it needs from the body tissues, and it can lead to dehydration. Whenever you take a saline laxative, you need to drink two or three large glasses of water to help your body replace the moisture it uses in making the laxative work. Second, saline laxatives have a high sodium content and should not be used by people who need to limit their salt intake—especially those with high blood pressure, kidney disease, heart disease, or edema. Also, these laxatives should never be used by those over the age of sixty.

Check the labels: Laxatives containing saline solutions list some kind of magnesium or sodium product as an ingredient. Laxatives containing only saline include Clyserol enema, Fleet enema, Milk of Magnesia liquid and tablets, Phospho-Soda liquid, and Sal Hepatica powder. Saline laxative ingredients are also found in combination in the following laxative products: with stimulants, Milk of Magnesia-Cascara Sagrada; with bulk-forming laxatives, Turicum emulsion; with lubricants and softeners, Ceo-Two suppositories, Haley's M-O emulsion, Milk of Magnesia liquid with mineral oil, and Vacuetts adult suppository; with both stimulants and bulk-softeners, Petrogalar emulsion.

Bulk-Formers. Bulk-formers expand and swell when they come into contact with water. When they encounter the moisture present in the digestive tract, they form a large mass that, in turn, stimulates the wavelike motions of the colon.

Bulk-formers should be taken with care. For one thing, they must *always* be taken with water. If you try to chew them or swallow them dry, they can cause serious obstructions of the throat or stomach. And keep drinking water after you've taken the laxative. The bulk absorbs water from body tissues as it travels through the digestive tract, leading to dehydration if the water is not replaced. Also, bulk laxatives cause an increase in gas, so you shouldn't use them if you already suffer from uncomfortable or painful gas. You shouldn't use them if you have any kind of intestinal disease, either, because they tend to form obstructions in the intestine.

Bulk-forming laxatives generally take twelve to twenty-four hours to work; in some cases, they may require three to four days. So if you need faster relief, you might consider using another kind of laxative or a bulk-former that has been combined with some other kind of laxative (such as a stimulant).

Laxatives listing agar, methylcellulose, guar gum, psyllium, karaya gum, or sodium carboxymethylcellulose work as bulk-formers. Laxative products containing only bulk-formers include Cellothyl tablets, Effersyllium powder, Hydrocil powder, Hydrolose syrup, Konsyl powder, L. A. Formula powder, Metamucil powder, Metamucil instant mix powder, Mucilose flakes and powder, Mucilose compound tablets, Plova powder, Serutan powder and granules, Siblin tablets and granules, and Syllamalt powder.

Bulk-formers combined with stimulants include Bassoran granules, Casyllium powder, Gentlax tablets and granules, Hydrocil Fortified powder, Imbicoll granules, Innerclean granules, Saraka granules, and Senokot with Psyllium powder.

Bulk-formers combined with lubricant-softeners include Agoral emulsion (plain-flavored only), Dialose capsule, Disoplex capsule, and Mucilose-Super powder.

Turicum emulsion is a combination of bulk-formers and saline; Dialose Plus capsules and Disolan Forte capsules combine bulk-formers with lubricant-softeners and stimulants.

Lubricant–Softeners. Lubricant–softeners aren't actually laxatives, because they don't really stimulate a bowel movement: They simply help the body form softer, moister stools that are easier to pass. This kind of a laxative is good for those who need to avoid straining during bowel movements—those with hernias, hemorrhoids, heart disease, or other medical conditions that may be aggravated by straining to eliminate hard stools.

There are two kinds of lubricants and softeners:

1. Those containing mineral oil lubricate and soften the stool, but they inhibit absorption of food into the intestines. Doses that are too large may cause oil to leak through the anus. Mineral oil slows the time it takes the bowel to empty, and it should be taken at bedtime instead of at meals. Mineral oil laxatives generally produce results in six to eight hours—overnight, if you take them right before going to bed.

2. Laxatives containing *dioctyl sodium sulfosuccinate* act as a wetting solution that enable water to mix with the stools as they form. You need to drink a lot of water throughout the day if you use this kind of a laxative. This type of laxative takes about one to three days to produce results, so you should consider something else if you need faster results.

You should use lubricants with caution. They can easily lead to dehydration; they can also interfere with the body's ability to absorb and utilize the food you eat. Mineral oil that gets into the lymph glands can cause them to get infected or inflamed. As you swallow a laxative containing mineral oil, it can coat the back of your throat, and droplets inhaled into the lungs can cause lipid pneumonia.

Laxatives containing lubricant–softeners *only* include Aquatyl tablets, Clyserol oil retention enema, Colace capsules and liquid, Coloctyl capsules, Dio-Medicone tablets, Disonate capsules and liquid, Doxinate capsules and solution, Fleet Enema Oil Retention, Kondremul plain emulsion, Magcyl capsules, Milkinol liquid, Mineral Oil liquid, Rectalad enema, Regutol tablets, Revac Supprettes suppository, and Surfak capsules.

Lubricant–softeners combined with stimulants include Agoral flavored emulsion, Correctol tablets, Disolan capsules, Dorbantyl capsules, Dorbantyl Forte capsules, Doxan tablets, Doxidan capsules, Gentlax-S tablets, Kondremul with Cascara emulsion, Kondremul with Phenolphthalein emulsion, Neo-Kondremul emulsion, Peri-Colace capsules and syrup, and Senokap DSS capsules.

Castor Oil. Although castor oil has been used as a laxative for years, its exact mechanism of action is unknown. However it is known that it does have an overall irritant effect which increases peristalsis (the wave-like movements that move fecal material along the intestinal tract). Castor oil is not generally recommended for laxative use because prolonged use may cause excess fluid loss, which can lead to dehydration.

For combinations with saline and bulk-formers, check the lists under the other categories.

Enemas. These non-oral laxatives may contain either saline solutions or lubricant–softeners. They may be used to treat constipation or to empty the bowel before and after surgery and prior to X-ray examinations. The enema is one of the best laxatives you can use, insofar as it works only at the end of the colon and does not disturb or affect any other part of the digestive tract.

Follow the instructions on the enema package carefully. The horizontal position is important. Many people give themselves enemas while they are sitting on the toilet. This only cleans the lower part of the colon. You should always be in a horizontal position, and the enema container should be held slightly above your hips to give the fluid sufficient force to flow freely through the tube and into the intestines. If the container is held too high, too much pressure is on the fluid as it enters the colon. If the container is at the proper height, there is less pressure, and the fluid flows freely through the tube and seeps into the colon. You should rarely need more than a pint of fluid.

Results are immediate.

Suppositories. These work much as the enema does—in the lower colon only—but they are much more convenient to use. There are three different kinds: stimulant, lubricant–softener, and saline/lubricant–softener. They are listed under the appropriate categories earlier in this section; you can determine their action by reading labels.

Some suppositories rely on glycerin to absorb water from the tissues (much like the saline laxatives work), thus creating more mass and stimulating expulsion. You should take care to drink adequate amounts of water to replace lost fluids.

CAUTIONS

Once you have used a laxative, get back to your own regular bowel habits quickly, and remember these things about the use of laxatives:

• Don't depend on a laxative for longer than one week. Try to identify the cause of your constipation, and take active nonmedical measures to correct it. The regular practice of taking laxatives is habit-forming.

• Discontinue use of a laxative if a skin rash appears. Phenolphthalein may cause this; it may also color the stool or urine an orangish or reddish color.

• Saline laxatives should not be used everyday, and they should not be given orally to children under 6 years old or rectally to children under 2 years of age.

• Overdependence on the stimulant laxatives may cause diarrhea, cramps, and dehydration. Other conditions affect the colon itself such as a loss of ennervation to the colon, atrophy of smooth muscle (which can produce a loss of intestinal muscle tone), and abnormal pigmentation of the colon.

• Enemas and suppositories should be administered properly to be effective.

- You shouldn't take an OTC laxative and a prescription drug at the same time because of the danger of ill effects.

DIARRHEA

Diarrhea can consist of watery stools, loose stools, or simply stools that are much too frequent. Fifty different diseases and disorders claim diarrhea as a symptom; some are serious, and some are not.[10] Because of the potentially serious illnesses that can cause diarrhea, you must know the causes of diarrhea before you can determine when it is safe to self-medicate and when you should see a doctor instead.

TYPES OF DIARRHEA

There are two types of diarrhea: acute and chronic. *Acute* diarrhea is identified by the sudden onset of frequent and loose stools accompanied by weakness. Acute diarrhea generally as other symptoms, such as gas production, pain, and often fever and vomiting. *Chronic* diarrhea is characterized by the persistent or recurrent passage of unformed stools. Diseases or other conditions producing both kinds of diarrhea are as follows:[11]

Acute

Amoebic dysentery	Medication
Antibiotic use	Radiation
Cancer	Salmonellosis
Cholera	Shigellosis
Diverticulitis	Staphylococcal infection
Escheria coli (bacteria) toxin	Ulcerative colitis
Food poisoning	Viral gastroenteritis

Chronic

Addison's disease	Irritable colon
Blind loops of the large intestine	Lactose deficiency
Brain disease	Malabsorption syndrome
Cancer	Intestinal stricture (narrowing)
Diabetic neuropathy	Surgery
Gastrointestinal hormone imbalance	Tuberculosis
Gluten enteropathy	Ulcerative colitis
Hyperthyroidism	Uremia
	Tumors of the intestinal villi

CAUSES

What kinds of body actions combine to produce diarrhea?[12] Diarrhea occurs when the large bowel doesn't absorb as much water from the food in the bowel movement as it usually does; the stools, then, are much more watery and loosely composed. Some diseases, such as cholera, result in increased secretion of water into the large intestine. Or, in some cases, the bowel movement moves too rapidly through the bowel to allow the intestine to absorb food and liquid it usually does.

What are the underlying causes of diarrhea? The more common causes include:

1. *Nervousness, tension, and anxiety.* Diarrhea caused by emotional upset is generally mild, occurs in an otherwise healthy person, and is related to a specific stress situation. The colon is highly affected by emotional stress. The diarrhea should clear up when the cause of the stress disappears or when the anxiety is relieved.

2. *Irritable colon.* This is the same culprit that can cause constipation, and it is most likely a result of long-term emotional stress. Diarrhea caused by irritable colon is characterized by pain in the lower left side of the abdomen; often the pain is relieved by having a bowel movement or by passing gas. Often diarrhea is intermittent with constipation; when diarrhea does occur it usually happens in the morning (before or after breakfast, or both). There is generally a lot of mucus with the stools; sometimes you might pass mucus without any stool.

3. *Virus.* A virus is the cause of diarrhea that accompanies flu, gastroenteritis, and other digestive disturbances. Diarrhea caused by virus occurs suddenly in an otherwise healthy person, and is characterized by frequent, watery stools and by the explosive passage of gas. Vomiting might also occur, and there is usually abdominal pain. Fever is sometimes present. Viral diarrhea usually disappears in two to three days.

4. *Food poisoning.* As the body reacts to spoiled food, diarrhea is generally brief and of mild intensity. Mild stomach cramps and other mild abdominal pains occur probably within twenty-four hours after you eat the suspect food. If you talk to others who ate the same food, and they also have diarrhea, your diagnosis is quite certain.

5. *Change in water.* When you travel to different areas of the country or world, you might not be accustomed to amoeba and other bacteria in the water. Your body reacts with diarrhea. The diarrhea does not begin

for two to three days after you drink the water (if the diarrhea is caused by salmonella); in some cases, it may not begin for three to five days (if it is caused by amoeba). It's self-limiting and runs its course, but it will probably take two or three weeks for you to return to normal.

6. *Drugs.* Some prescription or over-the-counter drugs can cause diarrhea as an unpleasant side effect. You should always call your doctor if you develop diarrhea while you are taking a prescription drug. Frequent culprits are antibiotics and some antacids.

7. *Allergies to food.* For some reason, an allergy to milk is particularly prone to result in diarrhea.

8. *Disease or other medical problems.* Diabetes, inflammations, tumors, and neurologic diseases are apt to cause diarrhea.

9. *Narcotic withdrawal.* Withdrawal from narcotics produces diarrhea as well as other symptoms like tremors, nausea, vomiting, hot and cold flashes, and hallucinations.

10. *Infantile.* It is usually difficult to identify the cause of diarrhea among babies, but in many cases it is caused by a virus.

TREATMENT
Nonmedicinal Treatment
Instead of or in addition to using an over-the-counter diarrhea medication, you can take the following steps to relieve or to avoid diarrhea:[13]

• Keep on a liquid diet until the diarrhea subsides. Drink warm and salty fluids; fruit juice and tea are both good. (Keep away from drinks with a high sugar content, such as cola drinks or sweetened tea.) Avoid eating heavy foods or rough vegetables. As the diarrhea improves, slowly add semisolid foods (such as jello and soup; bananas and rice may help to firm the stools). Return to solid foods gradually and with caution.

• Get plenty of rest.

• If you travel to a foreign country, drink only boiled or bottled water, bottled soft drinks, beer, or wine. Make sure that all the food you eat has been thoroughly cooked. Fruits and vegetables should be recently cleaned thoroughly and recently peeled. Make sure that the water you use to brush your teeth or the water you use for making ice cubes is also bottled or preboiled.

You can be safe in treating yourself for diarrhea under those circumstances:[14]

• Your principal symptom is the frequent release of watery stools.

• You have only mild abdominal cramping, vomiting, nausea, or loss of appetite.

• Your diarrhea came on suddenly, without prior warning of impending illness.

• You do not continue your treatment longer than 48 hours.

You should *not* attempt to treat yourself for diarrhea—but rather call your doctor immediately—in a number of circumstances:

• You have a fever over 100°.

• Your bowel movements are bloody, black, or tarry.

• The medication is for a child under the age of three.

• The medication is for a person over the age of sixty.

• Your symptoms last for over forty-eight hours.

• You have any acute or chronic disease.

• You noticed changes in your bowel habits before the diarrhea occurred.

• You have been taking prescription medications (especially antibiotics or antihypertensive drugs that may be affected by medication you take for diarrhea).

• You are pregnant.

• You are run-down or weakened (a number of disorders can cause a weak feeling and can also result in diarrhea).

• You suffer from diarrhea that occurs frequently or that lasts for long periods.

• You notice an excessive amount of mucus in your stools.

• You lose weight rapidly.

• Your diarrhea is accompanied by severe abdominal pain.

• Your skin or eyes take on a yellowish cast.

Elements of Diarrhea Medication

There are three main elements in over-the-counter diarrhea medication.[15]

Kaolin and Pectin. Kaolin, a gelling agent, is usually combined with pectin in diarrhea medication. The gelatin in kaolin helps you produce more solidly formed stools; the effect of the pectin is unknown.

Kaolin and pectin medications are generally mild, and they are not effective against severe bouts of diarrhea. Because of its mildness, kaolin/pectin medicine is particularly good for children, when the doctor authorizes it.

Take about two to four tablespoons each time you have a loose bowel; medications containing a kaolin/pectin combination include Kaopectate, Kalpec, Kao-Con, and Donnagel.

Because of their mildness, you should start treating diarrhea with kaolin/pectin mixtures. If they do not control your diarrhea in 24 hours, you should call your pharmacist and reassess the situation with him or her. A pharmacist is likely to suggest something a little stronger. You should take the stronger drug for another 24 hours, and, if your diarrhea is still not under control, you should call your doctor.

Paregoric. Paregoric, a mild narcotic preparation available in most states without a prescription, stops the propulsive, wavelike motion of the intestines.

Since paregoric is stronger than kaolin/pectin, you might try one to two tablespoons after each loose bowel movement for a couple of days. You should not use paregoric more often than four times a day without your doctor's permission. Paregoric can be taken in combination with medicines that contain kaolin and pectin; there is no side effect from either medication when the proper dose is taken.

Bulk-Forming Compounds. Diarrhea medicine that contains bulk-formers serves to increase the mass of the stools and to reduce the watery quality of the stools. Most of the medicines containing bulk-formers rely on psyllium; Metamucil is a common one. Psyllium is generally not very effective when used alone, so it's a good idea to use it in conjunction with some other medication or to find a medication that combines ingredients. There are no side effects when the medication is taken in the usual dose.

Picking Diarrhea Medicine

How can you choose the medicine that is best for you? Look for two important elements:

• Make sure that the label clearly lists all the ingredients in the medication; dont's use a medication that contains an ingredient you are unsure about or that you know may be wrong for you.

• Choose a diarrhea medicine that combines at least two of the common antidiarrhea medicines (such as a combination of kaolin/pectin and paregoric).[16]

Avoid diarrhea medication that contains adsorbents (such as attapulgite and charcoal), anticholinergics (such as atropine sulfate or homatropine methylbromide), and astringents (such as alumina powder or bismuth salts).

CAUTIONS

Besides being careful about when to use laxatives, two other precautions are in order:

• As soon as your diarrhea stops, stop taking the laxative. Overuse can cause constipation.

• Never administer a laxative to a child under 3 years of age, unless ordered to do so by a doctor.

HEMORRHOIDS

Most people over the age of thirty have them, and men and women are just about equally affected.[17] What exactly are hemorrhoids? The condition we have labeled as "hemorrhoids" consists of dilated veins in the anus and rectum like varicose veins that appear on legs. Sometimes they swell, itch, and bleed; other times they are virtually unnoticed. Most require no treatment or only mild home treatment; severe cases require surgery.

SYMPTOMS

Specific symptoms of hemorrhoids include:[18]

1. *A protruding mass from the rectum.* This symptom may especially occur following a bowel movement or some other strain, such as coughing or sneezing. Because of the sudden strain, the mass of engorged veins that normally sit just inside the rectum is pushed out. The protrusion is usually painless, but it is extremely uncomfortable. You can definitely tell that a lump is protruding from your anus. A protruding mass is sometimes accompanied by a leakage of mucus. Some hemorrhoids originate outside the anus as enlarged blood vessels just underneath a thin layer of skin; these, of course, are always outside the anus and do not protrude in a mass as internal hemorrhoids do.

2. *Bleeding.* Bleeding can result from both internal and external hemorrhoids, but it's more commonly a result of internal hemorrhoids. Bleeding most often accompanies a bowel movement, simply because that's when the most strain is put on the blood vessels. Bleeding can vary in intensity: Sometimes you may notice just a trace on the toilet tissue; at other times you may notice that your fecal matter is streaked with blood; occasionally you may experience enough of a "gush" of blood, which can be quite frightening, to turn the toilet water pink or red. The blood that comes from hemorrhoids, of course, is fresh, so it is bright red in color. Any blood that is dark red or black, or that appears tarry, has originated much higher in the digestive tract and is a reason for concern.

Bleeding *can* occur at times other than when you are passing a bowel movement; such bleeding can, of course, be very embarrassing. Any bleeding that results from hemorrhoids is usually intermittent, and it will generally go away after a few days.

Because rectal bleeding can come also from a serious medical condition like cancer, *you should see a doctor for any condition of rectal bleeding.* Then, if hemorrhoids are diagnosed, you can probably treat them yourself with the doctor's advice.

3. *Pain.* Pain is a serious complication of hemorrhoids, because it usually signals that the blood inside the hemorrhoidal veins has clotted. If you have developed a clot, surgery is probably necessary, so you should see a doctor if you develop pain.

4. *Itching.* Television commercials would have us believe that we are all half-crazed idiots, living for the chance to be alone even for just a few seconds) so we can scratch our—dare we say it?—hemorrhoids. Itching is not all that common with hemorrhoids; when it does occur, it is a result of the irritation caused by the protruding mass. Itching rarely occurs inside the rectum above the anal opening. We hate to tell the ad agencies, but there are many other causes for anal itching, most of them not very pleasant: Poor anal hygiene, worms, infection, tight underwear, and psychological problems can all cause an annoying itch at the anus.

CAUSES

Hemorrhoids can be caused by any one or combination of the following factors:[19]

• chronic constipation (since pressure is exerted on the rectal veins when you strain to pass a bowel movement, constipation can also increase the discomfort due to hemorrhoids);

• infection of the rectal/anal area (an infection may weaken the wall of the blood vessels and lead to hemorrhoids);

• diarrhea;

• occupations that involve constant standing (especially when it is combined with hard manual labor) or constant sitting;

• pregnancy;

• pressure in the abdomen resulting from disease or from some surgical procedure (such pressure, as in pregnancy, causes a backup of blood that causes the hemorrhoids to swell);

• unusual stress or tension;

• consumption of heavily spiced foods (especially those containing curry, pepper, or chili) that may irritate the rectum;

• abnormally frequent coughing and sneezing;

• diet deficient in fiber and bulk;

• inadequate fluid intake;

• failure to maintain good anal hygiene;

• frequent use of laxatives, suppositories, or enemas;

• hormones; or

• heredity.

TREATMENT
Nonmedicinal Treatment
You can treat hemorrhoids without medication by trying the following:[20]

1. Make every effort to keep your stools soft. Drink lots of water—at least a quart a day—and make sure your diet contains plenty of bran cereals and fibers (such as celery and apples).

2. Make conditions good so that the protruding mass will return. If it doesn't do so immediately, try soaking in a hot tub (or sitz bath) for a few minutes. The muscles around the anus will probably relax enough to permit the mass to slip back in. Or try lying down for a few minutes. If that doesn't work, you'll have to push it back in with your fingers:

Coat them with Vaseline first (or simple soap and water), and knead the mass gently until it returns to its proper position. (Don't worry—it won't hurt.) Then dry your rectal area thoroughly so that the mass won't slip back out again.

3. Use a sitz bath to soothe burning and itching, as well as to relieve minor pain.

Self-Treatment
You can treat your hemorrhoids yourself, after you have received a confirmed diagnosis from your doctor on the following conditions:[21]

- You are trying to get temporary relief from mild itching, burning, or soreness caused by simple external hemorrhoids.

- Your doctor explained that your hemorrhoids were uncomplicated.

- You do not feel sick in any other way, and you have no symptoms anywhere else in your body besides the ones at your anus.

- You can get relief from self-treatment in less than four days.

You should see a doctor immediately if any of these circumstances applies:[22]

- Your hemorrhoids are accompanied by excessive bleeding that does not go away after a few days.

- The blood that you pass is black, dark red in color, or tarry in appearance.

- An excessive amount of mucus is present.

- You have been taking any prescription antibiotic drugs (especially tetracycline, ampicillin, or lincomycin).

- You want to get long-lasting, permanent relief in the form of a cure (something that is not possible from self-treatment with over-the-counter drugs).

- You suffer from severe itching.

- You get dizzy or faint when you stand up.

- You experience shortness of breath or nausea.

- You experience pain at your rectum or anus that is continuous or throbbing.

- You are experiencing so much discomfort that it is difficult for you to participate in everyday activities like sitting, walking, standing, or lifting of light objects.

- You feel pressure within your rectum.

- You have been using hemorrhoid medications, and you have not gained relief.

- You can feel or see a protrusion of tissue from the anus that is painful before, during, or after you have a bowel movement.

- You experience a change in your bowel habits (especially if you start suffering from intermittent diarrhea and constipation).

- Your skin or eyes take on a yellowish cast.

- You experience swelling of your legs or abdomen.

- Your urine turns dark.

- You are unable to replace protruding tissue that has protruded from the rectum. (Most protruding tissue returns spontaneously; if it doesn't, try pushing it with your fingers. If you still can't replace it, call a doctor.)

Complications of Hemorrhoids
Although hemorrhoids are uncomfortable, they do not usually produce any complications. However in rare cases, three conditions may develop which complicate the original hemorrhoids:

- *Prolapse*, in which the hemorrhoids hang from the anus or rectum.

- *Thrombosis*, in which clots develop (due to the stagnation of blood in the vessels) and may occlude the vessels.

- *Irritation and infection*, which results when fecal material passes by hemorrhoids during bowel movements and bruises the hemorrhoids.

Surgery may be needed if your hemorrhoids become so large that they interfere with your ability to walk, sit, stand, or do other normal things. You may also require surgery if the mass protrudes frequently and resists efforts to push it back in. Surgery is also indicated if bleeding is severe enough to pose a danger from anemia. Generally, any time your hemorrhoids stubbornly resist treatment for a period of more than a few weeks, your doctor will probably recommend surgery. Most hemorrhoid surgery can be done right in the doctor's office or in an outpatient clinic; in many cases, anesthetic is not even required. A new treatment for hemorrhoids is to tie them off with a rubber band. This method cuts off the blood supply to the hemorrhoids and is less painful than surgery.

Forms of Delivery
You can get hemorrhoid medicine in three forms.[23]

Ointments. Ointments are the most effective, because they allow for direct application of active ingredients to the sites of external itch, inflammation, and pain. You should use an ointment if the cause of your discomfort is from external, not internal, hemorrhoids. Never insert the ointment applicator into your rectum in an attempt to soothe internal hemorrhoid symptoms.

Suppositories. These are best if you are suffering from internal hemorrhoids; inserted into the anus, they coat the rectal wall with medication. Suppositories are ineffective in treating pain and itch of external hemorrhoids, because the medication from a suppository never comes into contact with the external hemorrhoid.

Aerosols. Designed to treat external hemorrhoids, aerosols are generally ineffective because the delivery of active ingredients to the site is usually erratic. The only advantage of aerosols is that they keep fastidious persons from having to touch themselves.

Choose the medication that best suits your needs. Again, ointments (creams) are best for external hemorrhoids, and suppositories are best for internal hemorrhoids. If you are unlucky enough to have both, you should probably use a combination; buy both kinds and use them as needed.

Drug Classes
Hemorrhoid medications contain any one or a combination of these general drugs:[24]

1. *Anesthetics* create a numbing effect that helps relieve the pain and itching associated with hemorrhoids. Benzocaine is the most common one used.

2. *Astringents* constrict the swollen tissues and help combat inflammation. Zinc oxide is the most common.

3. *Antiseptics* work to kill germs and to prevent infection of the anal area.

4. *Lubricant–softeners* are added to the base of the cream or suppository to make it more smooth and nonirritating to use. Cocoa butter, castor oil, cod liver oil, eucalyptus oil, glycerin, and lanolin are all used to make the creams more silky.

5. *Auxiliary drugs* are added to some brands, which may contain live yeast cells, vitamins A and D, sodium extracts, or various healing agents. All should be listed on the label.

4

pain

INTERNAL ANALGESICS

The many different kinds—and intensities—of pain pose a particularly difficult dilemma to the person who wants to use over-the-counter drugs for self-medication. Pain is a symptom, not a disease, and it is often a signal that something is very wrong in the body's network. So, pain is a protection that tells you about some actual or potential damage to the body's tissues. By simply killing the pain, you may be masking a serious or even fatal disease. For that reason, it is important to see a doctor for most instances of pain.

TREATMENT

You can safely use a self-prescribed pain-killer that you buy over-the-counter if you are using it to treat any of the following:[1]

- tension or sinus headache (Each week 15 percent of the population experiences the pain of some type of headache. Tension headaches are caused by stress and fatigue. The pain, usually in the forehead or in the back of the head, may feel like a tight band around the head. Tension and sinus headaches should be treated as soon as pain begins. However, migraine headaches cannot be treated by OTC drugs);[2]

- muscle ache, soreness, or pain that you know is the result of menstrual cramping, a minor injury, or a slight strain;

• neuralgia;

• mild fever (under 100°) that you are certain is a result of a common cold or the flu; or

• any headache, muscle ache, or neuralgia that accompanies a common cold or the flu.

You should contact a doctor and avoid using over-the-counter pain medications in the following instances:[3]

• You are taking prescription drugs—especially those for blood clotting, diabetes, gout, or arthritis,

• You have asthma or you suffer from asthma-like symptoms.

• You are sensitive to or allergic to any drug (especially aspirin).

• You are suffering symptoms from arthritis or bursitis.

• You have experienced blood-clotting difficulties in the past.

• You have had, or have now, an ulcer.

• You are suffering from a migraine headache or a headache that starts deep within the skull (this kind of a headache is usually deep, aching, steady, dull, and prolonged).

• You have recently had a drink of alcohol or plan to have one soon.

• You are suffering from body aches, pain, or soreness that you can't relate to any known injury, stress, or strain.

• You develop nausea, vomiting, redness, itching, or gastric distress when you take the pain medication or after a week of self-treatment.

• Your symptoms have been around for a long time.

• Your symptoms are more intense than those the over-the-counter medication claims to relieve.

• You are anemic.

• You are taking anticoagulants.

• You are taking oral insulin.

Forms of Delivery
Over-the-counter pain-killers are generally aimed at relieving headache, muscle and body aches, fever, and inflammation. They come in several forms.[4]

Tablets. The most common form of pain medication, tablets are supposed to dissolve immediately when they encounter the watery environment of the stomach and small intestine. From there, they are absorbed into the bloodstream.

Timed-Release Tablets or Capsules. Following the same principle as ordinary tablets, these dissolve in the digestive juices and are absorbed by the bloodstream. Timed-release medication, however, is designed to dissolve at different rates to provide extended pain relief. Most timed-release products do not provide rapid relief, but they are good to use when you need extended relief (such as at bedtime to relieve pain throughout the night).

Effervescing Powders or Tablets. Dissolve these in water before you take them. They work faster and are more readily absorbed than tablets or capsules, and so they are better for the person who needs rapid relief. Most are buffered to prevent stomach upset. Unfortunately, however, they contain high concentrations of sodium, and they should not be used by people on a salt-restricted diet.

Coated Capsules. Surrounding the medically active ingredient is a protective coating designed to withstand dissolution until it reaches the small intestine. Capsules, then, do not irritate the stomach lining, because no medicine is released until the capsule leaves the stomach. The effectiveness of capsules is suspect, though: Their release action is erratic, and sufficient medication may not be released in time to be absorbed in the small intestine.

Liquids. The most readily absorbed of all, liquids present the least risk of upset stomach. They generally provide for the fastest pain relief of any of the forms of delivery of pain medication. Most of the liquids contain flavoring (sugar) and alcohol, however, which could create a problem for diabetes and those who do not want to take the alcohol.

Gums. Gums are yet another form for pain medication. Aspergum is a common brand of pain reliever in this form. Usually the concentration of pain reliever in gum is quite a bit less than in other forms, so this type of drug is not as effective in controlling pain.

TYPES OF PAIN-KILLERS

Your choice of a pain-killer depends on the nature and origin of your pain, your past history of allergy, whether or not you have a peptic ulcer, whether you have blood-clotting problems, and whether you are presently using other medications.[5] Pain-killers fall into several categories.

Aspirin. By far the most common pain-killer is aspirin, listed as either aspirin or acetylsalicylic acid on labels. Aspirin has been around for about a hundred years, and it is generally the pain-killer by which all other analgesics are judged. More aspirin is purchased than any other nonprescription drug: It seems to be almost a cure-all, relieving pain, cooling fevers, reducing swelling, and relieving the ever-elusive headache.

Yet even though aspirin is the most widely used nonprescription drug, we know very little about how it actually works. In fact, if it were discovered today, the Food and Drug Administration would probably classify it as a prescription drug. Ironically, aspirin's most famous effect—its ability to relieve pain—is the one we know the least about. Unlike other opiates and narcotics, aspirin produces no mental effects; so we assume that it must work on the central nervous system.

Unfortunately, aspirin has a number of bad side effects.[6] At least 10 percent of all the adverse drug reactions recorded in hospitals in the United States are caused by aspirin; one out of every five hundred people who take the drug have a bad reaction to it. Most commonly, aspirin might upset your stomach. If you have a headache *and* an upset stomach, choose an analgesic that also contains an antacid. If you don't want to risk the side effects of aspirin, take the time to find a pain-killer that doesn't contain aspirin.

Another very common symptom of aspirin intolerance is an asthma-like attack, complete with wheezing, gasping, and shortness of breath. It happens anywhere from fifteen minutes to three hours after taking the drug. And there's another problem—unlike wheezing caused by ragweed or pollen, the asthma continues even after the person has stopped taking the drug.

Aspirin intolerance can erupt suddenly in people who have taken the drug for years with no side effects; it can't be predicted by allergy tests, and it doesn't respond to allergy treatments. In fact, it probably isn't an allergy at all, but a metabolic disorder that may result from chronic stuffy nose, sinus infections, bronchial asthma, and growths in the membrane lining the nose.

Still another side effect is chronic hives. Over 22 percent of those suffering from hives experience a flare-up when they take aspirin; hives can occur even in people who have never had them before. Why? It appears that aspirin contains a contaminant (aspirin anhydride) that joins with certain elements in the blood to kick off the allergic reaction that causes hives.

A third side effect is loss of blood through the lining of the stomach and the intestine. Sometimes the blood loss is minimal, and sometimes it's massive. The blood loss occurs because aspirin prevents blood from clotting normally; it interferes with the aggregation of platelets, the elements essential to clotting. As a result, ruptured capillaries aren't able to clot quickly enough to prevent blood loss. If the ingestion of aspirin has not been great, the clotting occurs slowly; if more aspirin has been ingested and is in the bloodstream, the clotting may not take place at all. Long-term aspirin use may set the stage for serious bleeding which, when combined with other factors, can bring on a peptic ulcer. Victims of peptic ulcer, stomach disease, or gastrointestinal disease who take aspirin may be in for a big surprise—the loss of several pints of blood, enough to require a transfusion. Aspirin, then should not be taken for at least a week prior to surgery. People with a blood-clotting disease should avoid using it, as well as pregnant women. In fact, studies in Wales have even linked aspirin ingestion during the first trimester of pregnancy with certain kinds of birth defects. An interesting and hopeful sidelight: A Canadian study has indicated that because aspirin helps prevent blood clotting, it may be used to prevent stroke. This study showed that aspirin decreased the frequency of stroke and death by 19 percent.[7]

Large doses of aspirin (more than ten five-grain tablets a day) can also cause ringing in the ears, and hearing loss (hearing returns when aspirin use is discontinued).

All these side effects are more likely to occur in people who take large doses of aspirin or who use aspirin over long periods (such as the elderly who use it in the relief of arthritis). You should therefore not take more than a few doses of aspirin each day, and no more than once or twice a week, unless specifically ordered to do so by your doctor.

In choosing a brand of aspirin, consider three things:

• All aspirin has acetylsalicylic acid, and so you can safely buy the least expensive aspirin on the market and still get as effective a pain reliever as the more expensive aspirins.

• You should look for the initials U.S.P. (meaning "United States Pharmacopeia") on the aspirin bottle. This means there has been an adequate control on drug purity.

• If possible, you should smell the aspirin before buying it. If aspirin is old and no longer potent, it has a strong, acidic smell. This smell means the active ingredients have changed to acetic acid and are no longer effective for pain relief.

Salicylamide. Salicylamide can be considered a "first cousin once removed" to aspirin. Salicylamide essentially does the same job as aspirin.[8] It relieves pain, cools fevers, and reduces inflammation. And, because it has a slightly sedative effect, it is used in some sleeping pills. The two are chemically related, but salicylamide is metabolized (that is, broken down) by the body more rapidly and thus requires more frequent doses. There are other differences, too. Salicylamide does not have the stigma of many of aspirin's undesirable side effects: Specifically, it is safe for people who are allergic to aspirin, and it does not cause gastric distress or gastric bleeding, as aspirin does.

Unfortunately, there aren't many products on the market that contain only salicylamide—Sal-Eze and Zarumin are two. It is, for some reason, most commonly combined with aspirin in pain relievers such as Excedrin, Excedrin P.M., and B.C.

Phenacetin. Phenacetin, unrelated to either aspirin or salicylamide, reduces fever and relieves pain, but it is not effective in reducing inflammation. It doesn't have many of aspirin's side effects, either: It doesn't produce gastric bleeding or distress, and it can be used by people who are allergic to aspirin.

But, as discussed earlier, phenacetin has a serious side effect of its own. Taken in large doses for a prolonged period, it can result in serious kidney impairment and can cause or worsen kidney disease. Those with an existing kidney disease, of course, should not take phenacetin under any condition.

Your best chance of pinpointing phenacetin is by reading labels. It's listed on the labels of the pain-killers that contain it. Some of the more common include Empirin, A.P.C., Bromo-Seltzer, and Duradyne.

Acetaminophen. Acetaminophen is chemically related to phenacetin, but it is considered the safest of the four pain-killing over-the-counter medications. It reduces fever and kills pain, but it is not effective in treating inflammation. Safe for those who are allergic to aspirin, it produces none of the undesirable side effects that aspirin causes. It is the pain-killer and fever-reducer most often used in children's medications.

Again, you can identify products containing acetaminophen by checking labels. Some of the most common products that contain acetaminophen include Datril, Liquiprin, Percogesic, Tylenol, Tylenol Extra-Strength, and Bayer Non-Aspirin. Acetaminophen is included as an ingredient and is mixed with other analgesics (including aspirin) in products like Vanquish, Bromo-Seltzer, Excedrin, and Excedrin P.M.

When you are looking for a pain-killer that contains acetaminophen but that does not contain aspirin, be sure to read the label carefully.

Caffeine. Although it is not an analgesic, caffeine is used in many pain medications because of its effect on headaches. It constricts the blood vessels, providing relief for some forms of migraine headache.

Caffeine is always listed on the label; it is an ingredient in Anacin, Cope, A.P.C., Empirin Compound, Vanquish, Excedrin, and Excedrin P.M.

Some pain-killer medications contain combinations of these active ingredients, but they are kept in the prescription department. Most notable are the remedies for arthritis. As with all other nonprescription drugs, study the labels and select the ingredient that is best for you.

CAUTIONS

Some specific guidelines apply to all over-the-counter pain-killers that are taken for any reason:

1. *Follow label directions exactly*—especially directions that apply to spacing of doses, the amount of each individual dose, and maximum daily dosage (unless your doctor tells you to do something else). Be especially aware that children's dosages for pain relievers are less. For example with aspirin, children under 4 years of age should be given one children's tablet. Children 5 to 9 years of age should be given one adult aspirin tablet; and children 10 to 12 years of age may be given two adult tablets.[9]

2. *Don't use pain-killers on a long-term basis.* They're meant to relieve minor symptoms of temporary diseases (like colds and flu) or for temporary, emergency pain relief until you are able to see a doctor.

3. *Call a dentist immediately* if you get a toothache. Over-the-counter pain-killers are only for emergency relief only until you can get to a dentist. You can't cure tooth decay or disease with pain-killers.

EXTERNAL ANALGESICS

A variety of diseases can cause aches and pains for which external analgesics are appropriate—specifically, joint and muscle pain. We distinguish this sort of pain from the kind discussed in the previous section by the method of treatment. In this section, we wish to deal with pain that responds to external analgesics. For example, over 10 million people in the United States (it has been estimated) suffer from rheumatism.[10] Arthritis causes pain for and cripples many others in this country. (In fact, because of the great number of people affected, quackery is rampant in these two areas.) Besides sufferers from disease, weekend tennis players and golfers come home on Saturday night, open the door, and head for the nearest tube of Ben Gay or Mentholatum Deep Heating Rub. For varied reasons, muscle and joint pain is experienced by almost everyone at least once during a lifetime, and external pain relievers may be used to reduce the pain temporarily. However, some conditions, such as gout, neuralgia, or rheumatoid arthritis, should be referred to a doctor. Remember, no external pain relievers can cure these illnesses; they can only relieve the pain for a time. In most cases, even doctors cannot cure these diseases, but they can stop the disease from progressing any further and they can usually give you something to provide some pain relief.

CAUSES

Quite a variety of conditions can make your joints ache or your muscles sore. Some of them are:

- not being accustomed to strenuous activity (the weekend tennis player!);

- being in a fixed and uncomfortable position for a long period;

- undergoing tension and anxiety;

- occupational discomforts (painters suffer more muscle aches and pains, because they use their arms and hands so much, and because their job involves reaching and sometimes remaining in awkward positions);

- exposure to cold, dampness, temperature, and air currents;

- having poor posture;

- arthritis (a condition that results in swelling, pain, aching, stiffness, and inflammation of the joints);

- bursitis (inflammation of the membrane that surrounds the joint, resulting in local pain, tenderness, and swelling);

- sprains and strains;

- neuralgia (resulting in disturbances of the nerves in the arms, legs, and sometimes the chest);

- rheumatism (with pretty much the same symptoms as arthritis, only with no inflammation in the joints); and

- gout (whose symptoms are very much like those of arthritis). Although experts disagree as to just what causes gout, most agree that it is a build-up of uric acid crystals in the joints. Yet precisely what makes this happen is still controversial.[11]

TREATMENT
Nonmedicinal Alternatives
To aid in pain relief, measures may be tried in addition to or instead of external pain relievers:

- Rest the affected part; move it as little as possible.

- Apply heat, either moist or dry.

- Do controlled exercises to maintain flexibility and movement.

- Reduce body weight to reduce the strain on joints.

- Before applying creams or ointments, soak the area of application in warm water for 15 to 20 minutes.

Self-Treatment
Joint or muscle pains may be a symptom of something that is seriously wrong in the body, so it pays to be a little cautious when reaching for the tube of Ben Gay. If any of the following conditions occur, you should avoid self-treatment and see your doctor in the following instances:

- If your symptoms last more than one week.

- If you have arthritis and other symptoms appear, such as fever, sick feelings, eye problems, rash, and shortness of breath.

- Whenever there is swelling, pain, and redness of joints along with arthritis.

- If you have gout. There is no effective OTC drug for gout treatment.

- If you have rheumatoid arthritis. Osteoarthritis involves just the joints, bone, and cartilage, so it may be treated at home. Rheumatoid arthritis is a generalized disease and may affect other parts of the body than just the joints.

- If you have recurring attacks of muscular pain or arthritis.

- If pain radiates out into the arms and legs (whether the pain be mild or severe).

- If the arm and leg muscles begin to atrophy (or shrink in size).

- If aspirin, rest, and heat do not provide relief of the symptoms.

- If you have a sensitivity or allergy to aspirin.

- If children experience aches and pains in the joints. These are not "growing pains"; they could be symptoms of rheumatic fever, which can lead to heart problems.[12]

In cases other than these, treating yourself at home with remedies from your household medicine cabinet is all right.

Forms of Treatment

Besides internal analgesics, drugs may be applied to the outside of the body to treat pain, specifically joint and muscle aches. External analgesics, sometimes known as counterirritants, produce a local irritation where they are applied, which affects the ache in several ways. In one way, they dilate the blood vessels in the area, bringing more warmth to the painful area. The counterirritant can also produce an irritation that is more painful than the joint or muscle ache; this takes your mind off your original hurt because the second pain is worse. Counterirritants also provide relief because so many people believe in their properties. This reaction is like the old placebo effect: It makes you feel so much better psychologically just to apply Mentholatum Deep Heating Rub that your sore muscles feel better too.[13]

The counterirritants may appear on the shelves of your pharmacy in several forms, each with its own advantage.

- *Liniment*, for external use only, is rubbed or massaged into the skin.

- *Gels* produce a lot of warmth—more warmth, in fact, than lotions or ointment. For this reason, you have to be careful not to apply too much and burn the skin.

- *Lotions* are usually in a liquid form and may contain alcohol. They dry to form a protective coat over the area. Their advantage is that they cover rapidly and uniformly.

- *Ointments* may be absorbed through the skin into the bloodstream, a process that may be an advantage if medication needs to get into the bloodstream. Otherwise, it can be a disadvantage, and it could cause poisoning.[14]

Chemicals in Treatments

Some of the most common and effective drugs used in external pain relievers are listed below:

- *Methyl salicylate* (wintergreen oil), the most widely used, produces heat as well as possible analgesic effects after it is absorbed.

- *Camphor* generates a feeling of coolness when applied, also giving a mild, local anesthetic effect.

- *Menthol* (mint oil) has the same effects as camphor, a feeling of coolness and mild anesthesia.

- *Alkyl isothiocyanate* (oil of mustard) is exemplified by the common mustard plaster. You should be cautious, though, in your use of mustard plasters because they can burn and cause a rash and broken skin.

- *Clove oil*

- *Thymol*

- *Turpentine oil*

- *Cinnamon*

- *Wormwood*

- *Myristica*

- *Chenopodium*

- *Eucalyptus*

- *Methacholine chloride*

- *Histamine*

- *Dihydrochloride*

- *Triethanolumine salicylate*[15]

Some of the products on the market that are safe to use and that contain these ingredients are: Absorbine Jr., Absorbine Arthritic Pain lotion, Analbalm, Arthralgen, Bengay, Capsolin, Counterpain Rub, Exocaine (contains benzocaine also; see the section on burns for additional information), Ger-O-Foam (contains benzocaine), Guia-Camph, Heet (liniment and spray), Lini-Balm, Menthofax, Mentholatum, Mentholatum Deep Heating Rub and Lotion, Minit-Rub, Musterole (regular and extra-strength), Myoflex, Omegn Oil, Panelgesic, Penetro Quick Acting Rub, Sloan's Balm and Liniment, Soltice Quick Rub and Hi-Therm, Soltice Children's Mild Quick Rub, S.P.D., Surin.

Choosing a Treatment
There are many things to consider when choosing an external pain reliever, but the choice must take into account your type of pain and the following criteria:

- *Solubility.* Do I want a water-soluble or an oil-base product?

- *Stability.* How long will the product "stay put" and not have to be reapplied?

- *Staining.* Will the product stain my clothing, sheets, or other items it touches?

- *Tackiness and consistency.* Will the product be greasy or sticky?

- *Route and degrees of penetration.* How quickly will the product soak in, and will it reach my pain?

- *Allergies.* Am I allergic to any of the ingredients?

Remember that these self-treatment products only temporarily relieve the symptoms of aching and pain; they do not cure the underlying cause. Also remember that for arthritis, aspirin is the drug of choice because it reduces inflammation. However, allergies to aspirin may mean you have to use another pain reliever (see the section on "Pain and Internal Pain-Killers" in this chapter).

CAUTIONS
Cautions should be observed anytime a drug is used for self-treatment. In the case of external pain relievers, you should beware of the following:

- Don't apply any of these products to broken skin (irritation and infection may result).

- Because of their irritating effect, do not apply these products to mucous membranes (such as the lips or nose lining) or to the eyes.

- Do not use these products on infants and small children (except Soltice Children's Mild Quick Rub, which is designed for that purpose).

- Do not apply these products to large areas of the body; they should be used only on localized areas.

- If you see unusual skin reactions (such as a rash), stop using the product. Mustard oil, turpentine oil, and camphor—rubbed into the skin too vigorously—may cause blistering or rash. Oil of wintergreen does not usually cause this problem.

• Do not use these products if you are allergic to aspirin. Many of them contain aspirin and could be absorbed from the skin into the blood stream.

• Follow the directions on the package to be sure you apply the product often enough or to be sure you don't apply the product too often.[16]

Side Effects
Three side effects can occur when using an external pain reliever:

• *Allergic reactions.* Skin irritations or rashes may result from using these products. Also, as mentioned previously, aspirin allergies may occur when aspirin is absorbed into the blood stream; symptoms include skin rash and asthma.

• *Burning.* Some of these products may produce a lot of warmth, and, because of this, skin burns may occur.

• *Poisoning.* Many of these products are very pleasant smelling (such as methyl salicylate), and children may be tempted to swallow them. To avoid such tragedies, external pain relievers should be locked up or put in some other safe place.

MENSTRUAL PAIN

Menstruation is a natural cycle in females in which the uterus prepares itself for possible pregnancy by increasing its tissue and blood supply. If a woman doesn't become pregnant, the lining that has built up sheds itself. Many women experience pain and cramping during the first day or two of the menstrual period. This pain is usually sharp and intermittent, and it generally occurs in the lower, middle abdomen. Some women also have painful cramps in the lower back or (rarely) in the thighs or the vagina. Other symptoms may go with the cramps, such as headache, nausea and vomiting, joint pain, painful urination, or diarrhea.

CAUSES
No one is entirely sure what causes cramps, but there are theories:

• changes in hormone levels during the monthly menstrual cycle,

• emotional stress,

- muscle contractions in the uterus and changes in blood vessel structure (perhaps linked to the hormone changes),

- fluid retention (that occurs before your period begins),

- psychological factors (many women experience cramps because they think they will or because of their distaste for having periods),

- low pain threshold (some women cannot tolerate pain as well as others), and

- heredity (you have a better chance of having cramps if your mother did).[17]

TREATMENT
Nonmedicinal (and "Slightly" Medicinal) Treatment
Things other than OTC drugs can help to relieve the pain of cramps. Many women have found that heat (either in the form of a heating pad or a hot bath) can control the pain of their cramps. Some doctors recommend getting in the knee-chest position to relieve the pain); this position may look funny, but it works for some women. Lastly, mild exercise, such as walking, cycling, or swimming, helps some women—although usually the first problem is convincing yourself that doing something physical will really help those painful cramps. Most women think it would be more comfortable just to sit and endure the pain.

Of the many OTC products that relieve pain, some are more effective than others. Probably your best bet in a pain reliever is your old friend, the aspirin tablet.

Self-Treatment
Self-treating your cramps is all right if they are routine and mild to moderate. If they are severe or if you notice any change in them or unusual symptoms, however, see your doctor. Sometimes cramps are an indication of a more serious condition. If you experience any of the following symptoms, you should consult your doctor and not self-treat your cramps:

- new or unusual symptoms,

- stoppage of menstrual periods,

- unusually heavy bleeding,

- severe pain or nausea, or

- cramps that begin after age 20.

These symptoms could mean endometriosis, uterine hypoplasia, pelvic inflammation, pelvic neoplasm (cancer), and retroversion of the uterus.

If your cramps are not unusual, however, self-treatment is safe. Over-the-counter products to treat cramps are really varied; they run the gamut of ingredients.

1. *Analgesics* (such as aspirin, acetaminophen, phenacetin, and the rest) give some relief from cramps; however, they are more effective in treating headache and muscle pain. Analgesics tend to be fairly good for cramps because they are absorbed well and distributed throughout the bloodstream. They are also relatively safe to take.

2. *Diuretics* are often found in menstrual products, but whether they are very effective in treating cramps is doubtful. They seem to help, though, in preventing tension before the menstrual period. These products work by increasing sodium excretion (sodium makes you retain body fluid) or by preventing reabsorption of sodium and water in the kidneys.

3. *Antihistamines* help to relieve the nervousness and irritability that come before the menstrual period. However, most of these products do not contain enough antihistamine to be effective in relieving pain.

4. *Antispasmodics* reduce cramping.

5. *Cinnamedrine* causes blood vessels to constrict. It is also a decongestant.

Chemicals in the Treatments
When reading the labels, look for these chemicals:

- *Analgesics* (previously discussed in the first section on pain): Acetylsalicylic acid, acetaminophen, phenacetin, and salicylamide.

- *Diuretics:* Mostly composed of pamabrom, caffeine, and ammonium chloride.

- *Antihistamines:* Pyrilamine maleate, methapyrilamine fumarate, phenindamine tartrate, and phenyltoloxamine dehydrogin citrate.

Several brand name products that contain these ingredients or a combination of them are considered safe for use. Trendar tablets contain acetaminophen, pamabrom, and phenindamine tartrate, while Midol tablets contain a combination of aspirin and caffeine plus cinnamedrine. Cardui and Pamprin tablets contain salicylamide and phenacetin, plus pamabrom and pyrilamine maleate. Femicin tablets contain pyrilamine maleate and homatropine methylbromide. Last, but not least, Aqua-Ban and Pre-Mens Forte contain caffeine and ammonium chloride.[18]

Choosing a Treatment
To choose the right treatment, talk to your pharmacist. Give him or her a brief history of your problem: the severity of your symptoms and any other information regarding abnormal conditions that you may have; also any allergies to medications and any medicines (prescription and OTC) that you are taking. A pharmacist should be able to suggest an OTC product that will suit your needs and your symptoms. For example, if your only problem is pain, an analgesic will undoubtedly be suggested. If you are bothered by water retention and tension before your period, a product with a combination of ingredients will probably be recommended. Your pharmacist can be a real help in guiding you to a product that is most effective for you.

CAUTIONS AND SIDE EFFECTS
Like most OTC drugs, the primary caution with OTC medication for menstrual pain is *not* to take more of the drug than you are directed to do. Read the label carefully to know just how much you can safely take.

Remember also that antihistamines may cause drowsiness, so you should not drive or operate machinery while taking them. Even though the dosage of antihistamines is small in medication for cramps, there is still the chance that drowsiness could occur. It is better to be safe than sorry!

As previously mentioned, there is always the danger of allergy with aspirins. Aspirin allergies cause asthma-like symptoms and skin rash.

5

indigestion

At least 575 different powders, liquids, pills, gums, lozenges, and tablets compete on today's market for the opportunity to soothe our upset stomachs, abdominal cramps, bloating, heartburn, gas pains, and morning sickness. But there's a good chance you've only heard of a few of them: Fewer than a dozen brands account for almost all the advertising and sales in this over-$200-million-a-year market.[1]

CAUSES

Indigestion is a catch-all phrase that covers a variety of discomforts in the abdomen and stomach. Like any other "symptom," it can be a sign of a trivial illness or a serious condition that should get prompt medical attention. Some of the conditions that might cause an upset stomach (or "indigestion") are:[2]

- simple overeating, eating too much, eating too fast (which may include poor chewing habits or swallowing air), and eating something that doesn't agree with you (such as highly spiced foods),

- smoking or drinking alcoholic beverages,

- accidental poisoning from ingestion of toxic chemicals,

- food poisoning (the body's reaction to the ingestion of spoiled food),

- diseases of the esophagus (including tumors or reflux esophagitis),
- diseases of the stomach (including ulcer, cancer, hiatal hernia, and gastritis),
- diseases of the duodenum (upper section of the small intestine), including duodenal ulcer,
- diseases that affect the small and large intestines (including diverticulitis, diverticulosis, regional enteritis, and ulcerated colon),
- infection or disease of the gall bladder (including gall stones),
- infection or cancer of the pancreas (including stones),
- heart disease or heart attack (heart attack often begins with a feeling of heartburn or indigestion),
- nervousness, or
- taking aspirin.

You are generally safe in treating yourself with over-the-counter medications if you experience the following symptoms:[3]

- You feel full or uncomfortable (that is, suffer from heartburn or sour stomach) in the upper abdomen or under the breastbone from a specific cause, such as overeating or drinking.
- Your indigestion is the result of overeating.
- The symptoms that you suffer from after overeating are limited to heartburn or sour stomach.
- The symptoms occur very rarely.
- One of the symptoms is a headache (in this case, use an antacid combined with an analgesic).
- Your symptoms are accompanied by gas (in this case, use an antacid combined with an antiflatulent).

At other times, you should definitely *not* attempt self-treatment. You should contact a physician immediately under the following circumstances:[4]

- The general complaint of indigestion lasts for longer than two weeks.

• You vomit for more than two days (excessive vomiting can lead to rapid dehydration).

• There is blood in your vomitus (indicative of a bleeding stomach ulcer).

• You experience difficulty in swallowing (the early symptom of a number of esophageal diseases).

• You have a severe pain in your abdomen.

• You have a pain in the left side of the lower chest or stomach area that radiates either around your rib cage to your back or straight through your body from front to back. Also, the pain is persistent with no feeling of burning, and it is not alleviated by antacids.

• You experience rapid weight loss.

• Your abdominal pain is relieved when you eat.

• Your abdominal pain is brought on when you eat, or it is made worse when you eat (especially when you eat fatty foods).

• You experience diarrhea from no apparent cause, and the diarrhea lasts more than a few days (again, a danger of dehydration).

• You experience a sharp or dull pain when you manually depress the abdomen.

• You see blood in your stools.

• You see large quantities of mucus in your stools.

• You experience shortness of breath, sweating, or chest pain along with indigestion (indicative of a heart attack).

• Your stools are black and tarry.

• Your symptoms seem to be recurrent—you have them more than once or twice a month.

• Your symptoms follow a regular pattern (for instance, you may have the symptoms every time you eat).

• You or someone in your family (brothers, sisters, or parents) has a history of peptic ulcers.

• You have had previous heart disease.

• You have had previous kidney disease (including gout, kidney stones, and urinary retention).

- You suffer from hypertension.

- You notice swelling in the legs and ankles along with your indigestion.

- You suffer from constipation or diarrhea before you start the medication.

- Your symptoms are made worse from your efforts at self-treatment.

- You are taking *any* prescription drug. A number of antacids, for example, neutralize tetracycline, penicillin, sulfonamides, pentobarbital, some anticoagulants, isoniazid, and cortisone (or other antiarthritic medication). You should always check with your doctor or pharmacist before you take an over-the-counter indigestion aid if you are also taking a prescription drug.

TREATMENT
Nonmedicinal Treatment
If you have frequent problems with indigestion, you can do some things to lessen your discomfort,[5] without resorting to medication right away:

- See your doctor to make sure that nothing serious is wrong.

- Stay away from milk as a cure-all for indigestion. All food and drink causes an acid "rebound" in the stomach: Your stomach pumps out increased acid several hours after the food or drink arrives. It's better to take an antacid.

- Steer clear of bedtime snacks. The increase in acid occurs when you least appreciate it—in the middle of the night. Instead, take an antacid (and consider an extra dose) before bed if nighttime indigestion is a problem.

- Stomach acid is stimulated by caffeine, so stay away from coffee, tea, or cola drinks that contain caffeine. (And read the label on your antacid—some of them contain caffeine!)

- Stomach acid is also stimulated by cigarette smoking. If you have a real problem with indigestion, quit smoking.

- A big cause of stomach acidity is anxiety. You should do whatever you can to control your tensions and your anxiety; you might consider seeking professional help if you have a real problem.

If you suffer from ulcers, follow your doctor's advice completely, including his or her choice of an antacid. You can lessen your discomfort by regulating your diet (again, check with your doctor):[6]

indigestion **71**

• Eat several times a day.

• Choose nonirritating foods, such as milk, cream, strained oatmeal, refined cereal, soup, peeled potatoes, butter, rice, enriched white bread, white crackers, sugar, eggs, cooked vegetables, ripe bananas, fruit juice, lean fresh beef or veal, cream or cottage cheese, fresh fish, custard, cookies, gelatin, and plain cake.

• Avoid spices, highly seasoned food, fried food, carbonated drinks, coffee, alcohol, meat broths, strong cheese, pork, raw fruit or vegetables, whole-grain cereal or bread, nuts, olives, rich desserts, popcorn, and pastry.

Self-Treatment
Your self-treatment is supposed to do primarily one thing: neutralize or block the chemical activity of the stomach acid. "Antacids," as they are widely referred to, accomplish this task in one or more ways: They may reduce the acid in the stomach, coat the stomach wall, or reduce certain elements in the gastric juice (like pepsin). They come in a number of forms and contain a number of different chemicals; it is important, again, to be a conscientious label-reader. The best antacids on the market are those that act promptly, that neutralize a good deal of acid for their weight, that remain in effect for a long time, that are not quickly absorbed into the bloodstream, that have no side effects, and that are inexpensive.[7]

Forms of Antacids
You can take your antacid in any of several ways:[8]

• *Liquids and suspensions* offer the most rapid and the most certain relief, because their active ingredients cover the surface area of the stomach and provide a medium for immediate chemical interaction.

• *Tablets and gums* are a little less effective. They have to be *completely* chewed up and dissolved before they can work correctly on stomach acid. Since complete disintegration is uncertain, the antacid effects can be reduced.

• *Effervescent powders* carry with them their own side effect: gas. Make sure that you completely dissolve any effervescent powders or tablets in water before you take them. Don't drink the solution until *all* the gas production activity ceases. For example, don't take an Alka-Seltzer until the tablet is completely dissolved and no more bubbles are being produced in the water.

What Do Antacids Contain?

An antacid may contain just one or a combination of the following major ingredients:[9]

Sodium Bicarbonate. Sodium bicarbonate—ordinary baking soda—has been widely used for years as a home remedy for upset stomach and indigestion. Its advantages? It is fast-acting, effective, and acceptable for occasional, short-term use. But it has some disadvantages that you should be aware of, too. It shouldn't be used for a long time or with any regularity. Why? If you use it for a prolonged period, especially if you are also drinking milk (common among ulcer victims), it can lead to the formation of kidney stones. It has a high concentration of sodium, which is quickly absorbed by the blood stream—a dangerous implication for people with high blood pressure, kidney disease, heart disease, or just about any other medical problem. Some commercial antacids are particularly high in sodium—Rolaids and Phosphal-jel, for instance—while others are low—such as Di-Gel, Gelusil, Maalox, and Mylanta. One other drawback of sodium bicarbonate is that it can cause what is known as the "acid rebound phenomenon."[10] After the sodium bicarbonate has done its initial job of settling the stomach, it can stimulate further acid secretion in the stomach. This side effect can be compared to the effect of nasal sprays and drops in which they initially reduce the swelling of the nasal passages, but with prolonged use they can cause a rebound in which the linings swell again. Still another disadvantage is that sodium bicarbonate forms carbon dioxide in the stomach. Too much carbon dioxide may stretch the stomach walls, which may produce tears at the ulcer site.

Calcium Carbonate. Calcium carbonate is considered by many to be an extremely good antacid, but it also has its pitfalls. Again, it is not acceptable for long-term use. Unlike most other kinds of antacids, those containing calcium carbonate produce an acid "rebound"—the stomach is apt to produce even more acid once the effects of the antacid wear off. Eventually, you're worse off than if you'd never taken the medicine. The acid from the rebound can last up to several hours. Another unpleasant effect of calcium carbonates (such as Tums or Pepto-Bismol tablets) is that they are constipating. Calcium carbonates can also raise the body's calcium so that stones form in the kidneys; these can decrease kidney function.

Aluminum Hydroxide. Although it, too, has a constipating effect, aluminum hydroxide is the most widely used ingredient in antacid preparations. It is considered the best because it has no effect at all on the acid–base balance of the body. It is especially safe for people who suffer from peptic ulcers. In order to counteract the constipating effects, many antacids contain a combination of aluminum hydroxide and magnesium, which has a laxative effect.

Magnesium. Some studies show magnesium to have the greatest neturalizing capacity over long periods of use; products containing magnesium are expecially safe for victims of peptic ulcer (even more so than products containing only aluminum). It is also safe to take magnesium products for long-term use; they are prescribed for treatment of ulcers that may last for months or years. Because the magnesium has a laxative effect, some antacids containing magnesium—such as Phillips' Milk of Magnesia—are advertised as an antacid at a low dose and as a laxative at a high dose. Many antacids, as already mentioned, combine magnesium and aluminum so that the laxative and constipating effects of both chemicals can counteract each other.

Naturally magnesium has a few drawbacks. If it is taken too often, you may have problems with diarrhea which can eventually cause dehydration; so you're worse off than if you'd never taken the medication. Also, magnesium salts may cause drowsiness or kidney problems with overuse.

Dihydroxy Aluminum Sodium Carbonate. This fancy-sounding name simply means that the antacid effects of both aluminum hydroxide and sodium bicarbonate have been combined. The end result? Rolaids.

Simethicone. Simethicone is not an antacid; it's a defoamer or anti-flatulant, designed to help get rid of gas. It acts in the stomach to help break up mucus that may be trapping small pockets of gas. Products on the market that contain only simethicone include Mylicon tablets or drops, Phazyme-95 Plus Pancreatin, and Silain tablets.

Auxiliary Drugs. Antacid preparations may also contain:

- magnesium carbonate, which acts as an antacid;

- bismuth subsalicylate, which acts as a protectorant in coating the stomach,

- bismuth subnitrate, which acts as a protectorant,

- dicyclomine HCl, which suppresses acid secretion in the stomach,

- aspirin or some other analgesic, to aid in the relief of pain (useful when the indigestion is accompanied by headache, but not recommended for victims of peptic ulcer), and

• a small amount of digestive enzymes, which help the stomach to digest foods more effectively and thus limit such conditions as "sour stomach" or indigestion.

In addition to these drugs, manufacturers often include ingredients in antacids to make them taste better: citric acid, glycerin, mint oil of wintergreen, oil of peppermint, skimmed milk, or aluminum phosphate.

Choosing an Antacid
The antacid you choose depends on a number of things:[11] your general medical history (high blood pressure? a peptic ulcer?), whether you need it for short- or long-term use, what ingredients you need in your specific case, and which form you most prefer (liquid/suspension, tablet, gum, or effervescent powder). The label can give you all the information you need to make a good decision.

Products good for *short-term use only* include Alka-Seltzer (you can get it with or without aspirin), Bell-Ans tablets, BiSoDol powder, Citrocarbonate granules, Eno powder, Fizrin powder (contains aspirin), or Soda Mint tablets.

Products suitable for *long-term use* are available with a number of chemical combinations:

• *Calcium carbonate* antacids suitable for long-term use include Amitone tablets, Gustalac tablets, Krem tablets, Pepto-Bismol tablets (contain bismuth subsalicylate for coating protection), Ratio tablets, Titralac tablets and liquid, and Zylase tablets.

• Antacids containing only *aluminum* include Amphogel tablets and liquid.

• Those containing only *magnesium* include any brand of milk of magnesia.

Combination antacids are available in the following mixtures, safe for both short- and long-term use:

• *Calcium carbonate/magnesium:* Chooz gum, Dicarbosil tablets, and Tums tablets.

• *Aluminum/magnesium:* Aludrox tablets and liquid, Creamalin tablets and liquid, Delcid liquid (extra concentrated), Di-Gel liquid (contains simethicone), Di-Gel tablets (contains simethicone), Kolantyl liquid and wafers, Kudrox tablets and liquid, Maalox liquid, Maalox #1 tablets, Maalox #2 tablets (double-strength), Maalox Plus tablets and liquid (contains simethicone), Mylanta tablets and liquid (contains simethicone), Mylanta II tablets and liquid (both double-strength, both contain simethicone), Riopan tablets and liquid (tablets in both chewable and swallow form), Silain-Gel liquid (contains simethicone), Silain-Gel tablet (contains simethicone), Triactin liquid (contains dicyclomine HCl for stomach protection), and WinGel tablets and liquid. A slightly different form of magnesium is combined with aluminum in A.M.T. tablets and liquid, Gelumina tablets, Gelusil liquid and tablets, Gelusil-Lac powder, Malcogel liquid, Sippyplex powder, Tricreamalate liquid, and Trisogel capsules and liquid.

• *Calcium carbonate/aluminum/magnesium:* Al-Caroid tablets and powder, Camalox tablets and liquid, and Ducon liquid (features extra duration of action formula).

• *Calcium carbonate/magnesium hydroxide/magnesium trisilicate:* BiSoDol tablets.

• *Aluminum/magnesium hydroxide/magnesium trisilicate:* Gelusil-M tablets and liquid, Magnatril tablets and liquid, and Mucotin tablets.

Using Antacids the Right Way
Timing is extremely important in the use of antacids. For the best effects, take your antacid one hour after you finish your meal. The antacid stays in the stomach longer, and it is much more effective. Taking the antacid after meals is especially important for victims of peptic ulcer, who tend to have a rapid gastric emptying line.

It's a good idea to at least call your doctor before you launch a long-term program of antacid use. A doctor can help you rule out any serious medical problem that might be causing the indigestion, and further help you choose the brand that is best for you.

CAUTIONS
As with all medication, certain cautions and disadvantages might guide you in choosing a brand or deciding against self-medication.

Sodium Level
As already mentioned, sodium bicarbonate formulas contain a level of sodium that can pose a hazard to people with high blood pressure, heart disease, or kidney disease, and to anyone else who has been advised to restrict salt intake. Some heart patients are allowed only 1,000 to 2,000 milligrams of sodium daily. A *single dose* of Alka-Seltzer or Bromo Seltzer exceeds that limit.

Those with medical problems aren't the only ones who need to steer clear of sodium bicarbonates: People over sixty should not exceed 2,300 milligrams of sodium per day in any antacid. This limit allows for only one to two doses of either Alka-Seltzer or Bromo Seltzer in a day. If you need more than one or two doses, consider switching to an antacid that does not contain sodium bicarbonate.

Acid–Base Balance
Sodium bicarbonates tend to disturb the body's acid–base balance. Body fluids and tissues become more alkaline than normal, a condition that can lead to stone formation in the gall bladder, kidneys, and pancreas. It can also lead to nausea and vomiting, headache, confusion, and the inability and desire to eat. Many antacids contain large amounts of citrates; for example, the maximum daily doses of both Alka-Seltzer and Bromo Seltzer exceed the level designated as safe (8 grams) by the Food and Drug Administration.

Unnecessary Ingredients
Make sure the antacid you are using does not contain analgesics (such as aspirin) if you don't need them. Alka-Seltzer, for instance, contains aspirin that could aggravate a peptic ulcer. Bromo Seltzer contains phenacetin, an analgesic that can cause kidney disease over long-term use. Check for other ingredients, too; some (like Bromo Seltzer) contain as much caffeine as a brewed cup of coffee.[12]

Conflicting Ingredients
Often, antacids should not be used while you are taking other medication. They can decrease the amount of other medications absorbed into the blood stream. They can also combine with other drugs to make the drug ineffective in the body. For example, the body cannot use the combination of an antacid and the drug tetracycline.

Guidelines
To make your choice of antacid as safe and effective as possible, follow these guidelines:[13]

  • Don't use *any* antacid longer than two weeks unless your doctor has given you the go-ahead.

  • Use antacids containing sodium bicarbonate or calcium carbonate (such as Alka-Seltzer) only occasionally; if you need to take an antacid more than twice, switch to one that doesn't contain either of these ingredients.

• If you are on a sodium-restricted diet, stick to an antacid that is low in sodium; Di-Gel, Gelusil, Maalox, Mylanta, Pepto-Bismol, and Phillips' Milk of Magnesia are all low in sodium content (all below 9 milligrams). If you're unsure, ask your doctor or pharmacist for a recommendation.

• For the greatest effectiveness, use a liquid whenever it is possible and convenient. If you do use a tablet, chew it thoroughly.

• If a certain food or beverage consistently causes you stomach upset or indigestion, cutting out the offending item makes much more sense than constantly trying to mask its effects with medicine. If you can't identify the culprit, call your doctor.

• If you are pregnant, steer clear of antacids containing aspirin or a lot of sodium. You should check with your doctor before taking any antacid.

• If your indigestion lasts longer than two weeks, or if it gets worse as a result of your self-medication efforts, immediately stop taking the antacid and call a doctor.

• When asking your doctor or pharmacist about which antacid to use, tell him or her about any other medications you are taking.

• If you change antacids, notify your pharmacist or doctor.

• Remember that no antacid is entirely free of side effects.

6

burns
and sunburns

BURNS

Burns can be one of the most devastating types of injury that can happen to your body because the skin is such an important organ. It may surprise you to know that the skin is the largest organ of your body; it makes up one-sixth of your body weight.[1] About one-third of your circulation is contained in your skin, so your skin takes care of body functions such as maintaining the fluid, chemical, and temperature balances for most of the body. The skin also protects structures such as organs and bone that lie beneath it. It has nerve endings, so much of your power of sensation comes from the skin. The skin also secretes waste materials, water (in the form of sweat), and oils (to maintain smooth, soft skin).[2]

DEGREES OF BURNS
Burns may be classified by degree according to the amount of damage done to the skin and tissues directly under the skin.

• *First-degree burn:* The skin is red, and it may or may not be swollen. This type of burn tends to be quite painful and sore.

• *Second-degree burn:* Swelling is common, and blistering occurs because fluids leak into the layers of skin tissue. Deep reddening also indicates that deeper layers of tissue have been injured.

79

- *Third-degree burn:* The skin takes on a charred appearance. But more than the skin is involved in the charring; the burn may involve muscles, tendons, nerves, blood vessels, and, in extreme cases, bones.

The Rule of 9s

Assessing the severity of a burn is usually quite difficult at first, but you should use the Rule of 9s as your guide to make an initial judgment. The Rule of 9s assigns percentages to each area of the body to make your judgment more accurate. For example, 9 percent of the body has been burned if you have burned your head and neck or either arm and hand. You may estimate that you have burned 18 percent of your body if your chest and abdomen, entire back, or either leg and foot has been burned. And 1 percent of your body has been burned if the burn occurs in the genital area.[3]

CAUSES

Burns can be classified by the environmental conditions that cause them:

- *Thermal burns* are caused when you come into contact with something hot, such as a hot iron, a camp fire, or scalding water.

- *Chemical burns* occur as a result of such things as contact with strong acids or alkalis. The school chemistry lab is probably the most likely place for chemical burns to happen.

- *Electrical burns* may result when high-voltage wires come into contact with the body. Many electrocution victims experience deep burns as well as electrical shock.

- *Radiation burns* are pretty rare among the lay public, but they may be more common among those who work with atomic energy and nuclear power.

- *Sunburn* is common from mid-spring until early fall. Everyone at least one time in life has experienced the pain and redness that occur from a day of activity out-of-doors on a bright, summer day.[4]

TREATMENT

When treating burn victims:

- keep them warm, but do not overheat them;
- cover burn areas with a sterile dressing;

- give *conscious* burn victims as many liquids as they will take (never give them to an unconscious victim);

- don't attempt to remove cloth that is stuck to a burn (your doctor will do that); and

- do not open blisters that occur with a second degree burn.[5]

Self-Treatment
You should not attempt to self-treat, but should see your doctor, in the following cases:

- If more than 2 percent of the body surface is seriously burned (major second- or third-degree burn). Extensive and deep burns are referred immediately to the special burn service of the hospital serving your area.[6]

- If you are very young, elderly, or have a chronic disease (such as diabetes, alcoholism, obesity, or heart disease), you should see your doctor because you cannot tolerate burns as well as the general population.

- If you begin to develop an infection after a burn, medical help is encouraged so that the infection will not become serious or spread.

- If you have serious thermal, chemical, or sunburn. (Minor cases may be self-treated, as long as you avoid dehydration and infection.)

- If you have any kind of electrical or radiation burn.

Two dangers in serious burns can best be treated by your doctor, and these make it imperative that you get immediate help:

- Fluids are lost from the body in serious or extensive burns, and you can easily dehydrate as a result.

- Many times, infection can occur that may spread throughout the body. Burned tissue is an ideal breeding ground for all sorts of bacteria because of the injured tissue and because the body is in a weakened state and can't fight the infection as well.

As a general rule, though, it is perfectly permissible to treat first-degree and minor second-degree burns at home.

Forms of Treatment
Several avenues of self-treatment for burns are open to you.

1. *Cold or salt water compresses and ice* are probably the best and most convenient treatment items in your home. A minor burn may repair itself without further treatment when water or ice is used, because early cooling may reduce the extent of the burn. Tissue continues to burn even after it is removed from the heat source. Think back to the last time you barbecued a steak. If you took it off the grill and right into the dinner table, it was probably still sizzling as you sat down to eat. Your skin does the same thing: It burns even after it is away from the heat. Prompt cooling stops this secondary burning. Cold water and ice also tend to reduce the swelling that accompanies burns.

2. *Local anesthetics* come in a variety of forms: ointments, creams, sprays, and lotions. Creams, sprays, and lotions are your best bet in the anesthetic department because they are more cooling and because they are water soluble, which means they are easier to remove when the time comes. Ointments tend to be greasy and oily, which means they do not let the tissues breathe. This can increase burn damage. Ointments seal the skin, so to speak. The heat cannot escape, and so the secondary burning continues to cause more damage. Ointments also make a good home for bacteria because bacteria easily stick to the greasy or oily surface. Ointments are also harder to remove.[7]

3. *Antiseptics* may or may not be included with an anesthetic. The job of an antiseptic is to kill or retard the growth of those bacteria that cause infections. Antiseptics may also come in ointments, creams, sprays, or lotions.

Commonly Used Chemicals
The best way to find a good medication for burn treatment is to read the labels:

1. *Local anesthetic only.* The preferred chemical ingredient for a local anesthetic is 5 to 20 percent benzocaine. Other ingredients that are not as effective as benzocaine but may be used are butamben picrate, lidocaine, tetracaine, pramoxine, and debucaine. Anesthetics should be discontinued when the pain stops.

2. *Antiseptic only.* Antiseptics commonly include benzethomium chloride, methyl benzethonium chloride, oxyquinoline, iso-octylphenoxypolyethanol, phenylmercuric acetate, triclosan, chloroxylenol, and phenol. Common brand names that include these ingredients are Bactine liquids, Betadine aerosol spray, Noxema medicated cream, Sun-Ice cream, and Zemacol lotion.

3. *Local anesthetic/antiseptic.* Combinations of anesthetics and antiseptics may be obtained by the following products: Aerosept aerosol spray, Americaine aerosol spray (probably the best product because it contains the highest concentration of benzocaine), Bactine aerosol spray, Burn-a-way cream; Clean n' Treat medicated pads; Foille liquid or aerosol spray; Kip Sunburn spray; Medicone dressing cream; Medi-Quick aerosol spray; Noxema sunburn spray; Solarcaine cream, lotion, aerosol spray, foam; Unburn cream, lotion, spray; Unquentine first aid spray; Unquentine aerosol spray.

4. *Auxiliary drugs.* Sometimes other ingredients may appear in burn medications. Some of them produce a cooling effect or a pleasant smell such as camphor, menthol, clove oil, Eucalyptus oil, oil of spearmint, oil of wintergreen, and thyme oil. Other ingredients make the product easier to apply such as petrolatum, lanolin, propylene glycol, polyethylene glycol, wax or paraffin, and vegetable oil. Still other ingredients such as zinc oxide, sulfur, and allantoin promote healing and provide a mild antiseptic.[8]

Choosing a Treatment
The treatment you choose depends entirely on the type of burn you have, and the extent of the damage. The treatments given below are *only* for thermal, chemical, and sun burns.

1. For a first-degree burn, you should use cold water compresses and/or ice. A good compress can be made by soaking a towel in cold water and then applying it to the area. This should be done immediately to minimize damage to the skin. After the early stages, you can apply a local anesthetic to help the pain. Local anesthetics may be especially helpful at night when pain seems more apparent. Aspirin or some other pain medication may also relieve pain. An antiseptic may also be applied.

2. For second-degree burns that are minor and cover a small area, you should apply cold immediately. This may prevent blistering. Salt water compresses are best for use with second-degree burns. They can be made by soaking a towel in a solution of 2 tablespoons of salt to 1 quart of cold water. The compress should be kept wet and should be applied for 30 to 60 minutes three to four times a day. If the burn has been caused by hot grease, the grease should be gently washed off with soap and water. You may also use an analgesic and antiseptic with these types of burns to relieve pain and prevent infection. Again, you may take some other pain reliever, too, such as aspirin.[9]

3. For severe second-degree burns and third-degree burns, do not put anything on them. Merely cover them with a sterile dressing, and go to your doctor.

4. Caution must be used in treating chemical burns. If you use a neutralizing substance, you need to be very careful because a strong neutralizing agent can cause more damage than was done originally, or a neutralizing agent combined with the acid or alkali could produce enough heat to cause more burn damage. Generally, treatment for a chemical burn is as follows:

  • Remove all contaminated clothing and flood the area with water. Many chemistry labs are equipped with showers for immediate use.

  • After a thorough washing, if the burn was caused by an acid, flood the area with a diluted solution of 2 tablespoons of bicarbonate of soda to one quart of water. In the case of an alkali burn, the area should be flooded with a diluted solution of half vinegar and half water.

  • Use a water-soluble burn cream and apply it to the area. Afterwards, cover the area with a sterile dressing.[10]

CAUTIONS
Burns can be dangerous, and some cautions are in order.

  • Don't overtreat a burn; undertreatment is better than overtreatment.

  • Anesthetics may produce sensitivities and allergies, so you should use them sparingly and discontinue their use if anything unusual such as increased redness or rash appear.

  • Do not use home remedies such as butter, grease, and cocoa butter on burns. They just increase the burn damage.

  • Do not use tannic acid (one of the ingredients in tea) or jellies on burns.

  • Do not use absorbent cotton to cover burns. Particles from the cotton may come off and stick to the burn. It is painful to have them removed later.

The American Medical Association rang the death knell on millions of Americans sprawled across sandy beaches, soaking up the rays, when they told us that the benefits of the sun's rays are mostly psychological—and that the dangers of repeated exposure to the sun far outweigh the benefits.[11] Too much sun can cause anything from a simple sunburn to sunstroke, heat prostration, or cancer. The amount of skin cancer is higher in farmers, sailors, construction workers, and others who do a great deal of outdoor work. Long-term exposure also leads to premature skin aging; the skin loses its flexibility, becoming thinner, more wrinkled, and drier.

These recent medical findings have increased the importance of protecting yourself against sunburn. A number of precautions give you protection. Preventive measures include being sensible about your exposure to the sun, using the most effective sun protection lotions, knowing which drugs may increase your risk of getting burned, and seeking immediate medical treatment for a bad burn.

FACTORS THAT INCREASE YOUR RISK

Prime Burning Time. The sun is a tricky character, and you can get sunburned even when you'd least expect it. As the sun climbs higher in the sky, more and more ultraviolet rays penetrate the earth's atmosphere; so the sun is most wicked at midday.[12] Your chances for a burn are much greater in the summer, and they get worse as you get farther south. You can get burned even on a hazy or cloudy day; you can burn through clothing if it's not protective enough. If the sun is extremely bright and you're on the beach, you won't get protection even under a beach umbrella. And you can get burned even if you stay in the water.

Genetic Makeup.[13] People who have dark skin and dark hair won't burn as easily as people with fair skin, fair hair, and blue eyes. But watch out—even if your skin is black, you can suffer from overexposure. Your genetic composition determines *how* you tan and burn: whether you tan first, burn first, or don't tan at all.

Certain other factors—physical things—can increase your chances of burning:[14]

Certain Over-the-Counter or Prescription Drugs. Chief among these that increase your photosensitivity are oral contraceptives, tetracycline, and tranquilizers. Others include psoralens, sulfonamides (including penicillin), griseofulvins, phenothiazines, hypoglycemic agents, and diuretics containing thiazide. Read the labels!

Contact with Antiseptic Products. The antiseptics found in many soaps, detergents, first-aid creams, household cleaners, cosmetics, and shampoos can increase your likelihood of burning.

Perfume. The oils found in many perfumes—especially oils of lavender, lime, lemon, bergamot, and rosemary—cause you to burn faster and easier.

Contact with Certain Growing Plants. Growing foods like parsley, dill, carrots, parsnips, and citrus fruits not only make you more susceptible to burn, they cause a rash similar to that of poison ivy if you are exposed to the sun following contact. Other plants, grasses, and certain tars can also make you more susceptible, depending on your genetic makeup.

Several Diseases that Cause Photosensitivity. Many people with allergies find that they can't tolerate the sun in big doses. Another disease that causes photosensitivity is lupus erythematosus, a usually fatal disease that causes degeneration of the collagen (the body's connective tissue protein). Still another photosensivity-causing disease is prophyria.

AVOIDING SUNBURN

Sunburn is much easier to prevent than to treat. Even before you buy a sun protection product, you can take the following steps to help protect yourself against sunburn:[15]

1. Don't go out in the sun between 10:00 A.M. and 2:00 P.M. The sun might seem as bright at 4:00 in the afternoon as it was at noon, but it has less chance of burning you because the burning rays are considerably reduced.

2. *Acclimate yourself.* Start out with a very brief exposure to the sun—no longer than fifteen minutes your first time out. If you don't burn after fifteen minutes, increase your exposure time to thirty minutes after a couple of days. After several days at thirty minutes, you may increase to forty-five minutes if you still haven't burned. Keep increasing your exposure time slowly until you find out the limit. Then don't exceed the limit.

3. *Don't go by your own body temperature to decide if you're getting burned.* Your body plays tricks on you, especially if you are at the beach. The cooling effects of the water and the breeze make you feel cooler than you actually are (even chilly!), while you may be sustaining a serious burn.

4. *Don't think you are safe just because the sun isn't bright.* Some of the worst burns get to you through clouds, fog, haze, or pollutants.

5. *Don't think that the ones on the sand are the only ones getting burned.* The sun can penetrate water, and you can go home with a severe burn even if you stayed immersed the whole time you were in the sun.

6. *Beware June 21.* The sun is at its meanest on June 21; by all means, don't start your acclimation program on or near that date. If you can start acclimating yourself in mid-April, you will probably be able to tolerate the summer sun during all hours except those at midday by the time June hits.

7. *Acclimate yourself before an extended trip.* If you're planning a two- to three-week vacation that includes activities in the sun, acclimate yourself *before* your intended trip. Many a vacation has been ruined due to blistered shoulders, scarlet chests, and painful legs.

8. *Take extra care if you are currently taking over-the-counter or prescription drugs.* Some of them can increase your sensitivity. If you are unsure about the drug you are taking, ask your pharmacist or doctor.

9. *Cover yourself with clothing that offers good protection.* Avoid light colors, open weaves, and clothing that doesn't cover you completely. Remember that your head, hands, and feet can burn, too; so wear a hat, shoes, and gloves if you will be out in the sun for a long time. Construction and yard workers are good candidates for the glove-shoes-hat routine.

SUN PROTECTION PRODUCTS
Three basic products help block out the sun's burning ultraviolet rays.[16]

Sun-Blockers. These contain para-aminobenzoic acid (PABA), the most effective sun-blocking ingredient available in sunscreen and tanning lotions and creams. Sun-blockers absorb those wavelengths of ultraviolet rays that normally cause skin to burn. You should apply the lotion about thirty minutes to one hour before going into the sun. It's a good idea to apply it for several days before your initial exposure. Also, since PABA can cause an allergic reaction in some people, you should perform a patch test to determine if you are sensitive or allergic to the lotion.

Lotions that contain PABA and that act as sun-blockers include Block Out, Estee Lauder Ultra-violet Screening Cream, Pabafilm, Pabanol, PreSun, Solbar, Sun-Gard, and Uval. After conducting a study that determined how many of the ultraviolet rays were actually blocked, dermatologists named Pabanol the best of all sun products available on the market; PreSun received an equal rating. They were both rated far above other available products.[17]

Sunscreens. While sun-blockers allow for only a minimal amount of tanning, sunscreens allow good tanning but don't protect as well against burning. Sunscreens usually work in one of two ways:

- They may have a lower concentration of sun-blocking ingredients than sun-blockers, or

- they may absorb different wavelengths of ultraviolet light (which is why they don't protect as well against burning—the burning rays are allowed to get through to the skin).

The protective agent in sunscreens is benzophenone. This ingredient is less effective than PABA, and it loses effectiveness rapidly when you get wet or begin to perspire. Although none of the sunscreen products protect as well as the sun-blockers, dermatologists rated Sea and Ski Dark Tanning Oil as the sunscreen product offering the greatest protection. Others are: Avon Sun Safe, Bronze Lustre Extra Protective, Coppertone Suntan Oil, Revlon Sun Bath Moisturizing Tanning Lotion—Extra Protection, Sea and Ski Dark Tanning Oil, Sundare Clear Lotion, and Swedish Tanning Secret Extra Protection Lotion.

Sun Barriers. These provide maximum protection against sunburn, by setting up a mechanical barrier to the sun's rays. Maxafil Cream is the best one; others that provide excellent protection include Nos-Kote (especially good for protecting the nose and tops of ears), RVPague, and zinc oxide ointment.

A number of products on the market serve only to moisturize the skin or to provide an attractive appearance or scent while offering no protection from the burning rays of the sun. Those products include Sea and Ski Tanning Butter, Tanfastic Tanning Butter, Tanya Hawaiian Tanning Butter, and any brand of baby or mineral oil.

Using Sun Protection Products

When using any kind of sun protection product, you should remember several safety tips:[18]

1. *Make sure you use enough.* The best sun protection product in the world won't do much good if you don't apply enough of it. You should use enough to give yourself a good coat.

2. *Reapply the lotion or cream every time you come out of the water, and reapply it if you begin to sweat heavily.*

3. *Don't swallow the lotion or cream,* and don't attempt to use it internally.

4. *Avoid getting the lotion in your eyes.*

5. *Quit using the lotion immediately if any irritation or rash forms where you applied it.*

6. *Apply the lotion everywhere the sun can reach.* Make sure you cover places like the back of your neck, the backs of your hands, the top of your feet, and areas with especially sensitive skin (on the tops of the ears, behind the knees, and on any skin that doesn't get exposed to the sun on a regular basis).

TREATING SUNBURN

If, despite all your best effort, you get a sunburn, follow these general guidelines for treatment:[19]

1. *See a doctor if the burn is extensive* (that is, if it covers a large area of your body) or severe (if it develops extensive blistering or is extremely painful). You shouldn't attempt to self-treat serious burns.

2. *Don't put butter, lard, goose grease, or other nonsterile greasy substances on your burn.* Even though they relieve the pain, they can lead to infection.

3. *Put cold compresses on the burned area.* You can use plain tap water. Cold compresses cool the burning sensation and reduce the swelling of burned tissue.

4. *Don't break any blisters that form.* They can easily get infected. If you have many blisters, check with your doctor so he or she can prescribe an antibiotic or antiseptic spray to counter blister infection.

5. *Use sprays instead of creams.* Of all the products on the market that claim to aid in pain and irritation from sunburn sprays are less irritating to burned skin and are easier to use. Sprays also have less chance of rubbing off on clothing, and they generally last longer than creams.

Most of the ingredients in these products are safe to use as sunburn pain relievers. Check the labels for these safe ingredients: allantoin, aluminum hydroxide gel, calamine, cocoa butter, cornstarch, dimethicone, glycerin, kaolin, petrolatum preparations, shark liver oil, sodium bicarbonate, zinc acetate, zinc carbonate, and zinc oxide. Four ingredients are *not* safe and should not be used to relieve sunburn pain (again, check the labels): bismuth subnitrate, boric acid, sulfur, and tannic acid. Zinc acetate, shark liver oil, and products containing live yeast cell derivative should not be used on children under the age of two; and aluminum hydroxide should not be used on infants under the age of six months.

6. *If the sunburn is painful, take aspirin or some other analgesic* for the first twenty-four to seventy-two hours.

7. *Don't use Caladryl.* It contains the antihistamine Benadryl, which is prone to cause allergic reactions among a number of people.

7

other ailments

The eye is one of the most complicated—and miraculous—organs of the body. The part we can see and inspect in the mirror is like the tip of the iceberg—a mere fraction of the organ, representing only a tiny bit of the total miracle.

TREATMENT
Nonmedicinal Treatment
As always, you should try to treat simple eye problems without medication first. The following guidelines might help you when treating eye irritation:[1]

- If you can identify it, eliminate the cause of the eye irritation. Get away from the cigarette smoke, wear sunglasses in bright sunlight, and so on.

- If your eyes get tired and irritated, try splashing them with cool tap water—a treatment you can repeat as often as you want.

- Try changing, reducing, or temporarily eliminating eye makeup.

- Apply cool compresses to your closed eyes.

Self-Treatment

You can feel safe about treating your eyes yourself if you experience:[2]

- slight redness (of one or both of your eyes),

- mild itching,

- a mild amount of *clear* discharge,

- mild dryness and discomfort, or

- mild burning.

These conditions indicate a lack of sleep, a mild viral infection, an allergy, or an irritant like cigarette smoke, smog, wind, dust, toxic fumes, or the sun.

You should not attempt self-medication and you should contact a doctor immediately if you experience:

- blurry or cloudy vision (especially if the change is sudden and recent);

- pain in the eye (suggesting that there may be a problem with the internal structures of the eye);

- anything more than just a slight degree of redness in either or both eyes;

- a discharge of pus from the eye (with or without caking or sticking of the eyelids in the morning);

- an ulcer or sore in the eye;

- severe itching;

- persistent foreign bodies that you are unable to remove easily and painlessly;

- partial blindness in one or both eyes, or a blind spot in either eye;

- double vision;

- bumps or lumps on the eye or the eyelid (particularly on the inside of the eyelids);

- pale, itching eyes;

- an injury to the eye (or to the area immediately surrounding the eye); or

- redness that begins at the center of the eye instead of at the edges.

Types of Eye Medications
Three main kinds of eye medications are available for over-the-counter purchase.[3]

Vasoconstrictors (Decongestants). These medicines, most of them in drop form, contain many of the same decongestant properties used to fight the common cold. The vasoconstrictor shrinks the blood vessels in the eye, resulting in relief from congestion and swelling. This vasoconstrictor action is what "makes the red go away" by shrinking the size of the tiny blood vessels laced throughout the white of the eye. You should choose a drop containing a decongestant if your main problem is redness and irritation of the eye.

Vasoconstrictors have a number of disadvantages. For one, they reduce tearing. Prolonged and frequent use of vasoconstrictors may therefore produce dry eye. The vasoconstrictors also sometimes produce "rebound constriction," which means that, after the little blood vessels have shrunk initially, they may swell again. While they act to shrink the blood vessels, they have just the opposite effect on the pupils: They cause dilation. People with narrow-angle glaucoma should *not* use eye medications containing decongestants or vasoconstrictors, because dilation can increase the amount of intra-ocular pressure.

Decongestants are listed on product labels as phenylephrine HCl (the most common one), ephedrine, zinc (an astringent agent that also acts as a decongestant), tetrahydrozoline, and naphazoline. Popular brands that contain a vasoconstrictor or decongestant include Allerest eye drops, Clear Eyes, Murine 2, Ocusol, 20-20, Ultra Clear, and Visine.

Artificial Tears. Drops that act as "artificial tears" help people who suffer from irritation or dryness of the eyes by lubricating and soothing the eye. Medicines acting as artificial tears also contain preservatives, antiseptics, and viscosity agents (that help thicken the liquid).

Products that act as artificial tears include Aqua-Flow, Bro-Lac, Contique Artificial Tears, Liquifilm Tears, Murine, Tearisol, and Ultra Tears.

Eye Washes. Eye washes, like artificial tears, are used to lubricate and soothe the eye, but they contain no thickening agents. The fact that they are not as thick makes them better for irrigating the eyes and for washing out foreign matter.

Eye washes include Blinx, BufOpto Neo-Flo, Collyrium, Eye-Stream, Ibath, Iso-Lo, Normol, and Ocusol Eye Lotion.

Auxiliary Drugs. Eye drops contain a number of additives, most of which fall under three general categories:

• *preservatives*, to prolong the shelf life and to discourage the growth of contaminants;

• *viscosity agents*, to thicken the liquid and to increase the amount of time that it stays on the eye's surface; and

• *buffers*, to prevent eye irritation from the medication and to stabilize the pH level.

Some eye drops may contain camphor (for a cooling effect), salts, or other additives.

CAUTIONS

One of the most critical things to remember in self-medication of eye irritations is to keep the container's tip completely sterile. You can introduce harmful bacteria into your eye if you let the tip of the eye dropper touch *anything*, including the surface of your eye. You should also bear in mind that:

• it is not safe to continue treatment with eye drops for more than three days (use eye drops only two or three times a day);

• topical anesthetics were not made for use in the eyes;

• you must wash your hands before applying any medication in the eyes; and

• you should watch for discoloration or any other unusual thing in the solution, which may mean it is no longer potent.

EARACHES

How many times have you had an earache and frantically looked through the medicine cabinet to find something to ease the pain? Chances are that you've found nothing suitable, because earaches—especially if you are older—are not as common as other ailments. Yet earaches can be very serious. An earache may signal that something is seriously wrong with the body, or the earache itself may progress to something serious. Earaches, if untreated and serious, have the potential to cause deafness (both nerve deafness and conduction deafness—which means that something in the ear structure itself prevents you from hearing).

CAUSES
Earache can result from a variety of causes:

• Changes in atmospheric pressure can cause an earache. For example, if you travel from Denver, Colorado (the mile high city), to Death Valley, California (which is below sea level), the change in pressure that comes with the change in altitude could cause your ears to ache.

• Diving and swimming may force water into the ears, resulting in earache.

• Traveling in an airplane can cause an earache due to the pressure changes in the cabin.

• Earache may be caused by a plugged eustachian tube (the tube connecting the nose and the ear). Eustachian tubes become plugged usually as the result of a cold or some other infection.

• Diseases of the ear, or even of the head or nose, can cause the ears to ache.

• Putting a foreign object into your ear can result in an earache. Sometimes the "foreign object" is not put into the ear; an insect may fly or crawl into the ear.

• Impacted wax can make the ears hurt. This condition should usually be referred to a doctor for treatment.[4]

TREATMENT
Self-Treatment
Because earaches can signal more serious conditions and because an earache can have serious results, you should see your doctor in most cases. If you notice inflammation, heat, or redness around or in the ears, see your doctor for treatment. Also, a discharge from the ears should be brought to your doctor's attention. If you experience persistent pain that doesn't go away, with or without treatment, in one or two days, your doctor should know. Impacted earwax or other objects or debris should be removed by a doctor. A physician should also be notified in cases of deep cuts, bruises, and abrasions connected with the ears.

Self-treatment may remedy your situation if you are experiencing only minor pain or some other mild condition. It may also be good in cases where people use it for prevention of ear problems. Sometimes, for example, ear drops can be used to soften earwax so it will not become impacted.[5]

Forms of Treatment

The only product on the market today for ear problems is ear drops. The reason is that ear problems are generally regarded as so serious that ear drops are the only form that should be tried. If they do not work, your next step is to see your doctor.

Chemicals in Treatments

Ear drops that are safe for home use should contain one or a combination of the following products:

glycerin	ichthymol
propylene glycol	aluminum acetate
urea	olive oil
peroxide antipyrene	menthol
thymol	camphor
boric acid	benzocaine
isopropyl alcohol	

Products that contain carbamide peroxide, aluminum acetate, or acetic acid often impact earwax. To dry out the ear, you should obtain a product that contains at least 30 percent glycerin.[6]

Some products currently on the market that contain these chemicals are Auro ear drops, Debrox drops, Ear drops by Murine, Kerid ear drops, and Swim ear drops.[7]

Choosing a Treatment

You do not have much choice of treatment when you are limited to one OTC drug—ear drops. In turn, however, if ear drops don't solve your problem, you don't have to try a multitude of other products before you see your doctor. Ears are delicate and sensitive organs, and you need to take good care of them because of all the wonderful things in your life that are made better when you can hear.

Some other things you might consider when deciding between using an OTC drug or going to your doctor are:

• chronic disease you may have (such as diabetes), which may slow healing,

• deformities or scarring of the ear,

- recent ear injuries, or

- allergies you may have to chemicals in the ear drops.[8]

CAUTIONS
Although ear drops are quite safe to use, you should remember several things:

1. *Do not put ear droppers or other applicators far into the ears.* Drops can be administered by holding the dropper at the very entrance to the ear canal. You have to get the dropper close enough for a good aim, but you don't need to insert the dropper far into the canal. Ear drops may get into the ear better and in farther if you gently pull on the ear lobe. Also, a cotton plug keeps the ear drops in the ear longer. The plug may also help keep the drops warmer longer.

2. *The drops should be at body temperature and no higher.* This degree of warmth can be accomplished by holding the bottle of drops in your hand or by warming them in warm tap water. If you warm them in tap water, be sure to test them on the back of your hand before you put them into the ear. Drops that are too hot can be painful and cause burns on the inside of the ear.

3. *Do not use products that contain carbolic acid (phenol), boric acid, or benzocaine.* The first two compounds are toxic to the body when introduced into the ears, and benzocaine, an anesthetic, may numb the pain so much that you may not seek the proper medical aid for your condition.[9]

4. *When you have an earache, keep all water out of your ears.* Protect them when bathing or showering, and do not go swimming if your ears ache.[10]

5. *Keep your ears and hair clean.* Remember, though, that you should never put something smaller than your finger, covered by a washcloth, into your ears.

6. *Keep all ear infections and other infections in the head area under control.*

7. *Earaches can be dangerous.* They may signal a more serious condition, and they have the potential to cause deafness. Never take chances with your ears. Always see your doctor if you have not had relief of pain in one to two days after self-treatment. Consult your doctor, too, if your pain is severe. Hearing is one of your most enlightening senses, so take proper care of your ears.

OVERWEIGHT

With all the TV commercials telling us that fat is not beautiful, why are 40 percent of the U.S. population overweight?[11] What does "overweight" really mean? You are overweight if you have accumulated body fat in excess of that which you need to function normally. You are overweight when your weight in relation to your height is 20 percent above the ideal.[12] Are there, then, benefits to being thin or at an ideal weight for your height? Certainly. You tend to live longer and have better health. You have less chance of having hardening of the arteries, heart and kidney problems, high blood pressure, diabetes, gall bladder disease, arthritis, and varicose veins. Plus, there are other advantages to being thin. You look better, you can wear more attractive clothing, and you have a better chance of having a more satisfying social life.

CAUSES

What are the causes of the age-old problem of "ugly fat," which has beset men and women alike since the beginning of time?

- Taking in more calories than are expended (in other words, your input does not equal your output).

- Overeating certain food types (primarily the carbohydrates and fats).

- Endocrine gland disorders (everyone blames obesity on glandular upsets; yet, in reality, this cause is rare indeed).

- Brain lesions that affect the appetite center in the hypothalamus (one part of the brain); this would be a rare situation.

- A missing enzyme that breaks down triglycerides (fatty acids) in the body, not a common problem.

- An excess of fat cells in infancy (theory has it that infants who grow up to overweight adults are born with a greater number of fat cells that are larger).

- The widespread advertising of foodstuffs in America.

- Socioeconomic class (overweight problems are more common among the lower socioeconomic classes).

- Decreased physical activity.

- Mental depression and stress.

- Increased sensitivity to taste.

- Metabolism (overweight individuals have a slower metabolism) also rare.

- Heredity (if you have one parent who is overweight, you have a 40 percent chance of being overweight; if both parents are over-weight, you have an 80 percent chance of being overweight. Not terrific odds, are they?)[13]

- Family eating habits.

- Boredom.

TREATMENT
Nonmedicinal Treatment
Many more things than OTC drugs are involved in weight reduction and control. Actually, in the whole scope of things, OTC drugs should play only a small part in weight control. Other important factors are:

- a permanent change in lifestyle and eating habits,

- an appreciation of the caloric value of food types,

- a reevaluation of the psychological aspects of life that might encourage overeating,

- self-discipline,

- realization that there is no simple plan for dieting—dieting is just plain, painful hard work,

- taking vitamins if your diet is lacking in some area, and

- increasing physical activity.

Being overweight is a problem shared by many in the world, and no simple or magic solution will melt unwanted pounds away. You must remember, though, that danger can occur with dieting, so you should consult a doctor or pharmacist before you use any weight control product. Most of the over-the-counter drugs for weight control have not been proven really effective, so you should be cautious. In the final analysis, much of weight control depends upon your reestablishing eating habits and realizing that, to achieve a desired weight, your input must equal your output.

If you have mild to moderate overweight problems and have been given a clean bill of health by your doctor, you may treat your condition yourself. But you should discuss your intended diet program with your pharmacist and preferably with your doctor before beginning. If you are thinking of fasting, starvation, or "crash" diets, you should always be under a doctor's care. Ideally, regardless of which diet approach you use, you should not lose more than one to two pounds a week. If you have a severe overweight problem, you should never try to devise your own diet; your doctor should always be consulted first.

Forms of Treatment

There are probably almost as many diets in the world as there are people. The purpose here is not to list all the diets ever devised. Instead, the major diet groups are listed with an emphasis on over-the-counter weight control preparations:

- fasting, starvation, "crash," or "fad" diets;

- group therapy and behavior modification;

- decreased calorie intake and increased physical activity;

- intestinal bypass surgery (of all options listed here, this is probably the most hazardous);

- prescription drug treatment (most prescription weight control drugs are amphetamines, which work by suppressing the appetite center in the brain. Unfortunately, this effect is not long-term, and the amphetamines are noted for their abuse potential); and

- over-the-counter weight control drugs.

OTC Weight-Control Drugs

1. *Phenylpropanolamine.* This drug has a similar effect to that of the amphetamines. The *AMA Drug Evaluation* indicates that phenylpropanolamine is "probably ineffective as an appetite suppressant."[14] Its prolonged use may cause nervousness, high blood pressure, thumping in the chest, restlessness, insomnia, headache, nausea, and increased blood glucose levels.

2. *Bulk-Producers.* Bulk-producers add mass to the stomach. They produce a feeling of fullness in the stomach and decrease the desire to eat. Chemically, they are made up of the same ingredients contained in laxatives. So far, they have not been established as a useful diet aid because tests have shown that they are emptied out of the stomach in 30 minutes.

3. *Benzocaine.* Benzocaine is a local anesthetic (the same benzocaine that is used in anesthetics for burn treatment). Ideally, benzocaine should numb the mouth and change the taste of food, but it comes in the form of capsules or tablets that are swallowed so the mouth is not affected. As yet, whether benzocaine has a positive numbing effect on the stomach is not known.

4. *Glucose.* The theory behind glucose is that if glucose is taken before meals, blood sugar is raised, and the appetite center of the brain is suppressed.

5. *Low-Calorie, Nutritionally Balanced Foods.* These foods are low in sodium and contain approximately 20 grams of fat and 110 grams of carbohydrates. The most famous of these foods are Metrical and Sego.[15]

6. *Artificial Sweeteners.* The most widely used artificial sweeteners are saccharin, cyclamate, and aspartame. Cyclamate was banned because it produced bladder cancer in laboratory animals, and saccharin is presently undergoing scrutiny for similar reasons. Aspartame is a sweetener that cannot be used by individuals with PKU (a metabolic birth defect).

7. *Diuretics.* Over-the-counter diuretics tend to be dangerous and should not be used for dieting purposes.

Weight control products come in a wide variety of forms: liquids, powders, granules, tablets, capsules, timed-release capsules, wafers, cookies, soups, gum, and candy.

Chemicals in Diet Products
Phenylpropanolamine and benzocaine products contain those chemicals by the same name. Bulk-producers contain methylcellulose, carboxymethylcellulose, psyllium mucilloid, and agar. Brand name products contain these products singly or in combination. Some brands that you may be familiar with are:

• *Bulk only:* Konsyl, L.A. Formula, Melozets, Metamucil powder, and instant mix.

• *Glucose only:* Ayds and Dex-a-Diet (these both also contain vitamins).

• *Phenylpropanolamine only:* Hungrex, Permathene-12, (plus caffeine).

- *Bulk/benzocaine:* Dexule, Slim-mint, Pondosan, Reducets, Wey-Dex.

- *Bulk/phenylpropanolamine:* Slender-X.

- *Bulk/benzocaine/phenylpropanolamine:* Diet-Trim.

- *Low-calorie foods:* Dietine powder, Proslim, Sego, Slender, Metrical.

- *Artifical sweeteners:* Diacryst, Saccharin, Sucaryl, Sweeta (many of these come in both solid and liquid forms).[16]

Choosing a Treatment

Any over-the-counter drug should be used along with a weight reduction program of some type. You should always ask your pharmacist and/or your doctor about which OTC drug to use. A professional has the most up-to-date information about the safety and effectiveness of these products.

CAUTIONS AND SIDE EFFECTS

Since the use of OTC drugs in weight control is particularly tricky, some caution should be used. Weight-control products can be dangerous and produce serious side effects, especially if they are taken too frequently and in too high concentrations. Phenylpropanolamine can produce nervousness, restlessness, insomnia, headache, nausea, rapid heart beat and heart palpitations, increased blood pressure, and increased blood sugar. Bulk-producers can result in a laxative effect, blockage in the intestines, and obstruction of the esophagus. Benzocaine can produce cyanosis (a bluish tint to the skin) and allergies that can result in asthma-like symptoms. Sego's side effects are watery stools, diarrhea, gas, and occasional constipation. In general, take this advice:

- Never exceed the dosage prescribed on the package because of possible side effects.

- Do not take phenylpropanolamine if you have diabetes, heart disease, high blood pressure, or thyroid disease.

- Do not take prescription drugs and over-the-counter weight control products at the same time.

- Take bulk-producers with plenty of water. Some bulk-producers come in wafer form, and if they are not taken with plenty of water, they may get stuck in the throat and cause serious choking.

You've seen the commercials on television: A woman drifts peacefully off to sleep, a blissful smile on her face, while a miniature bottle of nonprescription sleeping pills glides across the screen to a lilting melody, "Take Sominex tonight and sleep . . ." In another, a woman, amidst a thousand crises, turns to the screen with a grimace on her face. Her hair is unkempt, her apron is soiled, and her eyes are brimming with tears: "You need help. Retreat to the comfort of Quiet World." About 50 percent of the American population experience insomnia at some time in their lives. A third of the population rate insomnia as an ongoing complaint.[17]

Sleeplessness and tension are related, primarily because one can cause the other and because both can result from the same causes. People who have trouble falling asleep are probably bothered by tensions that are preventing them from falling asleep; people who are unable to sleep or who awaken early usually get tense and preoccupied over the problem.

CAUSES

Any of a number of things can be at the root of your inability to fall asleep. Insomnia can be caused by:[18]

- too much caffeine (consumed in coffee, tea, or cola drinks or drugs that contain caffeine);

- prescription drugs that may cause stimulation as a side effect (your doctor can tell you which ones they are);

- alcohol;

- naps (too much sleep);

- a recent shift in the normal sleeping and waking pattern;

- unusual stress or tension;

- symptoms of a disease—especially the need to urinate frequently, pain, difficulty in breathing, or headache;

- lack of exercise;

- age (sleep cycles change with age, and the elderly awake frequently during the night or early in the morning, generally getting less deep sleep);

- depression;

- environmental physical conditions such as a distracting noise, a strange or uncomfortable bed, too hot or too cold a room;

- brain abnormalities;

- mental activity at night (bedtime is the most convenient time of the day to think, and many people find themselves re-hashing the day's routine and planning tomorrow's schedule); or

- the habit of sleeping poorly.

Insomnia is a lot like constipation. Many different things can cause it, and you have the power to eliminate the cause (and therefore eliminate the problem) without resorting to sleeping pills. Unless insomnia continues for a long period, it is not harmful to your health. Sleeping pills, however—like laxatives—can be dangerous: You can develop a dependence on them, and they can eventually prevent your body's own natural sleep mechanisms from working. So, like laxatives, sleeping pills should be used only on rare occasions and only after you have assessed the problem and its causes, determining that you actually need and should take a sleeping pill.

TREATMENT

If any of these causes apply to you, you've found the source of your insomnia, and you probably don't need a sleeping pill. If you've grown accustomed to a peaceful afternoon nap after the kids leave for a football game and before your husband gets home from work, skip the nap. You're probably oversleeping, and you aren't tired when it's time to go to bed. If you need to urinate frequently and keep waking up to do so, go see your doctor. You need help with your bladder, not a sleeping pill. If you have recently switched shifts at work, and you are now on the graveyard instead of the swing shift, it means that you have to go to sleep and wake up in a pattern that you're unaccustomed to. Give yourself time; it can take up to four weeks to adjust to a new sleeping pattern.

Nonmedicinal Alternatives

Do everything you can to avoid using sleeping pills.[19] The following suggestions might help you:

- Take a warm bath before bed—warmth relaxes.

- Don't drink beverages containing caffeine after 7:00 P.M.

- Don't take a nap during the day.

- Don't use alcohol as a "nightcap." Contrary to popular opinion, it *won't* put you to sleep; a hot drink, such as milk, makes a better nightcap.

104 other ailments

• If you can't fall asleep, don't fight it. Don't try to force sleep. Get up and watch television, read a good book, or work on a craft project until you get sleepy. Don't worry that you're not getting enough sleep; your body *will* sleep when it needs it.

• If you get up for something during the night and can't fall back asleep, get up and do something. Don't just lie in bed and worry about not getting your sleep.

• Create a comfortable feeling in the bedroom so you want to sleep when you enter that room. Lie down intending to go to sleep only when you're sleepy; go into another room if you're not sleepy.

• Cut down on spicy foods; they may cause indigestion.

• Learn to do relaxing exercises, and do them before bedtime.

If your insomnia becomes a chronic problem, and if you cannot get relief from over-the-counter medications, check with your doctor. You may require professional help to eliminate some underlying tension, or you may be unable to sleep as a symptom of a serious medical problem that should have professional attention.

When to Use a Sleeping Pill
You may feel safe trying self-medication if:

• you have only *occasional* trouble falling asleep, and

• you have only *occasional* trouble remaining asleep.[20]

You should *not* self-medicate with over-the-counter sleeping pills if:[21]

• your insomnia is so severe that it impairs your daytime activities;

• your insomnia has lasted for more than ten days (and it occurs every night for those ten days);

• it is some symptom of disease—shortness of breath, cough, asthma, indigestion, or frequent urination, for example—that keeps you from falling asleep;

• you are pregnant;

• you are nursing a baby;

• you have glaucoma;

• you have heart disease;

- you have a peptic ulcer;

- you have prostate difficulty;

- you are taking any prescription drug (unless your doctor okays the combination); or

- you are using alcohol, which depresses the central nervous system at the same time that you are having trouble falling asleep.

If you *do* decide to use a sleeping pill, regardless of its relative mildness, never give sleeping pills to a child under the age of twelve. They are designed for adult use only.

Classes of Sleeping Pills

Over-the-counter sleeping pills may contain any of the following elements.[22]

Methapyrilene. An antihistamine used in many cold relief medications, methapyrilene is valuable in sleeping pills because it causes drowsiness. Over 300 sleep aids/sedatives contain it. However, recent studies and research have revealed that methapyrilene is a potent cancer-causing agent. Tests showed that rats who were fed a combination of methapyrilene and sodium nitrates and those who were fed only methapyrilene experienced liver degeneration that often accompanies or precedes liver cancer.[23] As a result, there has been a massive recall of all sleep aid products. More than 600 products, at a cost of $28 million, have been recalled. These include: Nytol, Sominex, Sleep-Eze, Quiet World, Compoz, Cope, Sleepinal, Tranquim, Miles Nervine, Dormin, Sedacaps, and Somnicaps.

Scopolamine. Scopolamine, also used in cold medications to dry up runny noses, is included in sleeping pills because it produces drowsiness. It is mildly sedative because it produces muscle spasms and stomach acid production. After you take it, outside distractions just don't bother you, and you sleep a dreamless sleep. It is not particularly recommended for a sleep aid.

Products containing scopolamine mixed with methapyrilene include Compoz, Devarex (also contains salicylamide), Nite Rest, Quiet World (also contains aspirin and acetaminophen), San-Man, Seedate, Sleep-Eze, Sominex (also contains salicylamide) and Sominex Double-Strength, and Sure-Sleep (also contains salicylamide).

Bromides. Used for their sedative properties for almost two hundred years, bromides in single doses don't usually produce ill effects, but they should not be used by children, by pregnant or lactating women, and by people with kidney disease or damage. They are *not* recommended for long-term use, because they are excreted so slowly that they often cause kidney damage. The Alva-Tranquil products contain a mixture of bromide and methapyrilene.

Auxiliary Drugs. Included in a number of sleeping pills, analgesics or vitamins usually serve as auxiliary drugs. The label can give you all the information you need.

CAUTIONS
You should take the following measures before you choose a sleeping pill:[24]

> • Read the label carefully. The only thing you need in a sleeping pill is something to make you drowsy—an antihistamine. Choose a sleeping pill that has a *single* ingredient. Acquaint yourself with the possible side effects of antihistamines (listed later in this section), and discontinue use if you develop a side effect.

> • Don't use a sleeping pill that does not clearly list all its ingredients. Don't use a sleeping pill if you are unsure about one of the ingredients or if you are confused about what one of the ingredients does.

> • Don't use a sleeping pill that contains a bromide.

> • Don't use sleeping pills that contain extra ingredients, such as aspirin, unless you need the aspirin for pain relief of a headache associated with the tension.

As is the case with most other drugs, you need to take other precautions when taking sleeping pills:[25]

1. People over the age of sixty probably shouldn't use sleeping pills: Their effect is sporadic, and side effects are apt to be more serious in the elderly.

2. Only about a fourth of the people who try sleeping pills get any effect out of them. Too often the cause of insomnia needs the kind of treatment and attention that the sleeping pill doesn't provide.

3. People who do fall asleep as a result of a sleeping pill are likely to suffer from a "hangover" the next morning. The effects of the drug do not go away as soon as you wake up.

4. Tolerance to the drug develops rapidly. Those who do receive results from the sleeping pill at first build up a tolerance and do not receive results after using the pill for a short time on a regular basis.

5. Some sleeping pills contain double doses of antihistamines to make them more effective; while this does help increase effectiveness, it also increases the risk of side effects, which include:

dryness of the throat and mouth	tremors
inability to concentrate	loss of appetite
dizziness	nausea
incoordination	vomiting
ringing in the ears	heart palpitation
blurred vision	increased sweating
nervousness	

Side effects may also be found with scopolamine usage:

dry mouth and throat	blurred vision
lights that appear within the visual field	inability to urinate

The bromides are famous for their effects:

headache	stomach upset
dizziness	acne-like rash

6. Never exceed the recommended dosage listed on the label of over-the-counter sleeping pills.

7. Don't use the sleeping pills too often. They should never be used more than two or three times a week, and then only in periods of temporary insomnia. Most sleeping pills are classified as "not habit-forming," but they can become a habit.

8. Don't take any other drugs containing antihistamines (such as cold medications) while you are taking sleeping pills. You'll only double your dose of antihistamine and increase your chance for unpleasant side effects.

9. Don't use pain medication or drink alcohol if you are going to take a sleeping pill.

STIMULANT PRODUCTS

Stimulant products—medications that help you stay awake—are widely used throughout the United States, but they are used especially by students near the end of the term and by drivers who must drive long distances without many rest periods. These products are designed to promote wakefulness and to relieve the sense of boredom and fatigue that accompany tedious work undertaken for long periods of time.

The major ingredient of most stimulant products on the market today is caffeine. Over 7 million kilograms of caffeine are consumed each year in the United States, and most of the consumption is in the form of caffeinated beverages such as:[26]

Brewed coffee	100-150 mg./cup
Cola drinks	40-60 mg./cup
Decaffeinated coffee	2-4 mg./cup
Instant coffee	86-99 mg./cup
Tea	60-75 mg./cup

Generally speaking, caffeine in moderate doses produces the following effects: increased alertness and mental activity, improved skeletal muscle tone, stimulation of the central nervous system, and stimulation of the heart muscle (which in turn produces increased force with each heart beat, increased cardiac output, and increased heart rate). At doses of 50 to 200 mg., you commonly feel an increase in the conscious mental processes: Ideas become clearer, and your thoughts flow more easily and rapidly. You also notice a decrease in fatigue and drowsiness. At doses of over 250 mg., caffeine can cause insomnia, restlessness, irritability, nervousness, tremors, headache, and in rare cases (depending, of course, on the dosage taken) mild delirium.[27]

Treatment

Because of the possible detrimental effects that may occur with overuse or overdose of stimulant products, it is suggested that they be used only on an occasional basis. They may be considered safe and effective when they are used to reduce fatigue and boredom that accompanies long and tedious tasks.

In cases other than these, the use of stimulant products is questionable. Many people have resorted to stimulant products to combat the symptoms of a hangover. However, it should be realized by the consumer that stimulants do not promote a sobering effect.

If you do desire to use stimulant products in their proper context, you should choose a product that contains only caffeine. You should avoid all combination products, which typically contain secondary ingredients such as vitamin E, aluminum chloride, and ginseng.

Tirend and No-Doz are the only products that contain caffeine and no other active ingredients. Double-E contains caffeine plus thiamin (one of the B vitamins); Pre-Mens Forte contains caffeine and aluminum chloride (which serves as a diuretic); Prolamine contains caffeine plus phenylpropanolamine (an antihistamine); and Vivarin contains caffeine and sugar.[28]

CAUTIONS

Large doses of caffeine may stimulate the medulla of the brain, which may in turn cause a decrease in the force of heart contractions, a decrease in heart rate, and a decrease in cardiac output. Further, high doses may produce cardiac irregularities such as beat irregularities. Large doses may also produce severe constriction of blood vessels in the brain. It is advised, therefore, that persons with heart or blood vessel disease decrease or stop caffeine consumption.

Note that people who consume more than 1,000 mg. of caffeine a day manifest symptoms of a syndrome called caffeinism. Many who have caffeinism experience symptoms much like those of anxiety neurosis: They are extremely nervous, irritable, and agitated; they have headaches; they breathe more rapidly; they experience tremulousness and muscle twitches; they have sensory disturbances and experience insomnia. Because of the adverse effects of consuming large doses of caffeine, you should not consume more than 100 to 200 mg. of caffeine every 3 to 4 hours.[29]

Be aware that caffeine used over a long period of time can cause tolerance (which means that more of the drug must be used to produce the desired effect) and psychological dependence (you continue to use the drug because you like the effect or the lift that caffeine gives you). Those who say they experience "caffeine fits" are not addicted to caffeine; they merely like the effects it produces and so want to continue using it.

Stimulant products should also not be used in the following instances:[30]

- for treatment of hangover,
- in conjunction with caffeinated beverages
- for children under age 12, or
- for self-treatment that continues for over 7 to 10 days.

INSECT BITES AND STINGS

Certain reactions may follow the bites or stings inflicted by insects. Stinging insects include bumblebees, honeybees, wasps, hornets, yellow jackets, and ants. Although the venom injected by bees is highly toxic, only a small percentage of the population (10 percent) is acutely sensitive to the venom.[31] To those who are not acutely sensitive to bee stings, local reaction such as local pain, swelling, and itch may be the only side-effects associated with the sting. For those 10 percent who are allergic to the bee venom, reactions may include nausea, vomiting, fainting, breathing difficulties, heart failure, and eventually death (if emergency medical measures are not taken promptly).

Biting insects include mosquitoes, fleas, lice, bedbugs, ticks, and chiggers. These insects penetrate the skin and may temporarily or permanently attach themselves to a blood capillary—they feed on human blood. People do not manifest symptoms of acute sensitivity to these insect bites, but local reactions do occur. Generally, insect bites cause local redness, itch, and swelling.

Mites are not considered to be insects that either bite or sting, but they are classified as parasites. These insects produce a disease condition, known as scabies, which occurs when an impregnated female mite burrows under the upper skin layers using her mouthparts and first pair of legs. She then lays her eggs and continues to tunnel under the skin layers. Her eggs hatch, the new mites mate, and then they lay more eggs and tunnel under the skin. The symptoms of scabies are redness where eggs are laid and where tunnels occur, as well as itching. Scabies tends to be prevalent under unsanitary conditions, and the disease is contagious.

TREATMENT
It is appropriate to treat insect bites and stings at home in the following instances:

• If your irritation is only local, that is, at the site of the bite or sting.

• If your symptoms include nothing more than mild to moderate redness, itching, swelling, or pain.

• You can identify the offending insect.

• Your symptoms do not increase after you self-treat.

• You have no previous history of allergy to either bites, stings, or medications to treat such conditions.[32]

Nonmedical Treatment
There are several things you can do to treat the bite or sting before you try over-the-counter medications. It may be helpful to apply ice packs to the site of the sting or bite to reduce the swelling. To remove a stinger the proper way, you should scrape the stinger from the skin with your fingernail or some other flat or blunt object. There is a venom

sac attached to the stinger, and if you pull the stinger from the skin with tweezers or some other type of similar instrument, you merely serve to force more venom into the wound.

Avoid scratching or any other irritation of the injured tissue. Additional scratching or other irritation may merely serve to cause increased inflammation or the probability of infection.

Boil all clothing, sheets, and pillow cases if you suspect that your bites may have been caused by bedbugs or lice.[33]

Using OTC Preparations

Before using any over-the-counter preparations for insect bites or stings, you should identify the possible source of the insect bites or stings so that the pharmacist can help you select a product that will relieve your symptoms and that will further help in the destruction of the insect and its eggs.

Over-the-counter medications for insect bites and stings may come in several delivery forms: creams, lotions, liquids, ointments, pads, or sprays. It is advised that you stay away from using any oil-base ointment or cream because these products may complicate healing and may even promote secondary infection. Liquids, lotions, and sprays are less likely to produce these complications.

You can use nonprescription medications to relieve itch, pain, or irritation, to prevent secondary infections, and to protect the injured tissue.

Ingredients in insect bite and sting products include:

• *Local anesthetics:* The chemicals commonly used as local anesthetics include benzocaine, dibucaine, tetracaine, and other pain-deadening compounds. Brand names of products containing such local anesthetics include Anti-Itch Cream, Chiggerex, Chiggertox, Lanacane, Quotane, and Surfadil. These products commonly contain other ingredients, so they may be listed under several of the other categories of the over-the-counter preparations for treatment of insect bites. There is one caution to be aware of when using products that contain local anesthetics. They must penetrate the skin and reach the nerve endings to produce their anesthetic effect, and thus they may cause allergic reactions at the point of contact.

• *Antipruritics/antihistamines:* These chemical agents relieve mild to moderate itching. Antipruritics contained in these medications include menthol, phenol, or camphor, and common antihistamines employed in over-the-counter preparations are diphenhydramine, methapyrilene, phenyltoloxamine, pyrilamine, or tripelennamine. Brand names that contain antipruritics/antihistamines include After-Bite, Benadryl, Caladryl, Chiggerex, Chiggertox, Surfadil, and Rucks. It should be noted that prolonged use of these products may produce allergic reactions.

• *Astringents:* These agents are used to protect, dry, and toughen injured tissue. Common chemical ingredients that are astringents are benzyl benzoate, calamine, resorcin, zinc oxide, and zirconium oxide. Medications containing these chemicals are as follows: After-Bite, Caladryl, Chiggertox, and Lanacane. Note that use of the chemical zirconium oxide may produce skin nodules or lumps.

• *Antibacterials:* These agents reduce the possibility of infection that may result from irritation such as rubbing or scratching. Chemical agents such as benzalkonium chloride, ben zethonium chloride, hydroxyquinoline, and methylbenzethomium chloride may be included in some over-the-counter preparations. Chiggertox and Tucks are brand name products that contain antibacterials.[34]

CAUTIONS
It may be wise to avoid over-the-counter products and consult with your physician if the following conditions occur:

• You have a history of allergic reactions or sensitivity to insect stings.

• You suffer from asthma or have a history of allergy to dust, pollen, smoke, or skin medications.

• You do not know the origin of the bites, stings, or kind of insects that produced them.

• Your symptoms are in any way severe.

• You experience excessive sweating, shortness of breath, vomiting, feverishness, or fainting that is associated with an insect sting.

• Your symptoms are accompanied by fever, chills, headache, or muscular soreness.[35]

In these cases, seeking emergency medical treatment is critical. Postponement of such treatment may lead to death. If you have an acute sensitivity to insect stings, your physician may recommend that you carry an emergency kit. These kits are available by prescription only and may contain epinephrine HCl, isoproterenol tablets, epinephrine HCl aerosol, antihistamines, or steroids to help combat the allergic reaction that accompanies stings.

ATHLETE'S FOOT

CAUSES
Athlete's foot is caused by a fungus. Commonly, the disease may take two forms. In one form, it is characterized by vessicles, burning, itching, sweating, crusting after the vessicles dry, and dry, scaly lesions between the toes. The other form of athlete's foot produces soggy skin, itching, malodor, discomfort, peeling of the skin in scales, and reddened skin underneath the scales. The fungus grows and reproduces best under certain conditions, such as excessive wetness of the foot due to exercise and emotions, tight and occlusive footwear, hot and humid weather, poor hygiene, poor nutrition, and trauma to the foot. Any of these conditions may precipitate an attack of athlete's foot.

TREATMENT
Self-Treatment
You can reasonably treat athlete's foot under certain conditions:

- if your infection is only superficial and of recent origin,

- if your symptoms include mild to moderate sores and/or dry, scaly skin,

- if your symptoms include only moderate itching or burning sensations in the areas affected,

- if you self-treat your athlete's foot for no more than four weeks (and then you should seek the advice of your doctor), or

- if you practice good hygiene—especially good foot hygiene.[36]

Nonmedical Alternatives
You may help to eliminate fungus infections of the feet if you follow a regimen of good hygiene:

- changing shoes and socks at least once a day,

- washing and thoroughly drying your entire foot frequently,

- avoiding activities that produce excessive perspiration of the feet,

- wearing footwear that is light and not too tight,

- wearing footwear that is open, to promote good air circulation,

- avoiding walking barefoot in locker rooms or on swimming pool decks, which are prime breeding places for athlete's foot fungus.

The use of drying agents after bathing is also helpful. Agents, such as powders, may absorb the excessive moisture to prevent athlete's foot or to treat a condition that is already present.

OTC Athlete's Foot Products

Over-the-counter athlete's foot preparations generally come in several forms of delivery such as creams, liquids, gels, ointments, powders, and sprays. Generally, you should avoid using oil-base creams or ointments because they often complicate healing and may produce secondary bacterial infections. Even though powders are widely used, they tend to deliver their ingredients with less certainty than products that are used in the forms of liquids, gels, or sprays.

Athlete's foot products contain three general types of ingredients:

- *Fungicides:* These products control and, in some cases eliminate, fungus infections and the spores they produce. Chemicals contained in these products are generally various forms of undecylenic acid, acetic acid, caprylic acid, hydroxyquinoline, resorcinal, tolnaftate, and zinc compounds. Probably the most effective compound on the list is tolnaftate. The following brand names contain fungicides in one form or another: Campho-Phenique, Compounded Undecylenic Acid, Desenex, Foot-Guard, Fungacetin, Fungi-Spray, NP 27 Aerosol, Quinsana, Solvex, Sporonal, Tinactin, and Ting.

- *Keratolytics:* Keratolytics are skin-peeling agents. They are an important form of treatment since the tissue most often affected by the athlete's foot fungus is shed when the external skin layers peel off. The most common chemicals included in keratolytics are salicylic and benzoic acids. NP 27 Aerosol and Ting contain keratolytic agents as well as fungicidal products.

- *Other ingredients:* Other ingredients are often added to athlete's foot products: various alcohols, astringents, surface anesthetics, absorbents, detergents, and antibacterial agents. These products serve to cool, relieve itch, desensitize, dry, or prevent secondary infections that may arise. These ingredients generally perform a secondary function to other ingredients.[37]

CAUTIONS

It is wise not to self-treat but instead to see your physician for advice if:

• you suffer from excessive sweating, skin allergies, or chronic disorders, such as diabetes before the onset of the athlete's foot;

• your infection spreads around or under a toenail (in this case, topical treatment provided by over-the-counter drugs will probably be ineffective);

• the inflammation or swelling spreads beyond the skin between the toes;

• the eruptions are oozing and moist; or

• you are under a doctor's care for diseases where your normal defense mechanisms are impaired.[38]

part two

PRESCRIPTION DRUGS

8

reading
your prescription

Doctors are notorious for their bad handwriting, which makes it hard enough to read the prescriptions scrawled across that official-looking little white paper at the end of your office visit. But prescriptions are even harder to read, because most of the terms written on that paper are in Latin or in abbreviations of Latin. No wonder the thing looks like Greek to you and me.[1]

Hundreds of generic drugs—and literally thousands of brand names—are listed for prescription use only. You will probably encounter only a fraction of them during your lifetime, but you should know:

- how to read a prescription,
- what to expect of the prescribing doctor,
- how to get your prescription filled promptly, and inexpensively,
- using your medication safely, and
- a little about common diseases and typically prescribed drugs.

HOW TO READ YOUR PRESCRIPTION

Sometimes—usually if you talk to your doctor over the phone of if your doctor needs to talk to the pharmacist—your doctor may phone a prescription in to the pharmacy of your choice. Usually, however, the

119

doctor gives you a prescription slip, which you have to take to the drugstore and give to the pharmacist. Exactly what *is* that little white piece of paper that you carry out of the doctor's or dentist's office? In essence, it's an order placed by an authorized person for a certain drug. It's an authorization for you to buy a certain drug from a licensed pharmacist. Prescriptions need to be on this printed form; prescriptions scribbled on a piece of paper are not legal and cannot be accepted by a pharmacist. Also, this form should be filled out in pen or indelible pencil to avoid alteration by patients once they leave the doctor's office. Without one, you can't buy a prescription drug. It's against federal law for a pharmacist (or anyone else, for that matter) to dispense a prescription drug without a doctor's prescription—that little piece of paper.

It's important for you to be able to read and understand that prescription form.[2] It contains instructions. It contains the drug's name. It gives you the important information you need if you plan on shopping at different pharmacies and comparing prices. Let's look at an example of a prescription form.

HEADING

The heading is generally printed on the form; the doctor rarely writes it in. Most often it consists of the physician's name, office address, and office phone number. If he or she is authorized to prescribe narcotics, it will also list the narcotics number assigned by the federal government.

The heading also contains a blank, where the doctor writes your name. This blank should contain your full name to avoid confusion at the pharmacy and to avoid mistakes once you get the medicine home and put it into the medicine chest with all the other prescriptions for the other family members.

SUPERSCRIPTION

This is the famous "Rx"; in Latin it signifies, "Take thou." It also signifies the God Jupiter. In ancient times, each prescription began with a formal prayer to invoke a blessing on the remedy. To save time, the prayer was simply shortened to "Rx."[3]

INSCRIPTION

This is the actual name of the drug you are getting. The doctor asks for a drug either by its *generic name* (a name that is untrademarked and that covers a number of separate brands) or by a specific brand name. Ask your doctor to consider listing the name of the drug by its generic name. You get the drug for less money than if the doctor insists on a certain brand. (Generic listing also helps pharmacists; they don't have to stock large amounts of specific brands, and they can pass the savings on to you.)

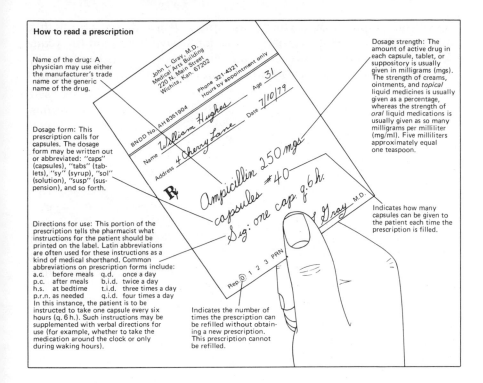

How to read a prescription

Name of the drug: A physician may use either the manufacturer's trade name or the generic name of the drug.

Dosage form: This prescription calls for capsules. The dosage form may be written out or abbreviated: "caps" (capsules), "tabs" (tablets), "sy" (syrup), "sol" (solution), "susp" (suspension), and so forth.

Directions for use: This portion of the prescription tells the pharmacist what instructions for the patient should be printed on the label. Latin abbreviations are often used for these instructions as a kind of medical shorthand. Common abbreviations on prescription forms include:
a.c. before meals   q.d.   once a day
p.c. after meals   b.i.d. twice a day
h.s. at bedtime   t.i.d. three times a day
p.r.n. as needed   q.i.d. four times a day
In this instance, the patient is to be instructed to take one capsule every six hours (q. 6 h.). Such instructions may be supplemented with verbal directions for use (for example, whether to take the medication around the clock or only during waking hours).

Dosage strength: The amount of active drug in each capsule, tablet, or suppository is usually given in milligrams (mgs). The strength of creams, ointments, and *topical* liquid medicines is usually given as a percentage, whereas the strength of *oral* liquid medications is usually given as so many milligrams per milliliter (mg/ml). Five milliliters approximately equal one teaspoon.

Indicates how many capsules can be given to the patient each time the prescription is filled.

Indicates the number of times the prescription can be refilled without obtaining a new prescription. This prescription cannot be refilled.

Your doctor may have a reason for listing a specific brand, though. He or she might want to be certain that the preparation is exactly right—down to the color, shape, and taste. Instead of writing out a complicated set of instructions for the pharmacist to measure and brew up, a physician can rely on prepackaged, commercial medications that have the needed ingredients.

SUBSCRIPTION

These are the directions—the instructions—from the doctor to the pharmacist. They tell the druggist what to mix, how much to include, and other important information.

The subscription is probably the hardest for you to understand, because it uses Latin abbreviations. To keep pharmacy a secret, ancient and middle age alchemists used strange symbols. Today, Latin abbreviations aren't part of a plot on the part of the medical industry to hide valuable information from patients. Rather, it's a kind of medical shorthand that allows a doctor to write instructions to a pharmacist in a quick way that the pharmacist is sure to understand. Latin is a convenient language to use on prescriptions because it is a "dead" language; it's not likely to be changed in any way, and it's meaning is exact and definite. The pharmacist usually translates part of the subscription into

English and types it onto your prescription label, if the information applies to you. But don't despair! You don't have to rely on the pharmacist to translate your prescription. The list of the most commonly used Latin abbreviations will help you understand the subscription.

Latin Abbreviation	Meaning
a.c.	before meals
ad	to, up to
ad lib.	as much as desired
alt. hor.	every other hour
b.i.d.	twice daily
c.	with
caps.	capsule
d.t.d.	give such doses
et	and
fl. or fld.	fluid
gr.	grain
gtt.	drop
h.s.	at bedtime
mist.	mixture
non r.	not to be repeated
O	pint
o.d.	right eye
o.s.	left eye
o.u.	both eyes
part, aeq.	equal parts
p.c.	after meals
pil.	pill
p.o.	by mouth
p.r.n.	as needed
pulv.	powder
q.	every
q.d.	every day
q.h.	every day
q.i.d.	four times a day
q.s.	as much as is required
s.	without
sol.	solution
s.o.s.	if needed (one-time only)
sp. frumenti	whiskey
ss	half
stat.	immediately

Latin Abbreviation	Meaning
tab.	tablet
t.i.d.	three times a day
tr.	tincture
ung.	ointment
ut dict.	as directed

Medicines are measured out using metric measurements, so abbreviations like gm. (gram), cc. (cubic centimeter), ml. (milliliter), and mgms. (milligrams) will appear in the subscription.

The subscription also tells the pharmacist how many pills or tablets to give you. For example, if you are getting 30 capsules, the subscription reads either "capsules No. 30" or "#30."

Refill information is also included for the pharmacist on the subscription. It can be either written or printed on the form. If your doctor writes it, it will probably say something like "Refill 2 x"—refill two times. In some forms, a line that reads "REP. 0-1-2-3 PRN" will appear in a lower corner. "REP." means repeat; the doctor simply circles the appropriate number, indicating to the pharmacist how many times to refill your prescription without requiring you to show a new prescription. "PRN" means as needed, that is, the prescription can be refilled as many times as you want to refill it.

SIGNATURE

The signature is the part of the prescription that the pharmacist types on the label and attaches to your medication. It is the set of instructions from the pharmacist and doctor to you. These instructions should be clear and complete. If the pharmacist types something obscure, such as "Take as directed," give the medicine back and ask him or her to type the complete instructions. If your doctor neglects to list them on the prescription form, ask the pharmacist to call the doctor and get the instructions.

Having the signature on the prescription label is quite important. Even those of us with excellent memories can forget exactly what the doctor said, especially if three months have elapsed and we are taking the medication for a recurrent problem. Also, following the instructions exactly is critical. Even things that don't seem important to you should be followed. For instance, if the directions tell you not to take a capsule that is cracked, make sure you don't. Don't take your pill with milk or coffee if the instructions tell you to take it with water. So seemingly unimportant parts of the instructions must be remembered and heeded.

SIGNATURE OF THE PRESCRIBER

Prescription drugs can't be dispensed unless prescribed by an authorized person. Your doctor *must* sign the prescription.

LEGEND DRUG

Finally, once you receive the prescription drug itself, look at its label. Along with the name of the drug—generic or brand—comes a *legend* that must accompany any drug sold only by prescription. This inscription is very meaningful. The label of every prescription drug must, under requirement of law, read: "Caution: Federal law prohibits dispensing without prescription." In other words, obtaining a prescription drug is illegal unless you have a legal prescription from your doctor for that drug; and sharing your prescription drug with someone else—even a family member—is also illegal unless the prescription designates that the drug is for that person too.

9

how the doctor
prescribes

You can take an active role in choosing which nonprescription drugs you buy over the counter, but there's no reason to think that you are totally helpless when it comes to prescription drugs. You can provide doctors with information—and you can ask them questions—that help them to prescribe the best medication for your individual needs and that help you utilize the prescription drug in the best way possible.

WHAT TO TELL YOUR DOCTOR

You should be sure to tell certain things to your doctor (even without being asked) before you accept a prescription:

1. *Mention all previous reactions to any drug, no matter what sickness the drug was for.* Name the ones that worked well. Also itemize those that did not, even if they seem to have nothing to do with the one the doctor wants to prescribe. For example, your doctor would be very interested in knowing whether you ever reacted adversely to penicillin; other drugs, closely related to it, could cause a similar reaction. To be

125

sure you name all your allergies, keep a written record of all drugs that you are allergic to or that give you a bad reaction. Do the same for members of your family, especially for the elderly and infirm.

2. *Tell the doctor about any food allergies.* You might not think a food allergy is related to an Rx drug, but it is. A good example is the fact that people who are allergic to eggs cannot get a swine flu shot, because it is cultured in egg medium. People who are allergic to *any* substance run the risk of a bad reaction that is four times greater than nonallergic patients.

3. *Advise the doctor of any other drugs you are taking—OTC medications or prescriptions from other doctors.* Certain drugs clash, so your doctor must know what you are taking. The easiest, safest, and most accurate way to inform your doctor of other drugs is to bring your prescription medicine to the appointment. If you are scheduled for surgery, tell your dentist, surgeon, or anesthesiologist about *all* the drugs you have taken for the prior several weeks.

4. *If you have a medical condition other than the one the doctor is treating you for, say so.* Prescription drugs that work well for one medical condition might be dangerous for another. One set of symptoms might disappear, but you might become even sicker with another.

5. *Tell the doctor whether you drink alcohol, coffee, or tea.* Alcohol and caffeine can greatly alter the effects of prescription drugs, even causing loss of consciousness or coma when mixed with certain drugs. Ask the doctor whether these beverages are safe to mix with the drug in question. You might have to skip your predinner cocktail or morning coffee for a while. Throughout *part two*, the dangers of driving while taking certain prescription drugs will be discussed.

6. *If you're pregnant or nursing a child, make sure the doctor knows.* Don't take any drugs while bearing or nursing, unless told to do so by a doctor. A nose, ear, and throat specialist, for instance, would probably not know that you're nursing a 6-month-old baby or perhaps that you're three months pregnant. If you get pregnant while you are taking any drug, inform your doctor immediately. Also, keep a written record of all drugs you take and all vaccines you receive during the entire nine months of pregnancy. Include the name of each drug, how much you took, the dates you took it, and why you took it.

You shouldn't just take your prescription slip meekly, and leave the doctor's office without a whimper. Many people don't get the benefit of their prescription drugs due to many reasons: They are careless in taking drugs, they are in a hurry, they are unable to understand directions, or they are forgetful due to memory lapses, inattention, or senility. You should ask your doctor questions that help you get the most out of your prescription. Don't let doctors brush you off simply by telling you, "This drug is going to make you feel better." Pin them down to specifics: Is it supposed to reduce your fever? Make the redness leave the area around your wound? Help you fall asleep? And so on. Ask your doctor questions if you are confused about *anything* pertaining to your illness or to your prescription. Ask him or her to write down information if it is unclear or if you think you will have trouble remembering it.

1. *When should I take the drug?* If your doctor tells you that you should take the medicine one hour before your meals, but you *never* eat lunch, say so and get more specific directions. Your doctor must know any of your daily habits that might influence your taking the drug: If you skip lunch everyday, the drug might have to be taken with food. The doctor can make that need clear to you, and you can plan to eat a light lunch while you are taking the medication. If the doctor says, "Take it four times a day," simply explain that you would be more comfortable if you had specific times—say, 8:00 A.M., 2:00 P.M., 8:00 P.M., and midnight.

2. *Should I take all the medicine?* Sometimes you can stop taking a drug when your symptoms disappear. In other cases (like antibiotics), the last pill is as important as the first; you should take all the pills in the bottle, no matter how much better you feel.

3. *How should I take the drug?* Different drugs work in different ways, and you should know how to take each one. Some drugs should be held under the tongue so that they are rapidly absorbed by the blood vessels there. Others should be taken with water to dissolve the pill; if you take it with milk instead, the dissolving process might be slowed down.

Make sure you ask for extra-clear instructions for use if the medicine is in an unfamiliar form. For instance, if you've never used a suppository, don't leave until the doctor has made completely clear to you exactly how to use it.

4. *Will I have to change my activities or my diet while I am taking this drug?* You'll need to know if the drug will make you sleepy, because you then know that you shouldn't drive or operate machinery. Some drugs (like some antibiotics) are neutralized if they're taken with milk! And while some drugs work better on an empty stomach, others work better if you have food in your stomach. Give your doctor a brief run-down of your usual daily activities.

5. *How soon will this medicine start to work?* Again, this question helps you to know whether or not your medication is working, and it will probably save you some worry and concern. Some drugs take a while before they start to work (most antibiotics take at least 72 hours); you shouldn't get upset if you aren't feeling better a few hours after you start taking the drug. Some antidepressants take up to three weeks to start working; if you don't know that, you might stop taking the drug after a week because you think it isn't working.

6. *Does this drug have side effects? Are they normal, or should I be concerned about them?* Every drug has potential side effects; that is, a drug can have unwanted results, other than those you are trying to achieve. Some of them are merely uncomfortable, and you should expect them and be prepared to keep taking your prescription even though the side effects might develop. In other cases, the side effects are a matter of real concern: If they develop, you should stop taking the drug and call your doctor. In some few cases a side effect might become so debilitating or potentially hazardous that you might have to go back to the doctor or to the emergency room at the hospital.

You shouldn't expect your doctor to rattle off every possible side effect, but you *can* expect a warning about the major ones: "You'll probably get a little nauseated from taking this drug, but be sure to call me if you start vomiting."

If you do start experiencing side effects, and they get intolerable— even if they are the "expected" side effects—don't suffer in silence. Call your doctor and explain the problem; often, he or she can switch to another drug that gives you the same benefits but that doesn't cause side effects.

Your question about side effects is particularly important if you are taking a long-term drug (for kidney disease or to prevent pregnancy, for example). Side effects of long-term drug usage are usually different from short-term drug usage, and they can be more serious. You should be fully aware of what to expect and which conditions to report to your doctor.

It would take a volume to list each drug separately, along with all the possible side effects. You can ask your pharmacist or doctor for the information concerning your specific prescription drug. In general, any of the side effects in the following list are a cause for concern. If any of them appear, you should call your doctor immediately.

increased frequency or severity of headaches

throbbing headaches

pulsating headaches

headaches made more intense when you lie down

a pattern of sudden headaches

increased frequency or severity of migraine headaches

forceful heart action

sudden dizziness

sudden changes in vision

sudden changes in hearing

difficulty in speaking

sudden weakness of any body part

sudden numbness

sudden tingling

sudden loss of feeling in any body part

"spots" before your eyes

blind spots in one or both eyes

flashes of light

reduces clarity of vision

inability to see in dim light

pain in the eyes

discomfort in the eyes

sense of pressure in one or both eyes

headache adjacent to the eyes

difficulty in focusing vision

loss of side vision

a "halo" effect when you look at light

faintness

soreness or tenderness of veins in legs

swelling of the feet

swelling of the ankles

sudden pain or pressure in the chest

sudden pain or pressure in the jaws

sudden pain or pressure in the shoulders

sudden pain or pressure in the arms

shortness of breath

nausea

sweating

cough (with or without bloody sputum)

acid indigestion

pain in the upper abdomen

vomiting of blood

blood in the stools

loss of appetite

fever

exhaustion

yellow coloration of the skin or eyes

dark-colored urine

light-colored stools

itching

pain, discomfort, or swelling in upper right abdomen

sudden abdominal pain

progressive fatigue

paleness

sore throat

abnormal bruising

nosebleeds

bleeding of the gums

bloody urine

evidence of bleeding or bruising without any cause

chills

7. *Can this prescription be refilled?* Your doctor might indicate on the prescription pad that the drug can be refilled, but you should find out whether you should refill it automatically or only if you are still suffering from the symptoms. Sometimes a doctor allows for a refill in case your symptoms are particularly stubborn but tells you *not* to refill the prescription if your symptoms are relieved.

Ask also whether you should save the medicine. The answer is probably no. Make sure you flush medications down the toilet when you dispose of them—don't just throw them into a trash can.

8. *Are you going to need to see me again? When should I call or come in again?* A doctor might need to check your progress midway through your drug therapy. Make sure you understand clearly when you should call or come back in. And follow the doctor's directions! If he or she tells you to come back in a week, don't wait for two weeks because you are too busy. Keep the appointment: Otherwise, the doctor will not be able to tell whether the drug is working.

9. *What should I do if I accidentally skip a dose?* It's only human to forget to take your medicine occasionally, and you need to know what you can do to correct the oversight. If you double up on a dose, for instance, you might accidentally poison yourself. With some drugs, though, you should take the pill as soon as you realize that you forgot it so that your blood level of medication does not drop so low that it affects your general treatment from the drug; oral contraceptives are a good example.

GENERIC VERSUS BRAND NAMES

Finally, you should ask the doctor whether the prescription can be filled by a generic rather than a brand name drug. The difference can save you money. Generic names are the simple, nonproprietary names for drugs, which are standardized by the American Medical Association, the American Pharmaceutical Association, the United States Pharmacopeial Convention, and the Food and Drug Administration. Generics are public domain, unprotected by patents, copyright laws, or trademarks. They are the "official" name for a drug, such as penicillin, tetracycline, and erythromycin. Brand names are the names we hear most often; they are usually trademarked and well advertised. In fact, pharmaceutical firms spend about $4,500 a year per physician, advertising and marketing their brand name drugs. As a result, the brand name usually winds up on your prescription—unless you ask.

How does this question save you money? As we shall see in the next chapter, the prices for brand name drugs vary widely, from $2.50 per hundred to $22.50 per hundred in one case, for the same drug manufactured under different brand names. Ask about a generic prescription. If you cannot have one, ask why not.

10

selecting a pharmacist

FINDING OUT ABOUT YOUR PRESCRIPTION

Once you get to the pharmacy, you can get more help from the pharmacist. Ask whether a *patient package insert*—a sheet of instructions and information for the patient—comes with the drug. Such an insert often accompanies a large quart-size bottle of tablets, but the pharmacist tosses it aside since the bottle's contents are going to fill forty or fifty small prescription bottles. Ask for it: You have the right to know. A patient package insert gives you the necessary information about the drugs you take. Or ask whether there are any written instructions that you could take home with you. Some pharmacies and doctors have developed instruction sheets for medications that they prescribe frequently; these save the time required to write instructions on each prescription each time the drug is dispensed. You are responsible for your own body, and you have a right to information that helps you carry out that responsibility.[1]

Insist on written instructions in some form—patient package inserts, mimeographed sheets, or the label on the prescription bottle. You should always insist that the pharmacist clearly label the prescription and put written instructions on the container. Then make sure that you never mix two different prescriptions in one container, and make sure also that you never switch containers. If you keep your medications organized, you'll always have a clear set of instructions with each prescription.

At one time, the consumer was pretty much powerless when it came to comparison shopping and saving money on prescription drugs. Consumer-oriented movements in the early 1970s may have changed all that, though. Consumers and their representatives spoke out about generic drugs, the posting of prices, and advertising—and won. As a result, we might all come out the winners.[2]

WHAT DETERMINES PRICE?

What determines prescription drug prices? Some of the price setting, of course, rests with the manufacturer. An antibiotic can be produced by a number of individual firms; tetracycline, for example, is produced by over *fifty* different companies. Some of those companies might charge your pharmacist a higher wholesale price than another company. Penicillin VK is a good example: in 1975, Eli Lilly and Company's product cost pharmacists $8.32 for 100 250-milligram tablets; Sherry Pharmaceutical sold the same size tablets of penicillin VK to pharmacists for $1.85. (One out of every five prescriptions filled in this country is for an antibiotic, so there's a real chance of making an impact with price differences like this one.)

Sometimes there is a wide price difference for the very same drug, manufactured by the same manufacturer. For example, Mylan Laboratories manufactures erythromycin (an antibiotic) in its final form for a number of firms, including Sherry, Smith Kline & French, Squibb, and Parke, Davis. But now look at what those separate firms charge pharmacists for 100 250-milligram tablets (of the *exact* composition): Sherry, $5.70; Smith Kline & French, $10.15; Squibb, $11.83; and Parke, Davis, $15.87.

Another thing that determines prices, of course, is the pharmacists' methods of computing their profits. Recent studies showed that most pharmacists didn't aim for huge profit margins; in fact, some were even operating at a loss on some items. Pharmacists use two general methods:

1. *Percentage markup:* No matter what the drug and no matter what the drug's wholesale cost, the pharmacist simply adds a set percentage—say, 3 percent—to the wholesale cost. So whatever you buy, you can figure it cost the pharmacist 3 percent less than the price you pay to stock that medicine on the shelves.

2. *Professional fee method:* The pharmacist estimates what is needed to cover overhead expenses, adds a little for profit, and

computes a flat fee for dispensing prescriptions. When you buy a prescription from a pharmacist who uses this method, you are paying the wholesale price plus the flat fee. There's an advantage for you in this method: Pharmacists who charge flat fees regardless of the price of the medication won't be as tempted to stock the shelves with high-priced brand names, because they're not getting a percentage of the price. Their cut is the same for everything.

GENERIC—BRAND NAME PRICE DIFFERENCES

Generally, you can save money if your physician prescribes a generic drug for you instead of insisting on a brand name. But keep in mind that doctors may have reasons for choosing a certain brand. They know that it is reliable, they are certain of its therapeutic benefits, or they know which auxiliary medications are added. So remember that they may not be willing to change to a generic brand. Don't be afraid to talk about it, though; they should be willing to give you their reasons for preferring the brand-name medication.

WHAT YOU CAN DO

What specifically can you do to save costs when you need prescription drugs? Follow these suggestions:

1. *Talk to doctors about prescription drug prices.* If they know that you are aware of price differences and that you care about them, they may make an effort to help you save money.

2. *Ask doctors to prescribe drugs under their generic names.* If they are unwilling to do so, ask them to explain why they think the brand-name medicine is best.

3. *Have doctors write out your prescription for the least expensive brand.* This alternative is even better than having your doctor write out a prescription for drugs under their generic names (as long as the doctor is aware of manufacturers' costs). Using the previous example, ask your doctor to prescribe Sherry erythromycin, representing a savings of over $10 when compared to the same medication from Parke, Davis. The following table lists fourteen of the most commonly prescribed drugs that are also available generically, with their brand names and what they do. If you are taking any of them under a brand name, you might save money by asking your doctor to prescribe a generic form.

FOURTEEN MOST OFTEN PRESCRIBED DRUGS THAT ARE AVAILABLE GENERICALLY

GENERIC NAME	COMMONLY PRESCRIBED BRAND NAMES	PURPOSE OF DRUG
Ampicillin	Amcill Omnipen Polycillin Principen	To fight infection (antibiotic)
Tetracycline	Achromycin V Panmycin Sumycin Tetracyn	To fight infection (antibiotic)
Acetaminophen/codeine	Tylenol with Codeine	To relieve pain, fever, and cough
Hydrochlorothiazide	Esidrix HydroDIURIL Oretic	For hypertension and edema (diuretic)
Penicillin V-K	Pen Vee K V-Cillin K Veetids	To fight infection (antibiotic)
Chlordiazepoxide hydrochloride	Librium	To relieve anxiety and tension
Propoxyphene hydrochloride, aspirin, phenacetin, and caffeine	Darvon Compound-65	To relieve pain (analgesic)
Erythromycin stearate	Erythrocin Stearate	To fight infection (antibiotic)
Amitriptyline hydrochloride	Elavil Enelep	To relieve symptoms of depression
Diphenhydramine hydrochloride	Benadryl	Antihistamine (also for motion sickness and parkinsonism)
Diphenoxylate hydrochloride with atropine sulfate	Lomotil	To help control diarrhea

selecting a pharmacist **135**

GENERIC NAME	COMMONLY PRESCRIBED BRAND NAMES	PURPOSE OF DRUG
Meclizine hydrochloride	Antivert	To control nausea and vomiting, and dizziness from motion sickness
Chlorothiazide	Diuril	For hypertension and edema (diuretic)
Erythromycin ethyl succinate E.E.S.		To fight infection (antibiotic)

From "Most Popular Generic Drugs Listed," FDA Consumer (June 1979), p. 25.

4. *Encourage your doctor to find out about drug prices and manufacturer costs,* if he or she is unaware of them. Of course, doctors are extremely busy, but they can have newsletters and price listings on hand to consult.

5. *If you are put on a long-term program of drug therapy, ask your doctor to prescribe large doses at once.* This method not only saves you the inconvenience of extra trips to the pharmacy, but it saves you money: Most pills, tablets, and capsules are less expensive when you buy them in lots of 100 or 500. You do need to take one caution: Check with the pharmacist and determine the drug's expiration date; many medications lose potency and effectiveness after a certain shelf life. If the drug expires before you are supposed to use it up, buy a smaller quantity, even if you have to pay more; the stale, ineffective drugs are a worse waste of money and will probably affect your health. Also, when you buy drugs in large quantities, ask your pharmacist for the best storage methods. You can take measures that ensure the freshness of your medicine until you use it up.

6. *Comparison shop!* There are wide differences in prices among pharmacies, even in the same city. To do a good job of comparison shopping, you have to have your facts straight. So ask your doctor to list the drug information on another scrap of paper, separate from the prescription form. Make sure you understand the name of the drug, the quantity prescribed, and the strength. For example, is it 250-milligram or 500-milligram? Find out what the form is, too; there are price differences among pills and capsules and liquids, for instance.

If you receive a prescription that you don't need to start taking right away, shop around before you have it filled. If you need to begin taking the prescription immediately, you'll have to go to a pharmacy and have it filled; that's where the extra scrap of paper comes in handy. When you have a free afternoon, visit a couple of different drugstores and pharmacies (or telephone, whichever allows you to cover the most ground). Tell the pharmacist exactly what you want, and ask how much it costs. Quite a few pharmacists used to refuse to release price information, but recent legislation requires them to do so if you ask for it.

If you do your homework right—and if you have the time and energy to repeat the experiment on a couple of different prescriptions —you'll find out which pharmacy or drugstore in your city has the least expensive prices. One survey of 147 different pharmacies in seventeen cities recently revealed startling differences in prices for the same product: Valium, for example, costs anywhere from $6.75 to $15 for identical brands. Tetracycline ranged from $2.50 to $20 in the same survey. Remember, these were comparisons of *exactly the same brand, quantity, and strength.*

If your doctor prescribes the drug under a generic name, ask the pharmacist what the least expensive brand costs; then ask what the most expensive costs. The difference gives you a good indication of your actual savings.

7. *Take advantage of prescription drug advertising.* Ads for prescription drugs used to be unheard of, but consumer advocate groups have succeeded in convincing some manufacturers to advertise. Some small cities don't yet have these services, but in some larger cities you can gain access to posters, listings, and ads that list all the price information you need. These posters and ads don't list unusual or atypical prescription drugs; if your prescription is for a drug that is not on the list, you have to ask the pharmacist for price information.

8. *Decide which services you need.* You might want to keep convenience in mind. Suppose you find a pharmacy that is generally a few cents less expensive than the one near your home, but the less expensive pharmacy is ten miles across town. Saving the crosstown trip is probably worth the extra price. (With today's crazy traffic patterns, a mile in downtown traffic could take as much time as ten on a freeway.) Service is important, too: Watch for long lines, crowds, and poor service during certain hours of the day when you prefer to shop—or an unfriendly pharmacist.

Sometimes it's worth paying a little extra to receive the service you demand. You'll probably pay a little more for pharmacies that offer credit, home delivery, and 24-hour service. If you need or would like those services, it's worth your money; if you don't, choose a pharmacy that doesn't offer extras and that passes savings on to customers.

9. *If you are over sixty, find out which pharmacies in your city give discounts for the elderly.* Some organizations, like the American Association of Retired Persons, have discount programs for prescription products, which enable you to save on your medicinal needs.

CHOOSING YOUR PHARMACIST

You have a regular doctor, a regular dentist, a regular hairdresser, a supermarket you prefer above others, and a plumber you like to call. Establishing "regulars" has real advantages: They get to know you, so they are apt to give you better service. They get to know your needs, so they can provide you with services that help you fulfill your needs. For the same reason, it's nice to have a regular pharmacist—someone who gets to know you, who can observe your general medical condition over a period of time, who knows which drugs you have taken in the past, and who is aware of any special needs you might have. A "regular" pharmacist, for example, knowing that you are in a wheelchair and can't make extra trips to the pharmacy, might arrange home delivery or help you consolidate trips by recommending purchases of nonprescription items at the same time you come in to buy a prescription drug.

How do you go about choosing a pharmacist? Besides proximity, price, service, and the other factors just discussed, many considerations have to do with the pharmacist as a person.[3] Look for a pharmacist who:

1. *Eagerly answers any questions you ask about the drug you are receiving.* A pharmacist who grudgingly answers questions or who refuses to answer questions at all is of no real service to you.

2. *Is friendly.* You don't need to put up with someone who is rude or apathetic. Remember: Without customers, a pharmacist is out of business. If you are treated rudely or with apparent lack of concern, simply take your business elsewhere.

3. *Keeps a medication record for regular customers.* This record has the effect of monitoring all the drugs you take; you'll have much less chance of taking drugs that won't interact smoothly and much less chance of accidentally getting a drug that you're allergic to. The medication record should list your name, age, height, weight, drug allergies, and sensitivities. You'll know someone is looking out for you.

4. *Is willing to counsel you on the purchase of nonprescription drugs.* Some pharmacists just shrug their shoulders if you ask them which brand of aspirin they'd recommend. Look for a pharmacist who tells you which one he or she prefers and why. (If your pharmacist tells you to see a doctor, take the advice.) A regular pharmacist can steer you away from over-the-counter drugs that might clash with your prescription drug.

5. *Gives you some instructions when handing the prescription across the counter to you.* A good pharmacist, for instance, tells you not to take your tetracycline with milk, iron supplements, or antacids—as he or she hands you your prescription.

6. *Serves the customers personally.* Steer clear of pharmacies and drugstores where someone other than the pharmacist (an assistant, clerk, or soda jerk) hands you your prescription. You have the right to see and talk to the pharmacist. In fact, it's against the law for anyone but a pharmacist to dispense a prescription drug.

7. *Unhesitatingly gives you information about prices.*

8. *Fills your prescription with a low-cost brand-name drug if your doctor prescribes the drug under a generic name.* A good pharmacist also tells you that the brand name your doctor has prescribed is much more expensive than others on the market and might offer to call the doctor while you wait to see if he or she would consider another brand.

9. *Offers extra services that you need or want* (if you are willing to pay a little extra for them), such as home delivery, around-the-clock emergency service, a charge account system of billing, or special discounts for the elderly.

A good pharmacist is as important to your good health as a good doctor or dentist. Finding one with most or all of the desirable qualities right away probably won't be easy, so be prepared to take your time and look around. You wouldn't stay with a doctor you didn't like or trust, nor would you put up with one you suspected didn't care about you or look out for your best interests. Do the same with your pharmacist. If you're not getting what you think you should, take your business somewhere else. *You* are the customer, and you have a right to demand satisfaction.

Take an active role in ensuring the success of treatment with prescription drugs. You can be just as informed about prescription drugs as you are about over-the-counter remedies—remember that. You're not in the dark ages any more.

You can do many things to make better use of prescription drugs by using them safely.[4] Consider the following suggestions:

1. *Tell and ask both your doctor and your pharmacist everything discussed earlier in this chapter.* Try not to miss any detail in taking the drug and in monitoring its effects.

2. *Don't pressure your doctor into prescribing something* if you don't really need it. No law says you have to leave the doctor's office with a prescription; there are many more ways to treat disease.

3. *Never take prescription drugs on your own,* that is, without authorization and instructions from the doctor.

4. *Don't take a friend's prescription drug* just because your symptoms are just like his or hers. Visit the doctor if you are sick, and take your own prescription drug.

5. *Don't give anyone else—even a family member—your prescription drug,* unless your doctor tells you to. It's against the law. And it's a dumb thing to do.

6. *Don't change the dose or timing of your drug,* unless your doctor tells you to. You might not like taking a drug, say, six times a day; it's probably more convenient to take it only three times, when you eat. So you decide to double up on doses and to take it only three times a day. Don't. You can seriously hurt yourself.

7. *Don't ever stop taking any drug without letting your doctor know.*

8. *Don't take more medications than you have to.* You might decide that taking aspirin or a cold medication would help speed recovery. Your doctor is the best judge. Generally, a prescription drug should be strong enough to act on its own; if it's not, your doctor can evaluate the need for additional medication. Don't risk possible bad reactions by mixing drugs without your doctor's recommendation.

9. *Never take any drug in the dark.* If you get up in the middle of the night to take your medicine, turn on the light and make sure you've got the right bottle.

10. *Don't mix medications in the same container.* Their potency may be destroyed. Also, if the medications look alike, you might take the same drug twice.

11. *Be especially careful when you take medicines that look alike.* You may get a double dose.

12. *Keep emergency drugs—such as nitroglycerin—on the night table next to your bed.* Keep all the rest in the bathroom or wherever you normally keep your medicine. It's best if you have only one bottle on your night table; then you won't grab the wrong one by mistake if you are panicked or ill.

13. *Learn the name and correct spelling of each drug you are using.*

14. *Follow your doctor's directions exactly.* If something happens that causes you to change your dosage or frequency, tell your doctor about it. Your physician can help you work out a new schedule.

15. *Shake liquids well before you take them.* Look at the liquid and make sure all the ingredients are mixed well.

16. *If you're taking a liquid, use a standard measuring spoon.* Your label might tell you to take two teaspoons, but a household "teaspoon" varies greatly in size. Use the same kind of teaspoon you use in measuring your cooking ingredients. Whatever you do, *don't* sip your medication from the bottle.

17. *Discard drugs that you won't be using.* Flush them down the toilet.

18. *Keep all your drugs out of the reach of children.* If you're done with a medicine, get rid of it. If you have long-term drugs that you need on a permanent or long-term basis, ask your pharmacist to package them in child-proof containers and take care to store them out of the reach of children. Lock them up if you can!

19. *Store drugs properly.* Read the labels on medication for storing instructions. Some medications need to be stored in a dark place; others need to be kept in a cool place.

THE ELDERLY AND DRUGS

The elderly present a special safety problem when taking prescriptions.[5] Because they sometimes have unsteady hands, poor vision and hearing, or unreliable memories, and because they may take a lot of drugs, the elderly may be more susceptible to drug overdose and accidental drug abuse. They also run the increased risk of complications with drug use because they usually have multiple medical problems requiring a number of drugs and because physiological changes take place within their bodies that influence the ways in which drugs affect the body. For example, decreased blood flow can impair absorption of a drug, and a drug's distribution can lessen throughout the body. Also, decreased kidney and liver functions can hinder waste elimination.

Doctors should therefore take special steps to ensure that elderly patients get the right medicine, in the right dose, at the right time, and with the right safety measures. Before giving an elderly person a prescription, doctors should assess their elderly patients in terms of what they can and cannot do functionally: What is the patient's physical status? Is he or she mobile and ambulatory? What is the person's current life style? Does the patient live alone? What medications is he or she currently taking? Also, to make sure the elderly do not accidentally take too much medication, the doctor can provide each elderly patient with printed information about the prescribed drug or drugs. The doctor might even tape a sample of the drug to the top of the sheet so that the drug is easy to identify. Another approach is to label cups with the times of the day that medication must be taken and then put each dose of medicine into its appropriate cup. A calendar might also be helpful. Elderly patients might write out what medication they take, when they took it, and the dosage each time. In this way, they don't double up on taking drugs. Sometimes, doctors have visiting nurses go to the homes of the elderly, educate and inform them about the drug they take, and help them measure out the proper dosages of medication. They may also help the elderly to create some memory device so they do not overdose.

11

common prescriptions

Of the thousands of prescription drugs available, a handful are quite common, and you will probably have occasion to take one or more of them during your lifetime.[1] The most commonly prescribed drugs are antibiotics; others that are common include pain killers, anticoagulants (to help those with heart disease maintain thin blood), anticonvulsants (used by epileptics), tranquilizers and sedatives, and antihistamines (to help in allergy control). You should be aware of the possible dangers of some prescription drugs—as well as of their effects, because all of them are not safe for all people. If you are aware of dangers and effects, you can help your doctor by providing him information if he prescribes a drug you don't think you should take.

EFFECTS AND DANGERS OF SPECIFIC PRESCRIPTION DRUGS

ANTIBIOTICS
Penicillin and Ampicillin
Used to treat bacterial infections, these two antibiotics are not effective against virus infections. You should generally take penicillin and ampicillin on an empty stomach one hour before or two hours after a meal. Do not take either of them with milk, milk products, or antacids; milk and antacids neutralize these drugs. Some types of penicillin are de-

143

stroyed by excess acid in the stomach, so fruit juices or any other drink that is high in acid should not be drunk while you are taking penicillin.

When taking penicillin, you should be alert for signs of an allergic reaction such as severe rash, a drop in blood pressure, and breathing difficulties. Many people are allergic to penicillin and to other sulfa drugs, and a severe allergic reaction can result in death. You should always inform your doctor of any suspected penicillin allergy or any allergic tendencies you have (hay fever, asthma, hives, eczema) before accepting a penicillin prescription.

These drugs should generally not be taken over a long period of time, because large doses can cause gastrointestinal, liver, or kidney abnormalities. Another major side effect from large doses is called "super infection,"[2] which happens when bacteria and fungi that are normally in the body in small amounts become resistent to penicillin and begin to multiply. Nausea and vomiting generally result.

Tetracycline
Also used to fight infection, tetracycline, unlike penicillin, does not kill the bacteria, but it does inhibit growth and multiplication. Also like penicillin, tetracycline is not effective against a virus.

Allergies and ill effects are not often seen in tetracycline use. Mild reactions are usually skin reactions of some kind (hives, itching, swelling), loss of appetite, nausea, vomiting, and diarrhea.

The more severe reactions are much like those of penicillin. It should generally not be given to children under the age of eight, because it often results in discoloration of the teeth in young children. Because it has recently been investigated for a possible link with birth defects, you should not take it if you are pregnant—especially in the first trimester. Nursing mothers should not take the drug either, because, passed to the baby through the mother's milk, tetracycline could have ill effects on the child. Even if not pregnant, women who take tetracycline are prone to develop vaginal infections (one type of super infection), characterized by severe itching and heavy discharge. While you are taking this drug, avoid direct exposure to the sun's rays; tetracycline sometimes causes a phototoxic reaction that results in swelling and redness of the skin. With long-term use, you will experience the symptoms of "super infection"—nausea and vomiting.

ANALGESICS
Darvon
Darvon is a widely prescribed and used pain killer marketed by Eli Lilly and Company. In 1975, 16.4 million new and refill prescriptions for Darvon were given. The key ingredient in Darvon is propoxyphene,

which is no more effective than aspirin in relieving pain, according to recent studies made by researchers at Georgetown University. Those researchers say that most of Darvon's effects come from two sources: (1) a placebo effect from the propoxyphene, and (2) an actual analgesic effect, which is no more effective than aspirin, from the other ingredients (caffeine, aspirin, and phenacetin).

The drug has a significant potential for abuse. In fact, one study in Milwaukee, Wisconsin, indicated that among young people, Darvon was the most abused drug in that area.[3] Darvon overdose is a common cause of death and suicide because many people who take it don't realize what a potent drug it is, especially if it is taken with alcohol. Tolerance to Darvon increases quickly, and more of the drug must be taken to produce the desired effect.

Darvon may make you drowsy and affect your mental alertness, judgment, and coordination; so you should not drive or operate machinery after you have taken it. You should not take Darvon at all if you are allergic to aspirin. Darvon should not be taken over a long period of time or in large doses, either, because of the kidney-damaging ingredient phenacetin. And do not use Darvon if you are trying to combat severe pain. Remember, Darvon won't relieve any pain that aspirin won't relieve. And aspirin is a lot less expensive.

Morphine and Codeine
These narcotic drugs are used to kill severe pain, and they also work to suppress anxiety. Because of their narcotic properties, both can be physically and psychologically habit forming. In addition, you should be alert to signs of allergic reaction commonly associated with these two drugs. Both morphine and codeine cause lightheadedness, dizziness, and drowsiness, so don't attempt to do anything that requires alertness (especially driving) while you are taking either. You might also have problems with nausea, vomiting, or constipation.

AMPHETAMINES
Dextroamphetamine or Benzedrine
Either is used to curb the appetite to lose weight. Unfortunately, the appetite-suppressing action of this drug does not last; the effects may disappear after a few weeks of use. Because the amphetamines build up tolerance quickly, you must take more of the drug to get the desired effect. Taking increasing doses over a long period of time can cause physical dependence on the drug. Taken over a long period of time, dextroamphetamine in particular can cause hives, headaches, dizziness, tremors, euphoria, dryness of the mouth, heart palpitations, and irregular heart action. Commonly, it also makes you nervous, increases

your heart rate, and causes insomnia. Because of these effects, you should not participate in hazardous activities, such as flying a plane, because your judgment may be imparied.

You should not take dextroamphetamine (or any amphetamine) if you have:

- an allergy to the drug,
- severe hardening of the arteries or any heart disease,
- high blood pressure or any thyroid disease,
- glaucoma, or
- severe anxiety or nervous tension.

Diet Pills
Like amphetamines, diet pills containing diethylpropion hydrochloride pose a real danger. Because people generally build up a quick tolerance for the pills' initial effects, they need more and more of the medicine to get any effect at all. In the doses required to suppress the appetite, the drug can lead to physical addiction.

People with heart disease should not take any kind of diet pill.

Many people who start on a regimen of diet pills are unable to continue taking them because they become so jittery and ill at ease. The most common side effect of diet pills is an increase in irritability, tension, inability to concentrate, anxiety, confusion, and delusions. Other side effects include nervousness, restlessness, insomnia, headache, chest pains, heart palpitations, and dry mouth.

ANTICOAGULANTS
Warfarin and Dicumerol
Useful in the treatment of certain kinds of heart disease, these drugs prevent the formation of blood clots. However, they can also lead to excessive thinning of the blood, with hemorrhage as a result. You should not take warfarin or dicumerol in the following cases:

- if you have any "bleeding" disorders (such as a bleeding ulcer or ulcerative colitis),
- if you have other blood disorders,
- if you have open wounds from surgery or injury,
- if you have liver or kidney damage or disease, or if you are pregnant (the drug could cause hemorrhage in the unborn child).

You should remain alert for the signs of hemorrhage or overthinning. Contact your doctor immediately in case of nosebleed, dark or bloody urine, bruises that you can't relate to any injury, blood in your stools (turning them dark, tarry, or black), or excessive menstrual bleeding.

ANTICHOLINERGICS
Atropine
This drug, which blocks specific nerve impulses, is used in several ways. It is given prior to a general anesthetic when you have surgery. It is put in the eyes prior to an eye exam to relieve discomfort. It is used to treat some gastrointestinal diseases, such as ulcers and spastic colon, and sometimes it is even used to eliminate bed wetting.

Naturally, atropine use must be accompanied with cautions. You should not use it if you have narrow-angle glaucoma or ulcerative colitis. If you are elderly, you may be more sensitive to the effects of atropine; in this case, take smaller doses of the drug. Taken in large amounts, atropine can have various side effects such as blurred vision, dry mouth and throat, constipation, hesitancy to urinate, dilated pupils, rapid pulse and heart irregularities, headache, and dry, hot, red skin. Atropine may also cause drowsiness, so you should not drive or operate machinery while you are taking it.

ANTICONVULSANTS
Dilantin
Also called diphenylhydantoin, this drug is used to suppress or control epilepsy or other diseases that cause convulsions.

Dilantin can cause many side effects: mental confusion, constipation, headache, slurred speech, nausea, dizziness, incoordination, double vision, swelling of the tongue, constipation, skin rash, blood abnormalities, and liver damage. The drug should not be taken by anyone with a liver or kidney disease. Dilantin also produces gum abnormalities within the mouth. The gums may enlarge and even cover the teeth. To reduce this enlargement, you should have good mouth hygiene; brush your teeth and massage your gums often. Dilantin may cause drowsiness, which, combined with incoordination and muscle weakness, makes it dangerous for you to drive or operate machinery. You should also avoid the use of other sedatives or alcohol, which may only increase the effects of Dilatin.

One other caution: You should never stop taking Dilantin suddenly. You may start to convulse.

ANTIDEPRESSANTS

Tricyclics

Commonly used to treat depression and other serious psychological illnesses, tricyclics are characterized by depression. You should not eat sour cream, cheese, chocolate, raisins, pickled herring, or canned figs; nor should you drink alcoholic beverages while you are taking a tricyclic. Taken in too large a dose, a tricyclic can cause cardiac arrhythmias that can lead to death. Other side effects include blurred vision, constipation, nausea and vomiting, headache, dryness of mouth, difficulty in urinating, impotence, tremors, delirium, and convulsions. Check with your doctor before you take any other drug—prescription or over-the-counter—while you are taking a tricyclic.

ANTIHISTAMINES

Actifed

This is the brand name for the chemical triprolidine, an allergy medication. It doesn't make your allergy go away; it simply relieves the signs and symptoms of the allergy, so that you can conduct yourself as though you do not have an allergy.

Antihistamines make you drowsy and may impair your alertness, judgment, and coordination. So you shouldn't drive a car or operate machinery while you are taking Actifed. However, coffee or tea may offset the drowsiness that some antihistamines produce. Taken in too large amounts, Actifed may produce the opposite symptoms: It may make you excitable, irritable, and unable to sleep. Besides drowsiness, the side effects of Actifed include dry mouth, dizziness, incoordination, unsteadiness, muscle weakness, upset stomach, and a feeling of tiredness. You shouldn't drink alcohol or take any other depressant drugs (like sleeping pills) while you are taking Actifed, because they will only increase the depressant action.

ANTIHYPERTENSIVES

Hygroton

This brand name for chlorthaldrine treats high blood pressure by causing fluid removal from the body.

Because hygroton is a diuretic, you should expect to urinate frequently. With the increased urine output, you can have a potassium loss. To offset this loss, you should include some of the following high-potassium foods in your diet: all-bran cereals, almonds, dried apricots, fresh bananas, beef, raw carrots, chicken, citrus fruits, rye crackers, dried dates and figs, fresh fish, beef liver, milk, peaches, peanut butter, peas, pork, dried prunes, raisins, and tomato juice.

Hygroton has other effects that you should be aware of. For one, it may produce lightheadedness or dizziness because of lowered blood pressure—especially apparent when you're getting up from a sitting or lying position. Alcohol should be used in moderation because it may increase the blood pressure lowering effect and thus the lightheadedness. Hygroton may also increase the blood sugar and uric acid levels, so it cannot be taken by diabetics or by those individuals with gout. You should also not take hygroton if you are allergic to any sulfa drug, if you have a history of liver or kidney disease or damage, or if you plan to have surgery in the near future.

SEDATIVES–HYPNOTICS
Nembutal
Nembutal, brand name for the chemical pentobarbital, is used as a mild sedative or as a hypnotic. *Sedatives* are used to produce a calming effect during the day, while *hypnotics* have their use at night as sleep inducers.

Nembutal has the potential for abuse, and so it should be used with caution. Besides physical and psychological dependence, the drug can also produce tolerance so that the dosage has to be increased. Alcohol and nembutal should never be taken together: Alcohol merely increases the sedative action, and brain function can be depressed. Driving or operating machinery while taking the barbiturates is not wise, because your thought processes may be impaired due to your drowsiness. The barbiturates should not be prescribed for long-term use because of their potentially deadly nature. The barbiturates are infamous for their abuse and for their connection with suicides and attempted suicides.

Aside from the desired result of drowsiness, nembutal produces the following side effects: mental and physical sluggishness, rash, dizziness, nausea, vomiting, and headache. High doses may cause vertigo, slurred speech, double vision, and impaired thought and judgment. The elderly may have quite a different experience taking Nembutal. The drug may produce agitation, excitement, confusion, and delirium with regular dosages.

Meprobamate and Valium
These sedative–hypnotics deserve brief mention. Both meprobamate (marketed as Equinil or Miltown) and Valium have effects, side effects, and cautions very similar to those for Nembutal. They, too, have the potential for abuse and can be habit-forming, both physically and psychologically. In fact, Valium is probably the most abused prescription drug on the market today.

HEART MEDICATIONS
Nitroglycerin
Nitroglycerin is used not only to blow up bridges in the movies; it is also used as a heart medication. Primarily, it dilates the coronary blood vessels so that the heart can have an increased blood and oxygen supply. Because nitroglycerin dilates blood vessels, it should not be taken by a person with glaucoma, because it may increase the pressure within the eye.

Nitroglycerin can produce various side effects: throbbing in the head, faster pulse, flushed face, and lightheadedness or dizziness (because of lowered blood pressure). Caution should be used in driving, operating machinery, and engaging in hazardous activity because of the lightheadedness and dizziness. If taken for too long, nitroglycerin may produce skin problems (such as rash or peeling), fainting, nausea, and vomiting. Nitroglycerin may also produce tolerance so that more of the medication must be taken.

Digitalis
A drug used to slow down and strengthen the heartbeat, digitalis is one of the most widely used and valuable drugs for treating congestive heart failure and other heart disorders that are indicated by irregular rhythms.

You should follow the directions for digitalis with religious care. Always take the *exact* dose prescribed, and take extra caution not to miss doses. *Never* take extra tablets; improper doses can cause dizziness, fainting spells, weakness, and signs of congestive heart failure.

One of the most uncomfortable side effects for men is painful swelling of the breasts. The general side effects include a loss of appetite, nausea, vomiting, double vision, flashing lights, moving spots, headache, fatigue, and drowsiness. So don't drive a car or operate machinery while you are taking digitalis.

HORMONES
Estrogens
These have been used for years to combat the annoying symptoms of menopause. In the female reproductive system, estrogen and its partner progesterone, play roles throughout a woman's lifetime. At puberty, estrogen secretion increases, and the female responds by developing breasts and other physical characteristics of "femaleness." During maturity, estrogen causes the lining of the womb to thicken in case of pregnancy, and it also helps to regulate the menstrual periods (during which the womb's lining is shed). At menopause, estrogen secretion decreases, and changes in the woman's body occur. She may have

vasomotor changes (the so-called "hot flashes"). The tissues of the vagina shrink. She may be nervous, tired, depressed, experiencing mood changes and insomnia. You should consider yourself a high-risk individual if you are obese or mildly diabetic; high blood pressure or a history of D and Cs also make you a high-risk candidate.

At the present time, estrogen therapy is under fire, and the question asked most is, "Do the risks outweigh the benefits?" Even the risks and benefits are controversial; no one is completely certain of either. The benefits of estrogen therapy are thought to be:

• Estrogen relieves vasomotor problems—specifically "hot flashes."

• It also reduces the shrinkage of vaginal tissues.

• In young women, estrogen stops bone loss (a condition known as osteoporosis).

• In aging women, estrogen therapy reduces the rate of bone loss.[4]

The risks of estrogen therapy are hotly debated, in a controversy that is still raging. Estrogen therapy, it is thought, may contribute to cancer of the uterine lining, high blood pressure, gall bladder disease, coronary heart disease, stroke, increased blood clotting, and breast cancer. So it is really a woman's responsibility to ask her doctor about the risks and benefits and then to decide for herself whether the benefits outweigh the risks. Someone in estrogen therapy may also experience salt and water retention, nausea, difficulty urinating, breast problems, fibroids in the uterus, inflammation of the uterus, vaginal spotting or bleeding, and abdominal cramps (very much like menstrual cramps).

Today, doctors are cautious in prescribing estrogen. They first make sure that their patient really needs it, and then they follow the warnings that appear on the estrogen packages. These warnings state that the drug should be used in the lowest possible dosage, that the woman should have a thorough pelvic exam every six months while on the drug, and that there has been a connection between the product and cancer.

SOME COMMON ILLNESSES

Some diseases require special consideration and special caution in drug use. If you have one of the following diseases, follow the ensuing guidelines and check with your doctor for further instructions.[5]

Diabetes

1. Test your urine for sugar more frequently when you are taking a prescription drug. Some drugs can affect your insulin output and interfere with your oral insulin therapy.

2. Adjust the amount of oral or injected insulin while you are taking prescription drugs. Ask your doctor to help.

3. Change your eating habits to compensate for any effect that the drug has on your sugar production. Again, ask your doctor for help.

4. If you need to, periodically adjust the dosage and frequency of any new drug that is added to your treatment regime. Let your doctor know your needs.

Epilepsy

1. Be alert to any changes in the frequency, intensity, or duration of seizures while you are on medication.

2. Ask your doctor to help you adjust the dosage of your anticonvulsants while you are taking a prescription drug.

3. If a new drug is added to your epilepsy treatment, adjust it periodically (with your doctor's help) until it best suits your needs.

Glaucoma

1. Have your doctor take regular readings of your internal eye pressure during the time you are taking prescription drugs.

2. Ask your doctor to help you adjust your glaucoma medication to maintain normal internal eye pressure while you are using prescription drugs.

3. If a new drug is added to your antiglaucoma regime, adjust the dosage schedule periodically (with the help of your doctor) to avoid over- or undertreatment.

Gout

1. Get your blood uric acid levels tested periodically to determine whether prescription drugs are affecting you; if they are, ask your doctor to help you adjust your antigout medication.

2. If you have an attack of acute gout while you are taking a prescription drug, contact your doctor immediately.

Heart Disease

1. Each time you take a prescription drug, ask your doctor to monitor your heart periodically for changes in rhythm, rate, and functional capacity while you are taking the drug.

2. Many prescription drugs contain sodium or other salt products (including potassium). Ask your doctor to help you determine how you should adjust your diet to compensate for the added salt in your system.

3. If you experience any side effect that could mean a derangement in heart action—faintness, weakness, lightheadedness, dizziness, shortness of breath, irregular heart rhythm, rapid or forceful heart action, or chest pain—contact a doctor immediately.

High Blood Pressure

1. Get blood pressure measurements regularly while you are taking prescription drugs; watch closely if any elevation is recorded.

2. Because so many prescription drugs contain sodium or potassium, ask your doctor to help you decide how to alter your diet to compensate for the added salt.

3. Call a doctor immediately if you experience sudden lightheadedness, weakness, faintness, recurring headaches, forceful heart action, agitation, or restlessness. These symptoms could signal either a significant rise or drop in blood pressure.

Peptic Ulcer

1. Make sure your doctor knows you have a peptic ulcer, and make sure that he or she doesn't prescribe any drug that might irritate your stomach lining or make your ulcer worse.

2. If, while you are taking a prescription drug, you notice any symptom that leads you to believe that your ulcer might be getting worse, call your doctor immediately.

3. If you have a peptic ulcer that has healed, immediately report to your doctor any sign that it might have reopened during your use of a prescription drug.

4. Watch your stools regularly while you are taking prescription drugs. Immediately report any sign of blood or dark coloration (dark gray to black) in your stools.

5. If you have had scar tissue form at the opening to your small intestines, it will make it difficult for your stomach to empty. A

number of prescription drugs can increase the difficulty of the stomach-emptying process due to scar tissue.

Take an active role in ensuring the success of treatment with prescription drugs. You can be just as informed about prescription drugs as you are about over-the-counter remedies—remember that. You're not in the dark ages any more.

part three

COSMETICS

12

using cosmetics safely

We're a beauty-oriented society. We are constantly being told by the television, the radio, and the attractive pages of magazines how to make ourselves more beautiful—how to have whiter teeth, fresher breath, silkier hair, cleaner skin; how to apply our makeup, get rid of dandruff, zap zits.

A *cosmetic* is anything that can be rubbed, poured, sprinkled, sprayed on, introduced into, or otherwise applied to the human body to cleanse it, beautify it, or alter its appearance. Cosmetics include things like lipstick, mascara, shampoo, perfume, soap, deodorant, and toothpaste.

You probably haven't considered cosmetics to be drugs, but they are. There is one important difference, though, between the toothpaste you use morning and night and the over-the-counter cold remedy you rely on for stuffiness: Conventional drugs (both over-the-counter and prescription) must be proved safe and effective by the Food and Drug Administration before they are put on the market. Cosmetics don't. So all kinds of products (posing all kinds of hazards) masquerade as cosmetics. Your only safety is in being a religious label-reader, because those that aren't safe or effective must, by law, contain a sentence on the label telling you that safety has not been determined.[1]

Most cosmetics are relatively safe because you apply them to the skin and hair and then wash them off a short time later. But you should be aware of general considerations that will help you make the cosmetics you use safer.

157

You can take an active role in protecting yourself against harmful agents found in cosmetics by taking extra cautions. The following suggestions should help:

1. *Be alert for irritating substances listed on the label.*[2] This is an important measure even with cosmetics that you just apply to your skin: Dangerous ingredients can gain entry through cuts, abrasions, or simple skin pores. If you're not careful, they can get into your eyes, mouth, or lungs. One example of an irritating ingredient is mercury, a common ingredient in many brands of cosmetics. In a minute amount, it won't hurt you. But as it accumulates in your tissues and blood-stream, it can cause neurological damage, kidney failure, and, if you get enough, death. Another irritating substance found in some cosmetics (such as nail-hardeners) is formaldehyde. Instead of hardening your nails, formaldehyde causes bleeding under the nails, discoloration of the nails, pain, and eventual loosening and loss of nails.

2. *Protect yourself against bacterial infection.* Creams, especially those found in facial cosmetics, are prolific breeding grounds for bacteria, especially in hot weather. Eyeliner and other eye makeup are especially vulnerable. Bacterial infections can include salmonella, staph, molds, and certain fungi. One particularly bad infection that results from bacteria in eye makeup can cause loss of sight within forty-eight hours if it invades the eyes.

Many cosmetics contain some preservatives that help prevent the growth of bacteria, but you need to take measures even with products that contain these preservatives. Wash your hands before you dip your fingers into a jar of cream or makeup. Don't leave jars sitting on your counter with the lids off; bacteria multiply rapidly in a warm climate. If the weather is really hot and humid, put your facial creams and other cleansers in the refrigerator; bacteria growth is severely retarded in a cool climate. One of the best protections you have is to keep your makeup and facial creams and cleansers to yourself. Letting other people use your cosmetics is a sure-fire way of spreading infection.

3. *Be careful with aerosol sprays.*[3] You can get quite ill from breathing aerosol fumes, and can cause serious respiratory damage. If you are using an aerosol product, make sure that the room is well-ventilated and that you have access to fresh air. If you are careless or inattentive when you spray your deodorant or hair spray, it might end up in your eyes or mouth. Aerosol contents are under extreme pressure. Never puncture an aerosol can, and don't expose one to temperatures higher than 120°; if you do either, the can is likely to explode and injure you. Finally, keep all aerosol products out of the reach of children.

4. *Pay attention to bad reactions to cosmetics.* Some cosmetic products are more likely than others to cause allergic reactions: deodorants, antiperspirants, depilatories, moisturizers, hair sprays, mascara, bubble bath, eye cream, hair dyes and tints, facial cream and cleanser, and nail polish.[4] These reactions are probably trying to tell you that you are allergic to the product. Listen to what your body is trying to tell you. If you experience visual damage when shampoo gets into your eyes, or if the shampoo causes scalp burns and hair loss, you're probably allergic to it. Watch out for swelling and rashes from any kind of cosmetic, especially underarm rashes. Change your eye makeup if you lose eyebrow and eyelash hair.

If you think you might be allergic to a cosmetic, perform a patch test. A rash, prickling, or burning indicates allergy. But the patch test isn't the final word: Some allergies don't show up in a patch test, or it's possible to build up sensitivity to a cosmetic you've used for a long time.[5]

Many companies offer products labeled "hypoallergenic." Before they can put the word "hypoallergenic" on their labels, manufacturers are required by the Food and Drug Administration to test their products and to prove that the drugs cause significantly fewer adverse reactions. So you can use these products with greater confidence.[6] Products that say "allergy tested" or "safe for sensitive skin" have also usually been tested and confirmed by the FDA.

5. *Read labels carefully, and follow the directions exactly.* Following directions is especially important when you are using antiperspirants, hair dyes and tints, home permanents, or hair remover for legs or face.

6. *If you get any kind of an adverse effect from a cosmetic (such as burning, breaking out, stinging, or itching), stop using it immediately.* If your reaction seems serious, call your doctor. He or she can help you identify the offending chemical and can let you know what other cosmetics contain it so you can avoid problems in the future.

7. *Also report adverse effects from a cosmetic to the manufacturer and to the local chapter of the FDA* (listed in your telephone directory under United States Government). You are doing other consumers a service by registering a complaint.

8. *Don't let children play with your cosmetics.* There are two reasons for this. First, you subject your cosmetics to bacterial infection: Children may not be careful with the cosmetics, may not wash their hands, or may use the cosmetics in conjunction with other substances (like cornstarch to gray hair), which might contaminate your cosmetics. Second, cosmetics aren't generally designed for the sensitive skin of children; many kids break out in a rash from your cosmetics.

9. *Be especially careful when you are using eye makeup.* You need a steady hand and an unrushed, calm application. It's easy to get hurried or startled and stick a mascara wand into your eye; careless application of eyeliner or eyeshadow can also injure your eyes.

13

dental hygiene

MOUTHWASHES

The American public yearly spends over $250 million on mouthwash products that promise to clean up breath, prevent sore throats, and make us attractive to the opposite sex.[1]

It's true: Our mouths are loaded with germs. But that's the way they're supposed to be. The thousands of species of flora and fauna in our mouths serve to aid in the digestion process, kill harmful bacteria, and do other good things for our bodies. Basically, mouthwashes are a joke. First of all, there is no way you could begin to kill even a fraction of the germs in your mouth with a few good gargles. Second, even if you did succeed in killing most of the germs, they'd be replaced when you took about five deep breaths or kissed a friend. Third—and most important—bad breath isn't a result of the germs in your mouth. So mouthwash that claims to kill germs really won't do a thing for your bad breath.

CAUSES OF BAD BREATH

What does cause bad breath? Bad breath is like indigestion—often a symptom of some other problem. The major culprit is poor dental hygiene—in other words, a failure to brush your teeth properly and completely. Bacteria can't cause bad breath unless it has food particles to act on, so instead of trying to kill the bacteria, it's a lot smarter and

161

easier to simply remove the food particles. Good brushing and flossing eliminates the problem. Bad breath can be caused by a number of other things, too; any of the following can contribute to or cause a mouth odor problem:

- mouth infection,

- gastric disorders,

- throat infection or disorder,

- canker sores in the mouth,

- decaying or abscessed tooth,

- diabetes,

- lung disease,

- liver disease, or

- strong-scented foods (garlic and onion, for example).

Obviously, mouthwash does nothing to cure or treat any of these causes. But not even onion or garlic? Won't mouthwash clean away the odor of garlic? The answer is no. The substance in garlic that causes the odor doesn't stay in your mouth: It is absorbed from your stomach into your bloodstream, where it circulates throughout your body, eventually reaching your lungs. And that garlic odor escapes with every breath of air you exhale. It would be ludicrous to believe that mouthwash could solve a problem that originates in the lungs! You really have only two recourses: Stop breathing entirely, or mask the odor temporarily until it can be worked out of your system. When you get right down to it, a stick of gum does a better job than mouthwash, and it lasts longer, too.

WHAT CAN YOU DO
TO FIGHT BAD BREATH?

Mouthwashes just don't cut it. You should try the following things if you are troubled by bad breath:

1. *Brush your teeth.* Do it after you eat and before you go to bed at night. Flossing helps, too. Keeping your mouth clean is the best way possible to fight bad breath.

2. *Pay attention to the condition of your gums and teeth.* If you notice the beginning of decay or gum disease, see your dentist immediately. It's always a good idea to have your teeth professionally cleaned on a regular basis.

162 dental hygiene

3. *See a doctor if you can't determine the source of your bad breath or if you have a sore throat or stomach upset that might be causing the problem.*

4. *Try chewing gum or parsley,* after you eat foods that might leave an offensive odor behind.

5. *If you need to gargle to soothe your mind,* try gargling with one-half teaspoon of salt in an eight-ounce glass of warm water.

MOUTHWASHES AND SORE THROATS

Mouthwashes that claim to kill germs have, over the past several years, claimed to cure or soothe a sore throat. Listerine was one of the most prominent, advertising effectiveness against winter colds and sore throats until the FDA made them admit that Listerine really has no such effect.

Why don't mouthwashes work on a sore throat? In the first place, most sore throats are caused by a virus, and viruses do not respond to either mouthwashes or antibiotic drugs. In fact, we haven't yet found a drug or medication that is effective against virus infection. Most sore throats that aren't caused by a virus are caused by bacterial infections, and the only way to fight them is to use an antibiotic drug, either taken orally or injected. And it is important that you determine the cause of your sore throat; a sore throat caused by a strep infection can lead to rheumatic fever if it is left untreated. You should see a doctor instead of trying to treat a sore throat with mouthwash.

Mouthwash manufacturers tell us that mouthwashes can at least soothe a sore throat because mouthwashes reduce the inflammation that accompanies sore throat. That claim is true: Most of them temporarily shrink swollen tissues that accompany sore throat. But the swelling tissues and the redness that accompany the swelling constitute the body's defense mechanism. It's the body's way of fighting the infection by rushing extra blood to the tissues, a process that speeds the body's healing processes. So by using mouthwashes and throat lozenges designed to soothe a sore throat, you are actually interfering with the body's ability to fight infection. In addition, a chemical found in many lozenges—benzocaine—is prone to cause an allergic reaction in many people.

The last straw is this: Most sore throats result from mucous membranes that are too dry. In fact, many colds are probably caused by mucous membranes that get too dry, which is why there are more colds in the winter than in the summer. Vigorous gargling with a strong mouthwash creates that condition: It dries up the mucous membranes in your mouth and throat, making them susceptible to invasion not only by bacteria but also by virus. Why? Most strong mouthwashes (those advertised to be most effective against bad breath) contain a significant amount of the drying agent, alcohol: Astring-O-Sol contains 70 percent, Dalidyne, 61 percent; Odara, 48 percent; Isodine Mouthwash/Gargle Concentrate, 35 percent; Oral Pentacresol, 30 percent; Listerine, 25 percent; Extra-Strength Micrin, 20 percent; Scope, 18.5 percent; Colgate 100, 15 percent; Cepacol, 15 percent; and Betadine Mouthwash/Gargle, 8.8 percent.

TOOTHPASTE

Tooth cleaners come in cream or powder form; powders are generally more abrasive than creams. Both forms of toothpaste contain abrasives, surface-acting agents, sweeteners, and flavoring.[2] Both are used with a toothbrush primarily to clean away food particles and the buildup of dental plaque from the teeth.

What about the toothpastes that promise to brighten your teeth and give you a whiter, brighter smile? Watch out—the brighteners aren't bleaching products, they're abrasives. You *can* heighten the brightness of teeth by polishing, but the most effective polishers on the market—Close-Up, Vote, Pearl Drops, and Macleans—are also the most abrasive. You can damage the enamel on your teeth by using toothpastes high in abrasives.

Some toothpastes—such as Thermodent and Sensodyne—advertise themselves as being suitable for people with sensitive gums and teeth. Neither Thermodent or Sensodyne, however, can stand up to those claims: Thermodent contains formaldehyde (which is dangerous to the sensitive tissues of the mouth and stomach), and Sensodyne is highly abrasive.

PLAQUE

Plaque, a buildup of bacteria on the teeth, is the main cause not only of periodontal disease but also of tooth caries among children. If they are left untreated, both periodontal disease and dental decay can result in the loss of teeth. Plaque forms all over the teeth, but most of it is removed by vigorous brushing. Some of it, however, can't be reached by a toothbrush—the plaque that forms between the teeth and near the gums. That's where flossing comes in.

You can test how well you are brushing your teeth by using a disclosing product, usually a tablet that you chew up and then swish around your mouth. Any plaque gets stained bright red, and you can see where the plaque forms and remains. You can use disclosing tablets in two ways. First, brush your teeth as you usually do; when you have finished, chew up a disclosing tablet, swish it around (making sure that you reach all the areas of your mouth), and spit out what remains of the tablet. You will have a vivid picture of your brushing skill; the places that you miss will be stained a bright red. Then try staining your teeth *before* you brush and floss: You'll get a good idea of what it takes to remove plaque. Try it a few times, until you get used to how much effort it takes to thoroughly clean your teeth.

WHAT ABOUT FLUORIDE?

Fluoride is definitely effective in fighting cavities and dental disease. It's most effective when included in the diet, by inclusion in water or some other means. It is less effective when applied directly to the teeth by a dentist or doctor. It is least effective—but still useful—when used as part of a fluoride toothpaste. Getting too much fluoride is impossible, so don't worry if your water is fluoridated. You can still benefit from topical applications and from toothpaste products that contain fluoride.

The only way to determine the effectiveness of a toothpaste is through clinical testing—the job of the American Dental Association. As of mid-1977, the only two toothpastes accepted by the American Dental Association as being effective in preventing tooth decay were Colgate MFP and Crest (both mint and regular flavors). Not as effective as Crest and Colgate—but still effective in helping to reduce dental disease—are A&P, Gleem II, Rexall, Safeway, and Worthmore.

HOW TO CHOOSE A TOOTHPASTE

For those under the age of twenty-five, Crest and Colgate MFP are the best choices because of their cavity-fighting properties. The child whose gums have started to recede prematurely should brush with a gentle toothpaste that is still effective against cavities; Worthmore is a good choice.

People over the age of twenty-five who have gum troubles, who use an electric toothbrush, or who have fixed plastic crowns should choose a gentle toothpaste that is near the top of the cavity-fighting ratings. Pepsodent or Craig-Martin are good choices. People over the age of twenty-five who brush manually, who have healthy teeth and gums, and who have no plastic bridgework can choose any brand of toothpaste that fulfills their personal needs. Since fluoride toothpastes prevent dental caries even among adults, however, a good choice would be Crest, Colgate MFP, or another fluoride toothpaste. Never use these conventional products on dentures (more fully discussed later in this section).

Toothbrushes come in all shapes, sizes, and colors. Some are electric—working with either an up-and-down or a back-and-forth movement—and others are designed to work with a little old-fashioned elbow grease.

ELECTRIC TOOTHBRUSHES

Electric toothbrushes make brushing your teeth more convenient, and they may prompt children to brush more often. In addition, they aid in the care of handicapped, ill people, or others who can't brush their own teeth. Some electric toothbrushes feature up-and-down movement of the brush, while others work from side to side. Both are effective, if used as directed, so the choice is yours. No electric toothbrush, though, can duplicate manual brushing. Other considerations include the convenience of the stand, location of the off-on switch, ease of cleaning, ease of brush replacement, styles and colors of brushes available, and power source. (Those who travel or camp a lot might prefer a toothbrush that operates on rechargeable batteries, as opposed to one that plugs in.) These are all factors influenced by your personal needs and desires.

The American Dental Association's Council on Dental Materials and Devices has approved five brands of electric toothbrushes, based on studies evaluating their effectiveness of cleaning, their safety from electric shock, and their freedom from harm to hard and soft oral tissues. Accepted and approved electric toothbrushes include Broxodent, General Electric, J.C. Penny Dual, Sunbeam Cordless Hygenic, and Water Pik Tough-Tronic. If you decide to use an electric toothbrush, choose from one of these brands.

MANUAL TOOTHBRUSHES

The kind of manual tooth brush you use depends on many considerations. Your dexterity and brushing method are two. The size of your mouth is another; certainly, you wouldn't choose a large brush for a small mouth. The flexibility of the bristles is important too, although the designations on toothbrushes are often unreliable. The designations "extra-hard," "hard," "medium," "soft," and "extra-soft" bear no relation to any universal standard. "Hard" by one manufacturer might be "extra-hard" or "medium" to another. Nonetheless, the sensitivity of your mouth is a consideration. A sharp angled brush can injure the delicate structures of your mouth.[3] In general, dentists advise patients to stay away from "extra-hard" and "hard" bristles. Too inflexible, they don't reach below the gum margin to clean away plaque and food particles. They can also actually damage gums. Comparing synthetic and natural bristles, the synthetic types seem to have the edge because they wear longer.

PROPER BRUSHING PROCEDURE

You may use any freestyle stroke that is comfortable, but you shouldn't use vigorous back-and-forth motions. Circular motions and short back-and-forth motions are best for cleaning plaque from the teeth.

Actually, the specific brushing method isn't nearly as important as the thoroughness of brushing. Work your way from one side of your mouth to the other, on both the top row of teeth and the bottom. When you finish, rinse well with cool, clear water. After you have rinsed all the residue from your mouth, brush your tongue. Use gentle motions to lightly cleanse the tongue of plaque buildup and any food particles. Use your toothpaste. Make sure that you don't scratch the tongue or harm it by brushing too briskly or by applying too much pressure. When you have finished brushing your tongue, rinse your mouth well again using clear, cool water. You may want to further discourage plaque growth by rinsing your mouth with a solution of warm water and baking soda.

DENTAL FLOSS

Since toothbrush bristles don't reach all the places in your mouth that can serve as hiding places for plaque, floss is available in four different forms, all considered equally effective in cleaning the teeth:

- *Unwaxed floss*, the most widely used type, cleans thoroughly in most cases.

- *Extra fine unwaxed floss* is a softer, thinner floss that spreads to provide a broad cleaning tool for the experienced flosser.

- *Waxed floss*, lubricated with wax, is easier for a beginner to use. The wax lubrication makes the floss slip easily between the teeth.

- *Tape floss* is flat, ribbon-like floss that is ideal for cleaning widely spaced teeth.

Your choice of the type of floss depends on which works best for you. Take into consideration the amount of experience you have had, the structure of your teeth (close together or spaced widely), and your personal likes and dislikes. If you are awkward at flossing techniques or if you don't want to put your fingers into your mouth, you can get a mechanical device that stretches a section of floss between two curved prongs. Threaders on these mechanical devices help you guide the floss under fixed dental bridgework.

HOW TO FLOSS
Follow this procedure for the most effective flossing:

1. Break off a piece of floss about eighteen inches long.

2. Wind each end of the floss two or three times around the middle finger on each hand. If you are just beginning or have trouble manipulating the floss in the traditional way, try tying it in a loop and holding the loop between your two middle fingers. You should have about two inches of floss between your hands.

3. Hold the floss taut. Use your thumbs and forefingers to guide the floss gently between your teeth.

4. Keep the floss pressed against the surface of your tooth as you move it back and forth and toward the gum. Slide the floss just below the gum margin.

5. Use a straight up-and-down cleaning motion to get rid of plaque that has settled between your teeth.

6. When the floss gets soiled, move to a new section until you have finished flossing all your teeth. Make sure that you get the area behind your back molars, too.

Never snap floss sharply or force it between teeth; you can cut your gums if you aren't careful.

DENTAL IRRIGATORS

Dental irrigators, devices that spray high-pressure streams of water aimed at dislodging food particles and stimulating gums, should be used to supplement regular dental care with a toothbrush and dental floss. They do not replace regular dental care.

In choosing a dental irrigator, you should pick from the brands recommended by the American Dental Association. The Association has approved several models on the basis of safety: Hydro Dent (manufactured by Hydro Manufacturing Company), Pulsar (McKesson and Robbins), and Dento Spray (Texell Products Company). Additional factors to consider are price, space required, provision for wall mounting, safety when immersed, ease of calibrating pressure, availability of rechargeable power sources, convenience of the off-on switch, and ease of changing tips.

Dental irrigators are good for some people, not for others. They should *not* be used by people who have periodontal disease, because the pressurized spray might force debris into pyorrhea pockets or under gum flaps. Others who should not use dental irrigators include those with bacterial infections of the mouth; bacteria can be forced into the bloodstream. Anyone with the tendency to bleeding gums, diabetes, or chronic heart disease should stay away from irrigators also. Dental irrigators *are* helpful for people who wear orthodontic appliances, because they help dislodge food particles that are difficult to reach with conventional brushing.

TOPICAL PAIN-KILLERS

The use of any topical pain-killer to ease toothache or some other painful problem in the mouth should be strictly temporary. In fact, you should use them only after you have called a dentist and are waiting for your appointment. Topical pain-killers should never be used as the sole treatment for a toothache; they can relieve the pain, but they do not heal the source of the problem. Any toothache that goes away by itself is a probable trouble spot: In most cases some destruction of the pulp has resulted in easing the pain.

Read the labels of products that work temporarily to ease toothache or mouth pain. The safest are the ones that contain benzocaine, lidocaine, and chlorobutanol. The most effective forms are the ointments, because they contain enough concentration of the medication to be effective in relieving pain. Other topical analgesics sometimes used can be dangerous and can worsen the problem instead of solving it. They include:

- *Oil of cloves:* The oil is extremely irritating, so you must be careful not to let it touch your gums or the mucous membranes of your mouth. To use it most effectively, dip a pledget of cotton into the oil, and use tweezers to place the pledget directly into the cavity.

- *Aspirin:* Never chew aspirin or place it on a sore tooth in an effort to ease the pain. Aspirin is *not* designed to be a topical pain-killer; it causes ulcers and severe burns in the mucous membranes of the mouth.

• *Teething lotions:* Researchers generally believe that teething lotions are ineffective, due to the fact that they do not penetrate deep enough into the gums to relieve the source of pain.

COLD SORES AND CANKERS
Special topical pain-killers should be used if you develop cankers or cold sores. The best medications to use are Orabase and Compound Tincture of Benzoin. Coat the lesions completely with the medications, and follow label directions carefully.

1. *Cankers* are shallow ulcers in the mucous membrane of the mouth. They generally have fairly even borders, and they are surrounded by redness and swelling of tissue. Most are extremely sensitive and painful. We don't know what causes cankers, but they seem to be aggravated by chocolate, nuts, citrus fruits, and other irritants taken into the mouth. Healing usually occurs spontaneously in three weeks and sometimes after one week. Treatment doesn't seem to shorten the length of the disease, but it can help to relieve the pain and discomfort associated with it.

2. *Cold sores* are acute viral infections that can be provoked by stress, exposure to the sun or wind, nervousness, minor infections, or fever. A cold sore usually lasts from one to three weeks, and it is normal and common for a cold sore to recur in the same location. Again, treatment does not seem to shorten the duration of the disease, but it can help to ease the pain.

SIGNS OF SOMETHING SERIOUS
Everyone gets a cold sore or canker once in a while, but you should be wary if yours does not go away within three weeks. It could be a sign of something that requires medical attention. Specifically, you should be aware of the signs of oral cancer so that you can call your doctor if you begin to have problems:

> • a sore on the lip or in the mouth that does not heal (the normal healing time for a canker or cold sore ranges from one to three weeks);
>
> • continued bleeding of the tissues in your mouth;
>
> • red spots or white patches in your mouth;
>
> • numbness or pain of tissues in your mouth; and
>
> • swelling that includes your palate or some other oral structure.

DENTURE CLEANSERS AND RELINERS

One of the most important factors in ensuring denture cleanliness is the use of a denture brush. Brushes should be larger than a normal toothbrush and conform to the shape of the dentures.

The type of cleanser, however, is also very important. Abrasive toothpaste, especially for dentures, should be used because regular toothpastes can etch the surface of dentures. Denture cleansers that claim to "foam away" stains and food particles without the use of a denture brush are pursuing the impossible. And the bubbling blue solutions that turn white supposedly when your dentures are clean aren't valid either. American Dental Association researchers point out that the color used in the tablets fade after a certain length of time has elapsed, whether or not the dentures are clean. One of the best solutions you can use to clean your dentures is simple Clorox, diluted in water. The taste may be difficult for you to tolerate, so you may want to make sure you rinse your dentures well after cleaning them with Clorox. Since Clorox damages metal, don't clean your dentures in a metal container of any kind.

If your dentures are going to be out of your mouth for a substantial length of time, store them in water. Water prevents warping, as well as the buildup of deposits on your dentures.

Reliners, denture pads, and other devices that cushion the dentures are frequently purchased in pharmacies by people who are dissatisfied with the way their dentures fit. Your dentist should be the only one to repair and readjust your dentures. The continued use of pads and reliners can cause bone damage and ruin the normal tissue structure that you rely on for a foundation.

14

skin care

The most commonly used cosmetic is soap, and the average American uses about 3.5 pounds of soap each year.[1] The basic ingredients of most soaps haven't changed for years: Most are still made from fat and lye. Soap works by using water to create suds that loosen and remove body soil, grime, body secretions, dead cells, bacteria and fungus, cosmetics, toiletries, and any medicine that you've applied to your skin.

There are two different kinds of soap: real and synthetic (usually called "detergent"). *Real* soap forms when lye (or other alkali) reacts with animal fat. *Detergents* are chemical combinations made from a number of synthetic materials. Detergents are generally a little milder than real soap, and they don't leave scum behind when used in hard water.

The most important consideration in choosing a soap is your skin type. There are all kinds of soaps on the market that are tailored for oily skin, dry skin, normal skin, and sensitive skin. You should take your age and occupation into consideration, too. A mechanic needs a soap that cuts through grease and oil; an elderly man needs one that is mild and that moisturizes aged, parched skin. A teenager who is fighting acne should choose an antiseptic soap. People over twenty-nine usually need a soap that contains some type of oil to moisturize the skin following cleansing. Take the weather and humidity conditions into consideration when you use your soap. In the summer, you need to cleanse carefully and daily to remove perspiration; perspiration contains salt, which can be irritating to your skin and which can plug up pores. In the winter, or when humidity is low and rooms are overheated, you should bathe more carefully to prevent removing too much of the outer skin layer—a condition that leads to chafing. Soaps that contain oils are good in cold climates and in climates with low humidity.

FORMS OF SOAP

Toilet Soap

Designed for all purposes, toilet soap is the most widely used variety of soap. It differs from plain old lye and fat soap by the ingredients that are added and whipped into it: all kinds of perfumes, colors, and deodorants.[2] Other ingredients include oils, moisturizers, or creams.

How effective are these ingredients? Least effective are the perfumes. A soap that may scent up your whole bathroom, as it sits innocently in the soap dish, probably won't leave enough scent on your skin to last until you get dressed. The deodorants in soaps are really not deodorants; most soaps that claim to be deodorant soaps contain only cover-up perfume. The best bet against body odor is still a thorough cleansing, and plain soap does that as well as any other. Few soaps on the market contain actual antibacterial agents that work as deodorants; this absence is due largely to the fact that the leading antibacterial agent, hexachlorophene, was removed from the market in the mid-1970s as a possible carcinogen.

You can get soap in just about any size; there are no standards of soap size regulating manufacturers. Commonly used bath soaps weigh anywhere from 2.2 ounces to 9.5 ounces—with 17 sizes in between! With so many different sizes, it's hard to compare prices, unless you compare a per-ounce price—which, by the way, ranges anywhere from 4 cents to $1.25.

According to *Consumer Reports*, there are some real differences among the brands of toilet soaps. The differences occur in the following major areas.

Lathering. Most of the toilet soaps on the market lather quite easily. Zest lathers best in hard water, and it produces the most lather from the least amount of soap. Lather is pretty hard to work up in hard water with Neutrogena, Safeguard, White King Lemon, and Truly Fine. Since lather is what cleans, you should keep the condition of your water in mind when you buy soap.

Shrinkage. All soaps shrink, of course, but some shrink much more than others in proportion to the amount of lather they produce. During a long shower or bath, soaps that shrink a lot are likely to clean only a little.

Soaps that tend to shrink less than normal include Lux, Caress, Dove, Phase III, Avon, Bronnley, Roger and Gallet, and Etherea. These soaps last longer and clean more per ounce than the soaps that are notorious for shrinkage: Kirk's Original Coco Hard-Water Castile, White King Lemon, and Neutrogena. Chanel No. 5 is one of the worst.

Apparently, shrinkage is somehow related to *shape*, which can also affect your ability to hang on to the soap. A sculptured bar, like Tone, is easy to hang onto. The number of times you have to retrieve your soap from the bath water obviously affects shrinkage! Shape determines how well your soap lasts in another way, too: Bars that are convex or concave allow air to circulate around it when you put it in the soap dish; so less goo forms on the soap bar. It lasts longer than a flat bar that gets all gooey and can't dry out after you use it.

Packaging. This fact has a big effect on the soap's price and on its attractiveness. But remember, attractive packaging doesn't get (or keep) you clean. You should decide what your best buy is, and you should probably steer clear of fancy packages. Soaps come packaged from the simple to the sublime: A&P Deodorant Bath and Beauty Soap consists simply of four to six naked soap bars in a plastic bag, and it costs 4 cents an ounce. Dial, at 6 cents an ounce, is in an individual paper wrapper. And for 7 cents an ounce, you can get Irish Spring in a cardboard box. Then there's the other end of the spectrum: For $1.25 an ounce (a whopping $7.50 a bar), you can get Etherea, which is wrapped in plastic and then set into a plastic soap dish with its own lid. The dish is covered with corrugated paper and placed into a cardboard box—which is then sealed.

Harshness. Real soaps sometimes contain too much lye for sensitive skins. You are the best judge of which soap is mild enough for you. Take the other factors (shape, shrinkage, lathering, and packaging) into consideration as you find a soap that is mild enough for your use.

Cost. Your best bet is to find the soap that cleans you at the lowest possible cost. After you take the other factors into consideration, keep these prices in mind:

- Soaps available for 4 to 5 cents an ounce include A&P Deodorant

Soap, Cashmere Bouquet, Ivory, Jergens, Nature Scents, Sweetheart Lime, Truly Fine, White King, and Woodbury.

• Soaps costing 6 to 7 cents an ounce include Camay, Dial, Irish Spring, Jergens Deodorant, Kirk's, Lifebuoy, Lux, Palmolive, Palmolive Deodorant, Safeguard, White King Lemon, and Zest.

• For 8 to 9 cents an ounce you can get Caress, Dove, Phase III, and Tone.

• Soaps selling for 10 to 50 cents an ounce include Yardley Oatmeal, Yardley Old English (lavender and herbal), Clairol Herbal Essence soap, Brut 33, Pears Natural Transparent Soap, Neutrogena, Avon Skin-So-Soft, Bronnley, Feminique Cocoa Butter, Roger and Gallet Savons, and Helena Rubenstein Skin Dew soap.

• The most expensive toilet soaps—selling for prices from 50 cents to $1.25 an ounce—include Germaine Perfume soap, Chanel No. 5 hand soap, and Etherea.

Superfatted Soap
Superfatted soaps act to moisturize by leaving a thin film of oil on your skin.[3] Most contain fine oils, cold cream, or lanolin, and they're a good bet if your skin suffers from dryness and scaling. They're especially good to use in the winter. Dove, Camay, Oilatum, and Basis are good examples of superfatted soap.

Deodorant Soap
Deodorant soaps claim to keep you odor-free by killing bacteria on your skin.[4] How well they work depends on what they contain. To be both safe and effective, soaps should contain germ-killing agents that kill the odor-causing germs without killing the other germs and bacteria that you need to maintain a healthy balance. Very few soaps on the market do what they claim.

Multi-Milled (French) Soap
This soap gets its name from the way it is processed and generally retains its scent to the last sliver. Yardley and Chanel are two.

White Floating Soap
These soaps—of which the best-known is Ivory—are good all-purpose cleaners. Why do they float? They are churned and impregnated with air, which makes them buoyant. The buoyancy doesn't improve cleaning effectiveness, but it can help you locate your soap easier if you drop it into the bath water.

Antiseptic (Medicated) Soap
Antiseptic, medicated soaps should be chosen by those who suffer from acne. Fostex is one of the best-known. Read the labels of these soaps: The most effective ingredients are benzalkonium chloride, benzethonium chloride, hexylresorcinol, and methylbenzethonium. Others have not generally been proven to be safe and/or effective.[5]

Transparent Soap
Transparent soaps are processed with only the purest fats and oils, so they are the most gentle soaps available on the market. Pear's and Neutrogena are two of the most widely available.

Heavy-Duty Cleansing Soap
Processed with pumice or other ingredients that work especially well in digging out grit and grease, heavy-duty cleansing soaps (like Lava and Fels Naptha) are abrasive and shouldn't be used by people with sensitive skin.

Being aware of all of these factors, you can choose the soap that best suits your needs.

MAKEUP

"She's lovely, she's engaged, she uses Ponds"—this was once one of the best-known advertising slogans in America.[6] Advertisers and cosmetic manufacturers continue to lure us with all kinds of promises of ravishing beauty and a changed lifestyle—if only we smear on their magic potions, contained in an array of tiny jars, tubes, and compacts. Many of us use cosmetics every day, but few of us understand exactly what is in our mascara, lipstick, and eye shadow.[7]

FORMS OF MAKEUP
Cold Cream and Other Cleansing Creams
Creams are used by women to remove makeup from the skin. Although soap and water generally do the same job, cold cream or a cleansing cream does it without drying out the skin and leaving it taut. Most have a softening effect on the skin that affords greater protection for dry skin. Most contain ingredients like beeswax, borax, mineral oil, and water. The beeswax works with the borax to keep the oil and the water together. Instead of beeswax and borax, some creams use either glyceryl stearate and woolwax alcohol or a chemical called sorbitan sesquioleate to keep the mineral oil and water from separating.

Lipstick

Nothing but oil, wax, artificial coloring, and perfume, most lipsticks are about 50 percent oil—usually castor oil—with enough wax added (generally beeswax, carnuba, or candelilla) to form a stick. Color additives must be approved by the FDA, and the additives tested for both purity and safety. Staining dyes, used years ago to produce bright red and vivid bluish-red lipsticks, are rarely used in today's lipsticks. Most of the dyes used today are derivations of bromo dyes; and, since each dye has its own peculiar qualities, two tubes of lipstick that look the same color in the tube can produce two very different colors on the lips. Guanine crystals, bismuth oxychloride, and mica coated with titanium dioxide are used to give lipsticks a lustrous pearly or glossy quality. Perfumes are also added, mainly to cover any fatty odor that might result from the castor oil. Antioxidants are used to prevent the development of unpleasant odors that can result when oils and waxes are combined.

Eye Shadow

Eye shadow comes in a rainbow of colors and can be purchased in powder, paste, or cream form. Many of the color additives that have been approved for other makeups by the FDA are not approved for use in eye shadow and in other eye makeup (such as eyeliner and mascara). The regulations are stricter for eye makeup because of the sensitivity of the eye area. With only a few exceptions, colors used in eye makeup have to be inorganic pigments. The main ones are ultramarines, iron and chromium oxide pigments, and carmine N. F. (made from the dried bodies of certain female scale insects). Ingredients in the paste and cream shadows include petroleum, lanolin, ceresin, carnauba wax, beeswax, stearic acid, isopropyl myristate, propylene glycol, gum tragacanth, water, and methyl cellulose. Most contain preservatives, additional ingredients to give a "pearly" look, and perfumes (based on natural oils and aromatic chemicals) to combat odor from the natural chemical ingredients.

HYPOALLERGENIC MAKEUP

The label on a jar of cream you're considering might boast that the contents are "hypoallergenic." A jar right next to it is labeled "allergy-tested." Still another on the same shelf says that it is "safe for sensitive skin." Still another says it is "less irritating." Which one should you buy? Is there any difference from one to another?

Not really. Products labeled "hypoallergenic," "less irritating," "safe for sensitive skin," or "allergy-tested" are products that are *less likely* to cause an adverse reaction among most people. The simple fact remains that it is impossible to create a cosmetic that does not adversely affect someone somewhere. A "hypoallergenic" cosmetic doesn't guarantee you won't have an allergic reaction; it just lessens your chances.[8]

Despite claims on the label, you should still perform a patch test of your own before using any cosmetic. Each person reacts differently to each chemical substance, and the only way you can determine your reaction is to test the substance yourself on your own skin.

USING MAKEUP SAFELY

You can guarantee the best results from your makeup if you follow these guidelines:

1. *Store your makeup in a cool, dark place, away from heat and sunshine.* This sort of storage increases their shelf life and prevents adverse reactions among the chemicals contained in the makeup.

2. *Wash your hands before you use your makeup.* Many times you can unthinkingly contaminate your makeup simply by using it before you wash your hands. Creams and cream-based makeups are marvelous breeding grounds for bacteria, especially in warm weather. Keep your makeup brushes and applicators clean, too.

3. *Don't pass your makeup around.* You can avoid serious infection (especially from contaminated eye makeup) if you keep your makeup to yourself and if you refuse to use someone else's makeup.

4. *Read the label and the directions for use carefully, and follow the directions.* Most labels list cautions that should be exercised and side effects that you should watch for. If you develop any of the side effects listed on the label, or if you develop redness, irritation, blistering, or a rash of any kind, discontinue use. If the redness or rash is severe, you should check with your doctor, who can help you isolate what caused the irritation so that you can avoid it in other products.

5. *Report your dissatisfaction to your local division of the FDA.* If you are unhappy with a cosmetic, or if you think it is unsafe for use because of some adverse reaction you developed, you protect other innocent consumers if you report it and complain.

DEODORANTS AND ANTIPERSPIRANTS

Everyone in the world perspires. Sweat is important: It helps us maintain our correct body temperature, and it helps wash waste products from our system. Most of us, under normal conditions, produce about one-half of a quart of sweat every day.[9] Sometimes we perspire more profusely than at other times. For instance, when we are under stress or tension of some kind or when we exercise heavily, we step up our production of sweat.

Not all perspiration produces an odor; in fact, only when it interacts with bacteria on the skin surface does it produce that telltale body odor. Whether perspiration takes on an offensive odor also depends on which gland secretes it.[10] *Eccrine* glands—located on the forehead, hands, soles of the feet, and in the armpits—excrete perspiration that is about 90 percent water and 10 percent salt. They respond to the body's normal cooling-down mechanism, and perspiration produced from these glands generally does not produce unpleasant body odor. The *apocrine* glands, however, found in the armpits and in some other areas of the body, become active and continue through old age. These secrete perspiration in response to tension, stress, emotional excitement, and emotional upset, and they are the culprits when it comes to offensive body odor. Perspiration from these glands mixes with bacteria on the skin's surface, and the result prompts us to be religious followers of the deodorant commercials on television and in the magazines.

PRODUCT TYPES
Two basic products control odor and wetness, and they work in different ways:[11]

Deodorants. Although they do *not* stop or control underarm wetness, deodorants do stop odor by controlling the bacteria on the skin's surface. In addition, most of them contain a perfume ingredient that masks odor. You can buy deodorants in sticks, presoaked pads, roll-ons, aerosol sprays, nonaerosol sprays, and creams. Most deodorants contain talc, perfumes, and an antibacterial agent such as kaolin, zinc oxide, or zinc stearate.[12] Remember, deodorants don't control wetness; you probably won't have an odor problem, but you *will* have wet armpits and stained clothing.

Antiperspirants. These work by diminishing wetness, and some can reduce perspiration by as much as 50 percent. They contain an ingredient to temporarily close the pore openings of the sweat glands— usually aluminum salts—and an antibacterial agent to check the spread and growth of bacteria on the skin's surface. Antiperspirants come in aerosol and nonaerosol sprays, creams, roll-ons, and presoaked pads.

CHOOSING A SAFE PRODUCT
As with all other cosmetics, some deodorants and antiperspirants are better for you than others. These guidelines help you stay away from dangerous or unsafe products and choose those that are safe and effective.[13]

1. *Don't use aerosol sprays.* They are bad for your lungs, especially if you use them in a closed room (like the bathroom, where most people apply their deodorant). It's better to use a presoaked pad, nonaerosol spray, solid stick, cream, or roll-on.

2. *Avoid using deodorants or antiperspirants that contain the antibiotic neomycin.* It has a tendency to sensitize the skin and produce allergic reactions, although some people can use it safely. Two deodorant products that contain neomycin are Hi and Dri and Top Brass.

3. *Avoid using products that contain zirconium,* a chemical that can cause inflammation and small benign growths on the skin. Secret, Secret Antiperspirant, and Sure Super Dry all contain zirconium. Because of its adverse reactions, few deodorant manufacturers use zirconium anymore.

4. Avoid deodorants that contain benzalkonium chloride. It causes skin irritation. But there's something worse: They become deactivated if you use them after you've washed under your arms, because they interact and neutralize when they come into contact with soapy residue left behind after showering or bathing. Products containing benzalkonium chloride include Clear Formula roll-on, Dainty Dry roll-on, and Mennen's Spray Deodorant. 5-Day pads and roll-on contain methylbenzethonium chloride, which reacts the same way with soapy residue.

5. *Avoid products that contain aluminum chloride or aluminum sulfate.* They become acidic when they contact water or sweat, and they are prone to cause redness, burning, and irritation. Even if you don't develop a rash, products containing this chemical can cause the fabric in your clothing to rot. Some of the products to steer clear of include Arrid Roll-on, Ever Dry cream, Fresh stick, and Super-Dry cream.

The most effective chemical contained in deodorants and antiperspirants is aluminum hydroxychloride; some of the products that contain it (and none of the culprits mentioned above) include: Allercreme, Aquamarine, Arrid Extra Dry aerosol or powder, Ban, Calm, Chantilly, Desert Flower, Dial roll-on or aerosol, Hour After Hour Antiperspirant, Manpower Super Dry, Right Guard Antiperspirant, and Dorothy Gray's Roll-On.

PRECAUTIONS
The way you use your antiperspirant or deodorant spells the difference between a happy, trouble-free experience and an irritated, sensitive pair of armpits. Follow these suggestions:[14]

180 skin care

1. *Don't apply an antiperspirant or deodorant right after you've shaved under your arms.* Post-shaving nicks and cuts can become inflamed and infected if you use deodorant. Even if you can't see any nicks, shaving with a safety razor has a mild abrasive effect on the skin. The best thing to do is to shave at night before you go to bed and then apply your antiperspirant in the morning.

2. *If you don't shave under your arms, make especially sure that the armpit area is clean.* Hair attracts bacteria and perspiration that can worsen your odor problem. Men who have a particularly stubborn problem with underarm odor should consider shaving under their arms.

3. *Use the same amount of antiperspirant year-round.* You perspire as much in the winter as you do in the summer.

4. *Switch to a different product if you notice a rash or stinging and burning after putting on your deodorant.* Deodorants and antiperspirants are especially prone to cause a rash or irritation.

5. *If use an aerosol, avoid inhaling the fumes.* If possible, use the aerosol in a room that has plenty of ventilation.

Remember, the best technique against body odor is clean skin. Never apply a deodorant or antiperspirant to skin that has not been washed; all you are doing is masking the real problem. If you let the odor go on long enough, even the best product won't be able to conquer it. Soap and water should always precede your deodorant or antiperspirant in your efforts to smell sweet and clean.

15

acne

No other complaint is as prevalent among adolescents as acne. At least two-thirds of all American teenagers between the ages of twelve and seventeen are afflicted with acne lesions. Most of them rely for treatment on over-the-counter drugs, which cannot cure acne, but which can reduce the symptoms.[1]

WHAT IS ACNE?

Acne, a common skin disease, can range anywhere from a mild, occasional blemish to severe formation of pustules that lead to scarring and disfigurement.[2] Sebaceous glands located under the surface of the skin are responsible for secreting *sebum*, a substance that all of us have but that we are still confused about. The theory is that free fatty acids are the main irritators in sebum. We don't really know what its function is, and we don't know how it is regulated. Some researchers believe that the increased production of hormones—especially testosterone—is responsible for the increased output of sebum, but further tests need to be conducted.

The acne lesion—called a *comedo*—is a sac-like structure that develops within the sebaceous gland follicle, usually along a hair follicle. The comedo is filled with masses of dead skin cells, lipids from the sebaceous glands, and colonies of bacteria. A comedo can be "open" or "closed":

182

1. An *open comedo* (a *blackhead*) is formed when the masses of flat, scaly, dead tissue work their way to the skin surface, dilate the follicle opening, and plug the pore. The sebum, combined with the other materials in the sac, turns black when it is exposed to air due to an oxidization process. The oily skin surrounding the lesion then attracts additional dirt and debris to the blackhead, which further hardens and plugs the follicle opening.

2. A *closed comedo (whitehead)* forms similarly to the open comedo, but the follicle opening is not dilated. Pressure that builds up from the bacterial action causes the whitehead to become raised above the skin surface.

The increased pressure under the skin's surface and the increased bacterial action that accompany whiteheads can enlarge the follicle. The follicle becomes inflamed, and the surrounding skin becomes swollen and tender. The lesions usually become filled with pus. The continued buildup of pressure can eventually lead to a rupture of the walls of the sebaceous duct; the sebum then spills beneath the skin. The surrounding tissue reacts by containing the infected material in a sac-like pocket called a *cyst*, which becomes hard and tender. Untreated or improperly treated, a cyst can lead to residual scarring and cellular destruction. At the same time the cyst is forming beneath the skin's surface, pus-filled infectious lesions form around the involved follicle on the skin's surface; these lesions are generally multiple.

WHAT CAUSES ACNE?

We aren't really sure exactly what *causes* acne, but we do know some of the things that may contribute to its severity:[3]

1. *Hormone production seems to be related to the activity of the sebaceous glands,* which in turn produce excess sebum that acts to clog pores. Androgens (or male hormones) seem to be the ones most closely related to producing acne. They increase the size of sebaceous glands and increase the secretion of sebum. Although these androgens are secreted by females in small quantities, females seem to have their worst acne problems right before their menstrual periods when their hormones are temporarily imbalanced.

2. *Heredity plays a part.* If one or both of your parents suffered from severe acne, the chances of your developing a bad case of acne are all the greater. In cases where acne is an inherited condition, it can't be cured—but it can be controlled.

3. *The cause of diet in relation to acne is a controversial issue.* We do know that the sebaceous glands are influenced by the kinds and amounts of food we eat daily, but we are not sure what that influence is. If you *already* have acne, chocolate, cola drinks, butter, milk, cheese, pork, French fries, potato chips, nuts, peanut butter, and foods you are allergic to can aggravate the acne and make it worse. Iodized salt and shellfish can also make an existing case of acne worse.

Although these foods possibly make acne worse, we are not sure that any of them *cause* acne to begin with. Proper nutrition is important, and you should not compromise getting proper and essential nutritional elements in your diet because you are afraid of causing or aggravating acne.

4. *Certain medications can aggravate acne.* Bromides—a common ingredient in many antacids—can make acne worse, as can medicine that contains iodides.

5. *Constipation can aggravate or possibly cause outbreaks of acne,* because it prevents wastes from being removed from the body on a regular basis.

6. *Emotional stress and tension can greatly aggravate acne.* The psychological stress and pressure encountered during adolescence, as teenagers try to adjust to new roles and demands, is probably a main cause of acne.

7. *The way you treat your pimples determines to a large extent whether they go away or spread.* Squeezing or picking pimples can spread the infection—leading to new lesions—and can result in scarring and disfigurement. Keep your hands away from your pimples. You hands are marvelous breeding grounds for bacteria, and they are bound to worsen any acne lesions.

8. *Environmental pollution can aggravate acne,* due to all the dirt and grease in the air.

9. *Acne can be caused by infrequent bathing.* Oils, bacteria, and dirt remain on the skin and produce both open and closed comedos. Related to this is frequent and prolonged sweating, which brings increased oils and dirt to the surface of the skin. Greasy hair oils also add to the oily condition of the skin and cause a type of acne known as "pomade acne."[4]

10. *Local irritation (such as wearing a football helmet strap or supporting the head with the hands) can cause acne or make it worse.* If you

184 acne

have a pimple that ruptures, protect it from further infection by applying an antiseptic and by keeping your hands away from it.

OVER-THE-COUNTER ACNE MEDICATION

Acne, left untreated, can cause increased infection, inflammation, permanent pitting, and scarring. So treat it you must.[5] Unfortunately, of the more than 150 over-the-counter preparations that are supposed to heal acne, few of them, when tested scientifically, do any good at all. Their ineffectiveness results in the waste of over $35 million each year, spent on over-the-counter preparations to clear up troubled skin. Actually, the aim of most acne medication is not to make blemishes less conspicuous, but to prevent scarring.

How can you tell which over-the-counter medications are effective? It's easy: Read the labels. The ingredient that has been found effective against acne is *benzoyl peroxide,* which works by drying and peeling the skin. Preparations containing benzoyl peroxide increase the growth of skin cells so that old skin is continually sloughed off. Some of the medications that contain it include Benoxyl, Loroxide, PanOxyl, Persadox, and Vanoxide. These preparations are pretty much equal in their acne-fighting abilities, so choose the one that is available in your area and that is the least expensive.

SAFETY MEASURES
With the goal of drying out the old pimples and preventing new ones from forming, you do need to take some precautions in using one of these preparations:

1. *Never apply it to your face while your skin is wet.* If you have recently washed your face, dry it thoroughly and wait thirty minutes until the skin has had a chance to dry out completely.

2. *Keep the medication away from sensitive skin.* Take extra care not to get the preparation near or in your eyes or near the sensitive facial tissue around your nose and around the corners of your mouth.

3. *Start the treatment slowly, and proceed with it gradually.* Medications containing benzoyl peroxide dry the skin and can cause redness and scaling; so you need to gauge how your own skin will react. Start by putting a thin layer on one small area on one side of your face. (Don't apply acne medication too vigorously because it is an irritant.) Repeat the application once a day for a few days. You should experience a mild redness and some irritation; but if the redness, scaling, or irritation is

severe, you are probably allergic to something in the medication and you should discontinue use. If the redness and irritation are only mild, extend application to the entire side of your face. Repeat those applications once a day for several more days; if you react well, extend the application to cover your entire face and other affected areas.

If you seem to tolerate the medication well, you can apply it more than once each day, but never apply it more often than three times a day. Don't stop using it when your skin gets dry—that's the whole idea!

Over-the-counter acne preparations that do not contain benzoyl peroxide are generally weak and usually have no effect on relieving the acne symptoms. PropaPH, Pro-Blem, Sebacide, Stri-Dex Medicated Pads, Tackle, Teenac, Therapads, and Ting are several of the brands that have been found to be ineffective against acne.

A Caution for People with Black Skin

Resorcinol, a chemical found in a number of over-the-counter medications for acne, causes discoloration and pigment changes in black skin.[6] If you are black, do not use Acne, Acne Aid, Acne-Dome, Acnomel, Acnycin, Bensulfoid, Cenac, Clearasil, Contrablem, Komed, Microsyn, Phisoac, Resulin, Rezamid, or Tackle.

PRESCRIPTION ACNE PREPARATIONS

If your acne is severe and if you decide to seek medical care from a doctor or dermatologist, you will probably get a prescription for any of a number of drugs and ointments used in the treatment of acne.[7] Common ones include the following.

TETRACYCLINE

Tetracycline works to control bacterial colonies that aggravate and worsen acne. Used in low dosages over a period of weeks or months, this antibiotic is usually prescribed in a full dose for about three weeks and then gradually tapered to about one-quarter of full dosage.

With any antibiotic, you should not continue use longer than is necessary, and you should not take larger doses than those recommended (see Chapter 2, "Prescription Drugs"). You should interrupt a regime of tetracycline periodically to see if the acne is clearing up on its own; if it is, you should discontinue use. Tetracycline can have a number of unpleasant side effects (including vaginal infections) if too large a dose is taken for too long. Also, don't take the tetracycline with milk.

ERYTHROMYCIN

This effective antibiotic works to keep bacterial growth in check. Doctors prescribe it as both an internal and an external medication in combatting acne. Internally, erythromycin is taken in low doses (like tetracycline) over a period of several weeks to several months. It is important that dosages be kept in check and that you be alert for the development of side effects. Externally, the erythromycin is combined with vitamin A acid in an alcohol base in an ointment or cream. These ointments, containing about 1 percent erythromycin, have achieved excellent results. We are not sure yet what their exact shelf life is, so you should check regularly for signs of rancidity (peculiar odor, change in color, change in texture, and so on), and you should ask your doctor to prescribe small quantities at a time so that you can easily keep them fresh.

As discussed in Chapter 2, there is a wide price differential in the brand name distributors of erythromycin. Ask your doctor to prescribe the drug under its generic name, and tell your pharmacist that you want the least expensive brand if you are taking the drug orally.

ESTROGEN

Because it reduces the amount of sebum produced by the sebaceous glands, estrogen has been used effectively in some cases to control acne. But because of recent findings linking estrogen to cancer (see Chapter 6), its use is limited in the treatment of acne.

Estrogen treatment has a number of other serious disadvantages. First, its effects are usually not seen for four to five months after therapy begins. While the estrogen does reduce sebum production for some time, sebum production usually returns to normal after about one year of treatment—even if you are still taking the medication. Estrogen works only for women; a medication with enough estrogen to work on a man would also have feminizing effects (loss of beard, a higher-pitched voice, and a rounder figure). Still another disadvantage is that estrogen is most often prescribed in the form of oral contraceptives. But most oral contraceptives also contain progesterone, which is known to *aggravate* acne, not heal it. In addition, oral contraceptives that contain norgestral, norethindrone, or norethindrone acetate may actually make acne worse rather than better. Also, oral contraceptives can be used safely for only a year; after that, use must be discontinued. They are not, therefore, good for those who need long-term acne treatment.

CORTICOSTEROIDS

Corticosteroids work to reduce severe inflammation that accompanies lesion formation beneath the skin's surface. Prednisone is the most widely used corticosteroid in the treatment of acne. Treatment with corticosteroids (especially oral medication) is not widespread, and your doctor will probably not prescribe it unless you are prone to develop quite a few stubborn cysts.

Corticosteroids can be administered two ways. (1) Taken *orally,* they work generally to control inflammation and help the lesions to drain normally instead of plugging up. (2) When *injected* into the cyst, the corticosteroid can prevent rupture, which otherwise leads to the spread of infection beneath the skin surface, severe scarring, and disfigurement. The corticosteroid is generally diluted heavily with a saline solution if it is to be used as an injection.

ULTRAVIOLET LIGHT

Because ultraviolet light has a drying effect on the skin, some cases of acne respond favorably to ultraviolet rays. The outer skin layer usually scales and peels off, the inner layer is softened, and the congested plugs of dead skin and bacteria are pushed out. Ultraviolet light is available in three main forms:

1. *The sun.* You can, with your doctor's direction and care, expose your acne-prone areas to the sun for a certain length of time each day at midday. This treatment is particularly hazardous and ineffective, because it is so difficult to regulate. It is easy to overexpose yourself to the sun, resulting in severe sunburn and other forms of skin damage.

2. *A sunlamp.* Again, this is a hazardous way to get your ultraviolet light. Because it is up to you to carry out the treatment at home, the doctor has little control or regulation over how you treat yourself. Burning yourself severely with a sunlamp is even easier than with the sun, because a sunlamp is so deceiving. It does not feel hot, and it takes only seconds to approximate minutes of exposure to regular sunlight. Because a sunlamp has a gentle warming effect, many people tend to fall asleep under a sunlamp, resulting in burns that require long-term medical treatment.

3. *X-rays.* This is the best form of treatment involving ultraviolet light, because the doctor can control the length and intensity of treatment dosages and can watch you closely for adverse side effects.

Most doctors steer clear of ultraviolet therapy, because recent medical findings emphasize the danger of exposure to too much ultraviolet light. Doctors have been able to link excessive X-ray exposure to cancer, and, as discussed in the previous section, overexposure to the sun can lead to skin cancer.

HOT COMPRESSES

Vleminckx's solution (containing a sulfurated lime solution) or White Lotion (containing a zinc sulfate and sulfurated potash solution) are both used frequently in hot compresses. Applied to the face for a certain length of time each day (by the patient under doctor's orders and direction), the hot compresses work to loosen and remove deeper pustules and cysts. They help prevent the dead tissue in the outer skin layer from adhering to each other, too, which prevents comedos from forming.

DERMABRASION

A surgical procedure, dermabrasion is generally prescribed for only the most severe cases. Dermabrasion consists of grinding down the outer layer of skin, helping to break open plugs, lesions, and cysts and promoting a natural draining and drying up.

Dermabrasion has several serious side effects and drawbacks. Once the outer layer of skin is ground down, the exposed layer of skin is susceptible to acute infection. Dermabrasion may cause pigment changes to occur in the skin, which results in a permanently mottled appearance and uneven facial coloring. In addition, dermabrasion is often unsuccessful the first time, and the procedure may need to be repeated several times.

VITAMIN A OINTMENT

Probably the singularly best treatment available for acne, vitamin A ointment is usually prescribed under the brand names of Tetinoin, Retin-A, or Aberel. This vitamin dries the skin, causes it to peel, and results in a sloughing off of the pimples that already exist. Those pimples that are under formation are brought to the surface and extruded.

For treatment with vitamin A ointment to be effective, you have to follow some simple guidelines, which your doctor will probably explain to you:

• Discontinue use of any other acne ointments or medication, especially over-the-counter ointments you may have been using (such as Tackle, PropaPH, or Stri-Dex). Let your face "recuperate" for a few days.

• Cut out the use of any antibacterial soaps that you have been using to wash your face. Switch to a mild, nonirritating soap, and wash only twice a day.

• Apply the vitamin A ointment only on a completely dry face. When your face is dry, the ointment penetrates more rapidly.

• Start the application cautiously. Apply the cream at first to only a small section of your face. A slight burning or stinging sensation is normal, but if it becomes severe or intolerable, you should discontinue use of the cream.

• After a few days, the section you are treating should turn slightly red. If your face is a bright red, you should apply the cream only once every other day. If you seem to be able to tolerate the cream quite well, apply it to your entire face right before you go to bed each night.

There are a few disadvantages to treatment with vitamin A cream. First, your skin doesn't get better right away. In fact, it gets worse: redness, scaling, and peeling reach a peak after about three or four weeks of treatment. Pimples that were forming below the skin's surface are forced to the surface, where they become painfully visible. But don't give up! It takes two to three months to notice improvement, but your skin should clear up completely as you continue treatment. In some stubborn cases, it may require several years of continued treatment to completely clear up all traces of the acne.

Because vitamin A cream creates photosensitivity, be careful about exposing yourself to the sun while you are using it. Use a strong sunscreen that contains PABA (para-aminobenzoic acid), and exercise the general precautions listed in the section on sunburns.

GENERAL TREATMENT TIPS

Besides using an over-the-counter or prescription formula for acne, a number of practices improve the condition of your skin and reduce your acne breakouts:[8]

1. *Wash your face often.* Washing helps to unblock the pores. It removes the dirt and bacteria that collect on the skin's surface and gets rid of the lipid buildup that is secreted from the sebaceous glands.

"Washing your face" sounds like easy instruction, but some cautions are involved. First of all, don't scrub too much; excess scrubbing can aggravate acne instead of clearing it up. And don't use a soap that is too irritating (like Irish Spring or Ivory), but stick with a soap that is mild and that doesn't irritate your skin. Second, don't wash too often. Acne can also accompany dry skin, and, if your skin is dry, use a superfatted soap (such as Dove, Tone, Caress, or Basis). If your skin is oily, try a soap like Neutrogena, Fostex, Acne-Aid, or Acnaveen. If your skin is sensitive or becomes reddened from the washing, reduce the time you scrub and switch to a milder soap.

2. *If your skin is dry, moisturize it after you wash it.* Remember, it's water—not oil—that keeps skin moist, so use a non-oil moisturizer. After you wash, rinse your washcloth in very hot tap water, wring it out, and spread it over your face. Leave it there for about a minute; it opens your pores and makes them receptive to the moisturizer. Pat your face dry, leaving a few beads of water, and then spread on the moisturizer. If your skin is dry or normal, try a moisturizer like Almay's Deep Mist Moisture Cream. If your skin is oily, you need to protect it from overdrying due to frequent washing; try a moisturizer like Ultra-Light Moisture Lotion.

3. *Shampoo your hair regularly.* Oily hair, especially hair that touches your face, can aggravate acne. Pay special attention to your scalp, too; it's another source of oil and bacteria.

4. *Use an astringent to cleanse your skin during the middle of the day.* The astringent cleanses surface bacteria from your skin and removes any oil that accumulates between washings. Some astringents come in a convenient form, such as thin pads soaked with astringent (such as Stri-Dex). While these cannot be expected to cure or clear up acne by themselves, they work as a tool in your cleansing regime.

5. *Modify your diet slightly.* If you are allergic to any food, make sure you avoid it strictly. If some food (such as greasy foods) seems to aggravate your acne, eliminate it as much as possible. Eat balanced meals, and make sure you get a nutritionally sound diet every day. Use un-iodized salt; iodine may increase sebum production.

6. *Drink plenty of water.* It keeps your digestive tract running smoothly and helps you avoid constipation, which can aggravate acne. If constipation is a frequent problem for you, increase the amount of bulk and fiber in your diet (see Chapter 3, "Constipation, Diarrhea, Hemorrhoids").

7. *Stay physically fit.* Your skin is a reflection of your general health. You need exercise, fresh air, sleep, fun, work, and a good diet to be at your healthful best. Once you reach the peak of good health, your skin glows in response.

8. *Learn to relax.* Avoid tension, try to steer clear of situations that encourage stress, and stop worrying. Some things that you worry about you can change; if you can change the things that are causing you worry, set about changing them. Other things will never change, no matter how much you worry about them. So stop worrying, and set about accepting them instead.

9. *Keep your hands away from your acne.* It's tempting to squeeze and pick, but don't. All you do is spread the infection and lead to the danger of scarring.

10. *Follow your doctor's advice.* Remember, if you are taking an antibiotic for the treatment of acne, don't take it with milk. Avoid dairy products in general while you are taking antibiotics of any kind. And don't take antacids or iron tablets at the same time; they neutralize antibiotics.

16

hair care

One of the most widely advertised cosmetics is shampoo, and we are promised all sorts of wonders if only we use the right shampoo. We can "step into a garden of earthly delights," the ads tell us, if we use Herbal Essence; Wella Balsam promises us that our hair will look like Farrah Fawcett Majors'. Yet, when you get right down to it, the purpose of shampoo is to clean your hair. Any product that does *not* clean your hair shouldn't be given a second glance; in addition to cleaning, you can find shampoos that also condition, leave a fragrance, and get rid of dandruff.

If the major purpose of shampoos is to clean, why don't we just use soap? The biggest reason is that soap leaves a film on the hair that dulls it, and the film is hard to rinse off, especially in hard water.[1] There's another problem, too: The chemicals in hard water react with the chemicals left behind in the soap film, and a residual scum is left on the hair and scalp. Nonetheless, soap is one of the major ingredients in most shampoos because it cleans well. When combined with detergents, you have a product that lathers easily (because of the soap), cleans well (due to both soap and detergent), and rinses easily and completely (thanks to the detergent). Detergent ingredients help make the shampoo more mild, so you run less risk of damaging your hair.

Some shampoos also contain a conditioner, a good idea in any kind of water. Not only do they cleanse the residual scum off the hair, so it is

193

really clean, but they also leave other ingredients on the hair shaft and scalp that help the hair to remain softer, easier to manage, and less prone to breakage. Conditioners are a good idea for you if your hair is dry or damaged from bleaching or dyeing. Make sure you choose the right kind of conditioner: Body builders coat the hair to make it thicker, and they don't really do much good in alleviating long-term problems. Therapeutic conditioners, usually applied to the hair for a certain amount of time and then rinsed out, utilize chemicals that help to moisturize and soften the hair, which generally gets to the source of the problem.

Because so many shampoos are on the market—and because the advertising claims can be quite fantastic—use your common sense in deciding which shampoo is right for you. Learn fact from fantasy. Some of the most common advertising pitches follow.[2]

LOW PH, NONALKALINE, PH-BALANCED

Scientists and researchers use the term "pH" to designate the relative balance of acid and alkaline. Something that is neutral—that is, neither acid nor alkaline—has a pH of 7. Things that are acid have a pH under 7; orange juice, for instance, has a pH of about 3. Things that are alkaline have a pH above 7; hand soaps have a value of about 9. Human skin and hair are slightly acid, so shampoo manufacturers have decided that we should use a shampoo that is slightly alkaline so that we can achieve neutrality. Yet most of the shampoos advertised as pH balanced (or slightly alkaline) have pH values anywhere from 5 to 8—not enough to make a difference. The highest one, Avon Protem Creme, scored in at 9—less than a plain old bar of Ivory soap.

PROTEIN

Human hair is made up almost entirely of protein, so the idea behind this advertising claim is to add protein to the shampoo. Hair then has more body, gets thicker and healthier, and self-mends its split ends—so manufacturers tell us.

Do they work? That depends on your definition. Most of the shampoos that claim to repair split ends *do* make split ends less of a problem; in actuality, they glue hair back together with chemical constituents, not with protein. Most of the shampoos claiming to build body with added protein simply coat the hair to make it thicker.

FRAGRANCE

Fragrance is added to shampoo for two reasons. First, it helps mask the odor of other chemicals that are in all detergents and shampoos. Second, fragrance sells. The fragrance doesn't do anything—good or bad—for your hair. In fact, it might as well not be there as far as effectiveness goes. (Interestingly enough, Clairol manufacturers admitted that Clairol Sunshine Harvest Shampoo in fresh peach, honeydew, and wild strawberry "flavors" were identical solutions except for the fragrance.)

DANDRUFF CONTROL

Dandruff is the flaking of cells that create white speckles through the hair. It won't cause baldness or disease, but it is a social stigma and is generally considered unattractive and undesirable. Dandruff can't be cured, but it can be controlled.[3] Medicated shampoos, lotions, and rinses that contain coal tar, resorcinol, salicyclic acid, selenium, sulfide, and zinc pyrithione are generally effective in controlling the flaking of dandruff.[4] They reduce the rate of turnovers of the scalp (so flaking is not as frequent), or they break up scale size so that they are less noticeable. As long as your shampoo contains one or a combination of these ingredients, you can make up your own mind about packaging, price, lathering properties, color, odor, and whether it's a liquid, cream, gel, or paste. Also, make sure you brush your hair daily to help distribute oil and mobilize flaking cells.

How do you choose a good shampoo? Price is certainly one consideration. Most shampoos cost between 15 and 25 cents an ounce. You can get plenty of good ones in that price range, so you shouldn't have to pay more. Aside from price, choose a shampoo that best suits your needs. Concentrated shampoos last longer than regular shampoos. Choose one based on your hair type (dry, normal, or oily). If your hair is extremely dry or if it has been damaged by the sun or chemical treatments, choose a shampoo that has a conditioner built in.

HAIR-COLORING PRODUCTS

Again, advertising plays a big part in convincing us to purchase and use hair-coloring products: You are told that your hair should be the same color as your two-month-old daughter's, that gray is something to be shunned, and that blondes have more fun. In reality, the dyes and tints and bleaches that millions of Americans use on their hair can lead to problems that are far from "fun."

A number of different coloring products are available for hair, and their effects range from temporary to permanent.[5]

RINSES

Rinses are temporary colors, which you can't use to lighten your hair color. They add highlights, improve the shade of gray hair, and blend the color of your hair if it's uneven now. Rinses also come out completely in one shampooing, because they never penetrate the hair shaft. For the same reason, they are easy to use; most of them are applied to the roots and then combed through the hair to the ends. However, you have to be careful with them. They are liable to rub off on pillowcases and clothing, and they might run if you are caught in the rain or if your scalp perspires heavily.

People who want to try on a new color before they do something permanent use rinses to see what they'd look like with different coloring. Rinses are also used by people in theatrical productions who need a temporary change in hair color. Sometimes they're used to tide people over between permanent hair color treatments.

SEMIPERMANENT HAIR COLORINGS

If you don't want something permanent, but you want something that lasts longer than a rinse, you can use a semipermanent hair coloring product. These products *do* penetrate the hair shaft, so they last for about four shampoos. The dye is applied to your hair just like a shampoo: It's rubbed in, lathered up, and rinsed out. It takes about four shampooings to get rid of a semipermanent product, but your hair loses color with each shampoo until the product is eventually gone.

Since semipermanent products don't foster a chemical reaction, they are milder than permanent dyes. This characteristic also means that you can't lighten your hair color with a semipermanent product; the change is generally a few shades darker instead. You can, however, use semipermanent products to improve white or gray hair, to add highlights to natural blonde hair, and to blend in colors of hair that has been streaked.

PERMANENT HAIR-COLORING PRODUCTS (DYES)

The harshest of the hair-coloring products are permanent ones—those that cause chemical reactions in the hair shaft. There are three general kinds of dyes, each with its own advantages and disadvantages:

1. *Oxidation dyes* are the only ones that can be used to lighten hair. They last longer than other kinds of dyes, and they offer a wider range of natural-looking shades. For all these reasons, they are the most popular and widely used. Oxidation dyes come in either a shampoo-in formula (the kind most often used by amateurs at home) and cream formulas (used in salons by professionals). Unfortunately, although organic dyes work the best as far as color is concerned, they also present the greatest probability of adverse reactions.

The effects of oxidation dyes depend on several different chemical reactions, and a certain amount of preparation needs to take place before the dye is ready to use. If you want a great deal of lightening (for instance, if you plan to go from brunette to blonde), you have to bleach your hair before you dye it. The bleaching process completely strips the hair of color so that it is able to accept the lighter dye.

What happens during the oxidation dye process? First, the hair shaft is caused to swell by an ammonia-type base in the hair dye soap. Once it has swelled, the hair shaft can absorb the peroxide and dye. The peroxide penetrates the hair shaft and bleaches out any old dye and some of the natural color. Hair dye chemicals penetrate the shaft and cause it to absorb the color. The coloring particles blend in a chemical reaction with the hair's own molecules. The larger-than-normal molecules that result "lock in" the hair color; it simply can't escape.

2. *Metallic dyes* are characterized by easy application and gradual color change. A small amount of the formula is combed into the hair each day; a metallic salt, usually lead acetate or silver, reacts on the hair. The byproduct is pigment product that coats the hair. This process is repeated until the hair is as dark as desired.

Metallic dyes, too, have their disadvantages. The color you get from them is usually unnatural. If you use them too long and neglect to taper off periodically, metallic deposits build up along your hair shaft and cause your hair to break when you comb it. Although allergic reactions are rare, metallic dyes may pose a danger from lead absorption into the scalp.

Remember one important thing about these metallic products: Your gray hair isn't mysteriously returning to normal. You're just coating your hair with color. Underneath it's still gray.

3. *Vegetable dyes* are not widely used. The most popular is henna, a compound composed of the ground leaves and stems of the henna plant. Usually it adds highlights to dark hair and adds color and interest to red hair. Henna's disadvantage, though, is an obvious one: Hair treated with henna for a very long period turns bright reddish-orange, looks unnatural, is stiff, and is extremely brittle and prone to breakage.

BLEACHING

As already mentioned, you need to bleach your hair—a process that strips your hair of all color—if you want to lighten it more than a couple of shades. Bleaching is rarely used alone as a hair color product, but it is generally used as a preparation for other hair-coloring procedures.

Never bleach your hair more often than once a month—and then restrict the bleaching to the new dark roots that have grown in. Once you have bleached your hair, you need to treat it with care, because bleaching breaks down hair fibers. Don't curl, tease, or use heat on hair that has been bleached. Treat your hair with conditioners that are designed specifically for bleached hair. They can't repair the damage done, but they can help soften it and moisturize it by coating the hair shafts with a conditioning formula.

Before using any kind of hair-coloring product, you should perform a patch test. Do it two ways:

• Select a tiny section of hair that is not visible, usually one underneath your other hair and near the neckline. Treat it; see how it reacts. If it turns brittle, breaks, or feels like straw, you shouldn't use the product on your entire head of hair.

• Put a little of the formula on a small area of your skin. Behind the ear or on the inside of the arm at about the elbow are the two easiest places to perform patch tests. Wait for twenty-four hours; don't wash the solution off your skin. If you see any redness, blistering, or swelling at the end of twenty-four hours, you are probably allergic to the dye or solution and shouldn't use it. Your entire scalp would look like that patch of skin.

In a word, hair dyes and tints and rinses can be extremely dangerous. The dyes that over twenty million Americans use each year can, in unusual cases, cause cancer and birth defects.[6] Researchers suspect other problems, too, making hair-coloring products a risky bet.

HAIR-REMOVAL PRODUCTS

You can get rid of unwanted body hair in a number of ways, which range all the way from the basic straight-edged razor, through complicated chemical products, to electric current. All are generally safe if they are used properly.

SHAVING
Shaving with a razor—either a safety or an electric—is the most common and widespread method of hair removal. You need water or some other moisturizer to prepare and protect the skin if you use a safety razor. An electric razor should be used on skin that is completely dry, to prevent the risk of electric shock.

You can do several things to make shaving more effective and safe:[7]

1. *Wash the area you are going to shave before you begin shaving.*
Body hair is normally coated with oil and debris that can cause the

razor to slip or that can prevent the razor from cutting the hair. Don't try to shave dirty hair.

2. *If you are using a safety razor, lubricate your skin completely.* You can use soap and water, shaving cream, or a moisturizer. Water alone isn't usually effective, because it evaporates too quickly.

3. *If an electric razor irritates your skin, use a preshave lotion designed for use with electric razors.* The lotion helps condition and moisturize the area to be shaved.

4. *Make sure your blades (in both safety and electric razors) are sharp.* Dull razors are the cause of most nicks and skin irritation.

5. *Keep your blades clean.* Rinse them under running water during the shaving process if hair accumulates on them. When you've finished using them, rinse them under cold water and let them drip dry. You will dull them if you wipe them. An electric razor, of course, should be cleaned with the brushes that are supplied with the razor.

6. *Shave in the direction opposite from hair growth.* Use long, even strokes; the short choppy ones give you problems.

7. *Don't be alarmed by profuse bleeding from a nick.* It looks much worse than it is. Moisten a piece of toilet tissue and apply it to the nick; bleeding should stop in about thirty seconds. If toilet tissue doesn't work, use a styptic pencil.

8. Don't apply deodorant to underarms right after you shave them, and don't apply perfume to areas you have recently shaved.

9. If you experience skin irritation from shaving, apply a medicated powder or moisturizing cream.

DEPILATORIES
These are chemical agents—usually alkaline—that cause hair to lose its elasticity and to absorb water so that a swipe of a washcloth or a quick shower removes the hair. Because the chemicals in depilatories can be harsh, you should perform a skin test before you apply the chemical solution to a large area of skin. Do the patch test on your skin: If the chemical affects your skin, you should not use it. Like shaving with a razor, depilatories only remove hair above the surface. Regrowth is usually quite rapid, and it tends to be bristly and stubbly.
     A number of different depilatories are on the market. Never use one

on facial hair unless the label specifically states that the product is designed and is safe for the removal of facial hair. Preparations designed for removal of leg hair are usually too harsh and would cause damage to the more tender facial skin. Several products are designed solely for use in removing facial hair; they are the best choices for a woman who wants to remove hair from her upper lip or elsewhere on her face.

WAXING

One of the oldest methods of hair removal, waxing involves combination of hot resins, oils, and several waxes. This concoction is applied to the skin, allowed to cool, and quickly stripped off in the direction of hair growth. The hairs are pulled out just above the root, and regrowth usually takes several weeks to appear.

You need to take certain cautions if you plant to use waxing. Make sure the wax solution isn't too hot; the oils and resins in most of the mixtures tend to hold heat, and you could give yourself a serious burn if you allow the mixture to overheat. Don't try to use waxing on large areas; it's meant for small areas, like the upper lip. Any bigger areas need to be waxed by a professional who has had training and experience.

There is one major disadvantage to waxing: The regrowth has to be pretty long before you can repeat the process, so you will have reasonably long hair quite a bit of the time if you choose waxing as your method of hair removal.

ELECTROLYSIS

In this process, an electrically charged needle carries a current of electricity along a hair root. The electric charge destroys the chemical makeup of the hair, and the decomposing hair dies and drops out. Electrolysis in some form or another has been used since 1875, but it was fairly dangerous until the 1940s. Today, schools across the nation train people in the science of electrolysis.[8]

Today's electrolysis machine is about the size of a short-wave radio. A rubber tube extending from it has a tiny needle at the end. A hand magnifying glass is used to locate the hair, and the needle is injected. A short burst of electricity—usually lasting about one-fifth of a second—is delivered through the needle and controlled by a foot pedal.

Most people aren't bothered too much by the pain, which feels similar to a pinprick. But you should consider other side effects and disadvantages before you decide on electrolysis:

1. *It's expensive.* It can run up to $40 an hour in large cities where many operators compete for your business. In smaller areas, with few operators, fees can be even higher. You can investigate local schools that teach electrolysis; some let their students experiment on patients for much less money.

2. *Some areas of the body are not suited for electrolysis.* The process is usually used on the upper lip, forehead, chin, and lower abdomen; in those places it is generally safe and effective. It should *never* be used on the hair in nostrils, on eyelids, or protruding from moles. Electrolysis performed on a woman's chest or on the insides of her thighs can result in tiny scars and raised nodules of skin.

3. *Completely destroying the hair takes a long time—and sometimes repeated attempts.* Because many hair shafts have been distorted by long-term shaving and plucking, it's hard for the electrolysis operator to get to the root on the first try. You can expect about one-fourth of the hair to grow back at least once. The area of the body, along with the texture and thickness of the hair, determines how long hair removal will take, but the average upper lip takes about twenty hours total. That's about $400 to $600.

4. *If you have sensitive skin, you might develop a rash after electrolysis.* These rashes usually disappear within a few days. You might try a medicated cream or moisturizer to help soothe the skin irritation. Scarring from electrolysis that is performed by a competent operator on sensible parts of the body is minimal.

part four

NONMEDICINAL TREATMENTS

17

home remedies

Folk medicine has a long history—much longer than that of contemporary, scientific medicine. The use of home remedies and herbs developed in the days when the scientific pharmacy was not available. A discussion of drugs and their use would therefore be incomplete without a brief look at the home remedies, herbs, and nutritional aids which may be used to treat certain discomforts and diseases when you choose not to use a synthetically manufactured drug. Remember, though, that many diseases are too serious to be suitable for self-diagnosis and medication. So *the information in this section is not intended to replace the services of a physician.*

Some home remedies of bygone eras may seem ridiculous by our standards, but apparently their use was widespread and accepted. We forget that home remedies saved many of our ancestors when doctors were few and far between and when doctors were not always trusted, usually because their mysterious remedies were not always understood.

Unquestionably, some home remedies are useless. For example, you might be interested in some of the common ailments and cures of the 1700s. Often the remedy was worse than the disease:

> To Cure Baldness: Rub the part morning and evening, with onions, till it is red, and rub it afterward with honey. Or, wash it with a decoction of boxwood. Or, electrify it daily.

A Cold in the Head: Pare very thin the yellow rind of an orange, roll it up inside out, and thrust into each nostril.

Settled Deafness: Take a red onion, pick out the core, and fill up the place with oil of roasted almonds. Let it stand a night then bruise and strain it. Drop three or four drops into the ears morning and evening, and stop it with black wool.

To Stop Vomiting: Apply a large onion, slit across the grain to the pit of the stomach.[1]

These home remedies probably do not sound appealing, nor are they likely to be successful at curing the ills for which they were intended.

We cannot, however, discount all the early home remedies as being of questionable value. Take, for example, the early cure for a tickling cough, which was to drink water whitened with oatmeal four times a day or to keep a piece of barley sugar or sugar candy in the mouth at all times. If you have ever had an annoying, tickling cough, you probably have successfully controlled it by having a piece of candy in your mouth until the tickling was gone. Or how about the eighteenth-century cure for extreme fat, which was to use a total vegetable diet? Although this is not a totally safe procedure for successful dieting, the underlying principle is probably acceptable: Vegetables have fewer calories than meats, many fruits, breads and cereals, and certainly desserts.

Other homespun treatments seem to have value also. For example, in 1864, *The Canada Farmer* noted that a nosebleed could be stopped by placing a folded piece of brown paper between the upper lip and the gum. How often have you heard that putting a piece of ice between the upper lip and gum stops a nosebleed? Many people testify that this works. *The Family Manual* in 1845 mentioned that for sprains and swelling, the affected part should be washed frequently with cold salt-water, kept as cold as possible, and elevated on a cushion. Also prescribed were a light diet and cooling medicine to be taken every day. When you have a sprained ankle, what is the first thing you probably do? Of course, you pack it in ice, elevate it, and stay off it. A lighter diet calorie-wise might also be part of the treatment, since you are not as active and are not burning as many calories. An early Texas remedy for sunburn was to apply thick, wet laundry starch to the area and let it dry. This treatment might not have done much to heal the burn, but it probably soothed the area and made it not quite so painful.[2]

So, our forefathers were not completely wrong in some of their ideas for home remedies.[3] Most home remedies, based on classical, traditional, or magical lore, may be founded on scientific principles. In fact, many folk cures practiced by the old crone are offshoots of early scientific practices. Many of the successful home remedies have endured from earlier times for several reasons. They are well-known, accessible, trusted, and inexpensive. They also solve everyday health matters. Alex Comfort has said, "Healing, as expounded by the 'healers' of folk medicine, is in fact the distinguished ancestor of modern medicine, which later generations have put in mothballs."[4] He further explains that folk medicine may have more value than we give it credit for because it treats both the mind and the body. The success of many home remedies is based on their psychological assurance. Folk medicine is, in essence, a combination of psychiatry, medicine, and magic; and some forms of it are reputable.

Because they are so close to our hearts, their future—like their past—seems assured: "Home remedies probably always will have a place in the treatment of mankind's aches and pains. Physicians do not expect and do not desire that patients shall dash to the doctor with every minor discomfort, every trifling injury, every small ache or pain."[5]

COMMON AILMENTS

You might consider using home remedies yourself for occasional aches or pains that you don't want to treat with drugs. Some of the more common treatments are explained here.

Bee or Insect Stings
Mix one quarter of a teaspoon of meat tenderizer with two teaspoons of water, and apply the mixture to the sting as soon as possible. The substance should have a paste-like texture, and you should rub it into the area surrounding the sting site. Another paste, made of baking soda, vinegar, and salt, may also be applied to the sting site to relieve pain and swelling. Another helpful treatment is to put moistened tobacco or its leaves on the sting site as a poultice. You can also put a cupful or two of quick starch or minute oatmeal into bathwater and bathe in this mixture.

Mosquito Bites, Poison Ivy, Fleas
You can get relief from itching caused by these and a number of other causes by applying hot water (about 120° to 130° Fahrenheit) several times during several hours. You can use either running water for a body part that you can conveniently stick under a tap or a hot washcloth for other areas. You should never treat an extensive area of skin in this

way, nor should you use hot water as a treatment for poison ivy that has caused blistering. If the itching is prolonged, see a doctor; hot water should be used only for occasional, short-term minor problems. Another home remedy to relieve itching from mosquito bites is to rub toothpaste on the area.

Insect Repellent
Try using vitamin B1 (Thiamine). You'll need about 200 milligrams a day, so you shouldn't use it for long. And don't rub it on; take it orally.

Hiccups
Swallow one teaspoonful of dry granulated white sugar. Believe it or not, this method worked in nineteen out of twenty cases. Twelve of these cases had had the hiccups for more than six hours, and eight had suffered for up to *six weeks* with the same bout of hiccups! If two tries don't work, swig down a jigger of vinegar.

Burns
Immerse the burned area immediately in cold water. Don't use ice, because it can damage the skin, and don't try to treat anything other than a simple first-degree burn. Don't treat a first-degree burn if it involves an extensive amount of skin. And, whatever you do, *don't* use baking soda, butter, or any other kind of grease. Cold water used immediately after you get a first-degree burn can not only relieve the pain, but it can actually stop the burning. It cools the skin to prevent the burning from continuing.

Sprains
Both heat and cold should be used in the treatment of minor sprains, but only in the proper order. Apply ice packs or cold water first; make sure that the ice does not contact the skin directly, since it can cause frostbite. Use the cold for up to two days, or until the swelling decreases. Don't apply ice or cold water for longer than two days; if the swelling hasn't reduced somewhat, see a doctor. After the second day, apply heat to relieve pain. Again, make sure that your skin is protected against the possibility of a burn.

Arthritis and Bursitis
Cold, not heat, should be applied to stiff joints and painful muscles. Make sure you protect the skin beneath the cold pack from frostbite. Or you can make a liniment to relieve soreness by thoroughly mixing two parts of sunflower seed oil and one part of turpentine.

Frigid Headache

The headache that you get from eating your ice cream too fast or from slurping down a glass of cherry slush too quickly can be immediately relieved by curling your tongue back and pressing it against the roof of your mouth.

Athlete's Foot

The symptoms can be relieved by placing small pieces of lamb's wool between the toes.

Toothache

An aching tooth should always be seen by a dentist. Any home remedy should therefore be considered temporary. One home treatment is to put oil of cloves on a swab and to rub it onto the painful area.

HOME REMEDIES AND COMMON SENSE

In using any home remedy, you should use your intelligence and your good sense. You probably have a batch of others that have passed down through your family—mustard plasters for congested lungs or cough syrups made from honey and butter—and you may have picked some up along the way from roommates or friends. Just remember that a home remedy is just that: a remedy that can be used to treat a malady that is safe to treat at home. You should never try to treat any serious condition—including headaches and toothaches—with a home remedy. A minor scratch can be treated successfully and safely at home; a laceration, on the other hand, can lead to serious infection and may need stitches. You can treat a minor sprain at home, but, if it doesn't respond immediately, you need medical attention. It might be a torn tendon or a broken bone. And, as mentioned in Chapter 1, never treat a toothache itself at home. Any remedy that you concoct out of the kitchen cupboard should be only a temporary measure to relieve pain while you are waiting to see the dentist.[6]

CAUTIONS

Far from soothing your symptoms, a home remedy may do nothing to treat a condition. It may even aggravate a condition if it is used improperly. It could also mask the symptoms of a more serious condition that should be seen by a doctor if treatment is to be effective. Home remedies may delay needed treatment to the point where permanent damage or death could result.

In a day when many people are going back to natural foods, many also desire natural medicines, in the forms that remedies took in their great-great-grandmother's day. You should be cautious, however, and use home remedies only to treat temporary and minor complaints. To be safe, always refer more serious conditions to your doctor.

18

herbs

An herb is commonly thought of as the leafy part of a plant that is grown in the temperate zones of the world and that is valued for its medicinal, savory, or aromatic qualities.

Historically, the oldest uses of herbs were medicinal: "The use of plants by man to cure his ills dates back to hoary antiquity."[1] In Egypt, as early as 2000 B.C., over two thousand physicians had abandoned the practice of magic in healing and used plants instead in their medical practices. Hippocrates, the father of medicine, was a herbalist of sorts. He made a list of four hundred herbs which he used. Surprisingly, one-third of these are still used today for one purpose or another. Aristotle had a garden of more than three hundred plants reputed to have medicinal qualities. Other references to herbs appeared in the literature of the day and even in the New Testament.

The Greeks passed their knowledge about herbs on to the Romans, who in turn passed their practices on to the Christians. The monks became the experts in herbal activity during the Dark Ages. In fact, the following joke circulated throughout the medieval world: "If you want to be cured of I don't know what, take this herb of I don't know what name, apply it I don't know where and you will be cured I don't know when."[2]

The influence of herbs spread so that by the Renaissance, individuals all over Europe had herb gardens much as we have vegetable gardens. In the Renaissance, herbs became the focus of illustrations and elaborate ornaments. At this time Nicholas Culpeper, probably the most famous herbologist of all times, introduced his doctrine of signatures; the medicinal purpose of plants, he maintained, could be determined by some element of the plant's appearance. "The spotted, lungshaped leaves of the liverwort indicated to the ancients that it was good for curing diseased or spotted lungs. The hollow stalk of the garlic showed it was a remedy for windpipe ailments."[3]

Later, the Englishmen who sailed to the New World took herbs with them. These settlers found that the natives of America already had a vast herbal knowledge of their own. About that time, arboretums (places where herbs and other plants are grown) were established, and some herbs received medical recognition as being successful for treatments. In fact, "fifty years ago, every physician practiced herbal medicine."[4]

HERBAL HEALING AGENTS

Now, in the twentieth century, the majority of our drugs are synthetic pharmaceuticals, but "it has been estimated that more than half of the prescriptions written by American physicians today contain a plant-derived drug: a drug that comes from a plant or one that has been synthesized to duplicate (or improve on) a plant substance."[5] In fact, many of our most important medical discoveries have come from plants, as shown in the following table.[6]

PLANT	MEDICATION	TREATMENT OF
Poppy	Morphine	Pain
Autumn crocus	Colchicine	Gout
Foxglove	Digitalis	Heart disorders
Ephedra	Ephedrine	Asthma
Willow	Aspirin	Pain, fever
Ipecacuanha	Ipecac	Amoebic dysentery
Snakeroot	Reserpine	High blood pressure
Chincona bush	Quinine	Malaria
Belladonna	Atropine	Relaxes eye muscles, dilates pupils

The Berkeley Holistic Health Center suggests that besides having herbal healing agents in the home, you also need an herbal first aid kit. This organization suggests that the following agents be put into such a kit:

- Charcoal to be used externally for its drawing properties
- Oil of garlic
- Cayenne
- Herb salve, eucalyptus oil, or tiger balm
- Cascara extract for constipation
- Peppermint for nausea
- Sweating herbs: ½ elder flowers, ½ peppermint
- Composition powder: 1 oz bayberry bark, 2 oz ginger, 1 oz white pine, 1 dram cloves, 1 dram cayenne. This composition powder should be taken hourly during the acute stage of a disease. To prepare it: Steep 1 tsp of the ingredients in a cup of boiling water for fifteen minutes; cover the cup. Drink the liquid that results— not the sediment.
- Antispasmodic tincture: 1 oz powdered lobelia seed, 1 oz skullcap, 1 skunk cabbage root, 1 oz granulated gum myrrh, 1 oz black cohosh, ½ oz cayenne. To prepare it: Steep powdered herbs in one pint of boiling water for one half-hour; strain the resultant mixture; add one pt of apple cider vinegar and bottle the result.
- Jethro Kloss's All-Purpose Liniment: 2 oz powdered myrrh, 1 oz powdered golden seal, ½ oz cayenne, 1 qt apple cider vinegar. To prepare it: Mix all the ingredients, shake the mixture every day for one week, strain the mixture, and bottle it.[7]

Other herbal preparations may be helpful for various first aid treatments:

- *For drawing out infections:* Make a poultice out of three parts mullein, comfrey, and marshmallow root to one part lobelia plus a pinch of cayenne. Take equal parts of wheat germ oil and honey, and blend all these ingredients until a paste is formed. Put this mixture on a piece of gauze and apply it to the affected area. Cover the gauze with plastic and leave it on the area for 24 hours.[8]
- *For spider or other venomous bites:* Wet some carbonate of soda and apply it to the affected area. It neutralizes the venom in the bite or sting.
- *For frostbite:* Use an Indian meal poultice covered with young hyson tea. Soften the poultice with hot water, as hot as the patient can stand.

• For *poison ivy*: Boil ½ pt of shelled oats until the water is very dark. Use this oat tea to wash the poisoned area.

• For *nettle sting*: Rub the affected area with rosemary, mint, or sage leaves. This treatment should stop the pain and itching.

• For *bee sting*: Wet salt and vinegar to make a poultice. Apply it to the sting.

• For *sunstroke*: Wear a cool cabbage leaf inside the hat to protect the head from too much sun and heat.

• For *sunburn*: Wash the body and the affected area with a strong sage tea.[9]

As well as the many herbs that are purported to have healing qualities, many people believe that many of the foods in our cupboards and refrigerators have healing values. Some of the common healing agents present in the home, along with their claimed healing properties, are as follows:

Vegetables
• *Beets*: Liver cleanser, red blood cell builder, fibrin dissolver (helps to dissolve blood clots), menstrual regulator, diuretic.

• *Carrots*: Cleanser of bile and moribund matter impacted in the liver.

• *Celery*: Leaves contain a small amount of insulin; stalk contains organic sodium, which helps the body eliminate calcium deposits.

• *Spinach*: Stimulates peristalsis in the digestive tract, which in turn relieves digestive upsets and disorders.

• *Potato*: Raw potato cures gastritis; boiled potato is an emergency poultice.

• *Corn*: Soothing qualities, relieves skin irritations.

• *Cucumber*: Hand lotion.

Fruits
• *Apples*: Digestive aid, cleanses the intestines.

• *Apricots*: Builds red blood cells, helps build strong bones, teeth, nails, and hair.

• *Berries*: Cleansing properties.

• *Grapefruit*: Dissolves inorganic calcium in the body, which aids in the relief of arthritis, reducing fevers.

• *Lemons:* Helps maintain the body's acid–base balance; alleviates the symptoms of the common cold; stomach cleanser; sweetener; used in the treatment of sore throat and upset stomach; tonic.

• *Papayas:* Appetite stimulant, meat tenderizer.

• *Pineapple:* Digestive aid; reduces edema and swelling in the body.

• *Grapes:* Diuretic.

• *Pears:* Laxative.

• *Pumpkin:* Prostate and urinary disorders.[10]

While a book on prescription and over-the-counter drugs should not extensively treat herbal remedies, you should be aware of some of the things that herbs are believed to do—rightly or wrongly—medically or cosmetically.

The following list contains some commonly used herbs and beliefs about their powers:

Alfalfa systemic alkalyzer, calcium assimilation, corrects hypercalcemia and osteoporosis, promotes growth (because of its influence on the pituitary), arthritis, colic, lesser duration of colds, affects parathyroid gland, mild laxative, tonic, stomachic, diuretic.

Almond warming properties, removes phlegm, quiets cough, lowers excessive energy, lubricates the intestines, dyspnea, asthma, constipation.

Aloe vera vulnerary, emollient, purative, insect bites, cuts, rashes, burns, suntan preparation, shampoo, soap, lotions, laxatives, open infected wounds.

Asparagus diuretic, gentle laxative.

Black cohosh hormone-type herb, antispasmodic, diaphoretic properties, helps control nervousness associated with menstrual periods, "female complaints."

Burdock fever, detoxifies, dispels wind, influenza, tonsilitis, boils, abscesses, pertussis, aperient, alterative, diuretic, blood-builder, skin problems, laxative, hair rinse.

Chamomile antispasmodic, tonic, nervine, emmenagogue; inflammation and abscesses, hair wash, blond dye for the hair, insect repellent, stomachic, stimulant, aromatic, anodyne, vermifuge, colds, bronchitis, bladder troubles, jaundice, typhoid fever, rheumatic pains, headaches, hysteria, sleep inducer, mild sedative, wash for sore or weak eyes, open sores or wounds, gargle, poultice (pains, swelling, gangrene).

Catnip   colic, tonic, stomachic, nervous headache, promotes perspiration.

Cat-tail   promotes diuresis, reduces swelling, promotes pus drainage, blood in sputum, blood in vomited material, nose bleed, bloody stools, blood in the urine, vaginal bleeding, bleeding hemorrhoids, cystitis, urethritis, menstrual irregularities, leukorrhea.

Cayenne   powerful natural stimulant, fevers, sore throat, hangover remedy, internal disinfectant, liniment, toothache, irritant, rubefacient, appetizer, digestive, sialagogue, antiseptic, tonic, rids the body of excess mucous, localized muscle pain, stopping internal or external bleeding, alcoholic gastritis, healing ulcers, expectorant, arthritis.

Celandine   ringworm, eczema, herpes virus, warts.

Celery   helps eliminate calcium deposits, contains some insulin, reduces fever, detoxifies, stops bleeding, epidemic influenza, jaundice, blood in the urine, irregular menstrual bleeding.

Cloves   warms body center, alleviates pain, vomiting, hiccups, pain in the heart and abdomen, hernia.

Comfrey   arthritis, astringent, demulcent, pulmonary ailments, soothing, internal hemorrhage, chronic catarrh and nasal congestion, poultice for sprains, swelling, bruises, skin ulcers, cosmetics, pectoral, vulnerary, anodyne, emollient, refrigerant, coughs, consumption, ulceration or soreness of kidneys, stomach or bowels, bloody urine, rheumatic pains, eczema, anemia, dysentery, diarrhea, leukorrhea, colitis, gall and liver diseases, hemorrhoids, cleanses entire system of impurities, strengthens the blood, boils, carbuncles, sore breasts, headache, gargle, mouthwash, tones the skin, whooping cough, cancer.

Dandelion   diuretic, laxative, hepatic, antiscorbutic, sialagogue, tonic, aperient, alterative, stomachic, cholagogue, kidney and liver disorders, jaundice, skin diseases, scrofula, loss of appetite, dropsy, fever, inflammation of bowels, rheumatism, gout, stiff joints, increases the activity of the liver, spleen, pancreas; poultice for snakebites, warts.

Deer's tongue   diuretic, anticoagulant, emetic, emollient, breast complaints.

Elder   dropsy, insect repellent, colds, flu diaphoretic, diuretic, sore throat, cough, healthy elimination, colic, diarrhea, kidney problems, antiseptic wash, ease inflammations of the skin, softens skin.

Fennel stimulates energy, promotes digestion, resolves phlegm, stimulates milk production, gastroenteritis, hernia, indigestion, abdominal pain.

Flaxseed used as setting lotion for hair.

Garlic blood cleanser, digestive stimulant, systemic cleanser, diuretic, beneficial to lymph system, cleanser of mucous membranes, antibiotic, high blood pressure, may have some effect against cancer, neuralgic complaints, skin disorders, external use, ringworm, scabies, lice, catarrh, asthma, TB, difficult breathing, regulates blood pressure, heart weakness, internal ulceration, kills parasites or expells worms, diuretic, stimulant, expectorant, sweat promoter, bubonic plague, antiseptic, stings, loosens congestion, opens vessels, antibiotic, cleanses the intestines, diarrhea, dysentery, colds, cough, boils, abscesses, antispasmodic, insect repellent, whooping cough, prevent aging and promote rejuvenation of the body.

Ginger diarrhea, colic dysentery, muscular rheumatism, toothache, headache, neuralgia.

Ginseng prostate problems, allay fears, general tonic, increases circulation to the brain, overcomes nervous prostration, reactivates sex glands, antispasmodic, fatigue, reflex nerve diseases, whooping cough, asthma, TB, fevers, weaknesses of all kinds, digestive disorders, stimulant, anodyne, slight laxative, diaphoretic, carminative, alterative, strengthens heart and nervous system, resistance to disease, strengthens endocrine system, acceleration and acquisition of learning, colds, coughs, rheumatism, neuralgia, gout, diabetes, anemia, insomnia, stress, headache, backache, double vision, normalizing menstruation, easing childbirth, rejuvenation, antitumor value, periodontal disease, supplements energy, produces saliva, stimulates the appetite, deficiencies of blood, internal injuries caused by worry.

Golden Seal tonic, astringent, emmenagogue, oxytonic, gastrointestinal and nasal catarrh, mucous membrane irritation, external ulcers, dyspepsia, erysipelas, typhoid fever, torpor of the liver, ophthalmia, ulceration of the mouth, spermatorrhea, natural insulin, diuretic, antibiotic, stops internal bleeding and swelling; gives strength to the veins, helps correct hyperglycemia and hyperinsulinism, inflamed eyes, mouth sores, acne, eczema, stomach and liver problems, superficial cataracts, tonic, laxative, alterative, detergent, antiseptic, deobstructant, antiperiodic, mucous membrane problems, spinal nerves, and meningitis, biliousness, increased bile and gastric juice secretion, gonorrhea, leukorrhea, syphilis, ulcerations of the stomach and bowels, morning sickness, vaginal and uterine inflammation, pyorrhea, sore gums.

Goldenrod aids digestion, relieves intestinal gas, expels worms, clears fever, detoxifies, influenza, headache, sore throat, malaria, measles, gastric pain, vomiting.

Hemlock astringent.

Hops antiseptic, digestive problems, insomnia, tranquilizer, earache, wounds, heart disease.

Kelp hypo- or hyperthyroidism, antiseptic, corrects nervous conditions, promotes moisturization, softens hard and enlarged lymph nodes, tumors, edema, congestion, painful testicles.

Lady slipper relaxant, antispasmodic, nervine, tonic, acts on medulla to regulate breathing, sweating, salivation, and heart function.

Licorice colds, sore throat, sexual vigor, strength, endurance, Addison's disease, acts like a steroid, allay thirst, demulcent, expectorant, female hormonal properties, laxative, pectoral, emollient, diuretic, bronchitis, irritations of bowels and kidneys, duodenal and peptic ulcers, blood purifier, supplements energy, detoxifies, loosen phlegm, splenic and gastric imbalance, abdominal pain, vomiting and diarrhea, productive cough, swollen abscesses.

Lobelia muscle relaxant, stimulant properties, poultice, asthma, emphysema, TB, nervous disorders, drug withdrawal, clears fever, detoxifies, resolves bruises, promotes diuresis, heals sores and abscesses, poisonous snake bites, tooth abscesses, ascites, traumatic injuries.

Mullein demulcent, emollient, soothing infusions, relieve cough, ease expectoration, ease throat congestion, anodyne, pectoral, antispasmodic, hemorrhoids, bronchial complaints, lung troubles.

Myrrh antiseptic, astringent, stomachic, tonic, stimulant, expectorant, emmenagogue, vaginal douche, accelerates healing, disinfectant.

Nettle rheumatism, cough, shortness of breath, consumption.

Parsley builds the optic system, inflammation of the kidneys, bladder, urethra, and genitals, digestive stimulant, regulation of the liver and spleen, dropsy, gall bladder problems, gallstones, gravel, menstruation obstructions, jaundice, intermittent fevers, hepatitis, insect bites, swollen glands, swollen breasts, cancer, difficult urination, syphilis, gonorrhea, anemia, TB, arthritis, obesity, high blood pressure, bad breath, rids the body of vermine.

Peppermint stimulant, stomachic, carminative, aromatic, vermifuge, anodyne, antispasmodic, cholagogue, tonic, liver complaints, intestinal gas, nausea, seasickness, vomiting, chills, colic, fevers, dizziness, diarrhea, dysentery, cholera, influenza, heart problems, insanity, convulsions, spasm in infants, nervous headache, toothache, burns, rheumatism, colon troubles.

Plaintain   drawing, blood purifier, diuretic, external pain reliever, reduces inflammation.

Poke berries   arthritis.

Quince   used as setting lotion for hair.

Raspberry leaves   flu, fevers, digestive disorders, female genital problems.

Rosemary   used as a shampoo for dry hair, heart tonic, headache, colic, colds, nervous diseases, astringent, rheumatism, high blood pressure, stimulant, emmenagogue, ecphalic, aromatic, memory restorer when taken with sage, mouthwash, pyorrhea, toothpaste.

Saffron   corrects stomach acidity, dysentery, scarlet fever, jaundice, rheumatism, snake bite, gout, stops lactic acid build-up, resolves bruises, stimulates tissue regeneration, emmenagogue, unexpelled dead fetus, prolonged post-partum discharge.

Sage   intestinal gas, indigestion, ulcerations of the mouth, toothache, hair dressing, meat preservative, sore throat and gums, skin eruptions, astringent, nervine, colds, coughs, tonsilitis, tiredness, fever, thrush, summer complaint, worms in children.

Sarsaparilla   diuretic, alterative, demulcent, stimulant, carminative, tonic, impotence, spasmodic pains following childbirth, physical debility, weakness, psoriasis, syphilis, increase the body's natural defense mechanism to disease, rheumatism, gout, skin eruptions, ringworm, scrofula, intestinal inflammation, catarrhs, fever, colds, dropsy, blood purifier, eye wash.

Sassafras   diaphoretic, antiseptic, ant repellent, inflamed eyes, mild diuretic, tonic, blood purifier, chronic skin problems, emmenagogue.

Slippery elm   demulcent, emollient, pectoral, diuretic, nutritive, expectorant, tonic, food for weak people and convalescents, ulcers, soothes mucous linings of internal organs, diarrhea, dysentery, bronchitis, lung bleeding, cough, douche, poisoning, chapped skin, wounds, boils, tumors, burns, inflammation, and skin infections.

Strawberry   mild astringent, diuretic, tonic, diarrhea, dysentery, night sweats, liver complaints, gout, jaundice, blood purifier, eczema, sore mouth and throat.

Sweet basil   cold, headache, urinary distress, respiratory infections, snakebite, consumption.

Yarrow diaphoretic, blood purifier, nervine, glandular complaints, menstrual troubles, stimulant, tonic, astringent, vulnerary, diuretic, mucous membrane problems, bleeding from the lungs and urinary organs, diabetes, bleeding hemorrhoids, dysentery, stomach disorders, typhoid, colds, diarrhea, measles, smallpox, chickenpox, Bright's disease, colic, rheumatism, constipation, toothache, earache, leukorrhea, astringent, mild aromatic, emmenagogue, cramps, excess bleeding, used to correct oily hair (yarrow tea).

Yucca arthritis, intestinal disorders, soap.

Specific organs and systems of the body are affected by herbs. The following lists the areas of the body and which herbs affect them:[11]

Hair rosemary, sage, henna.

Brain lily of the valley, ginseng, gotu kola.

Ears eyebright, Golden Seal.

Nose for the sinuses, make a snuff of one part powdered bayberry bark and three parts Golden Seal root powder.

Mouth and Gums tincture of cayenne rubbed directly on the gums for any gum infection; the more you do it, the quicker the relief. Bayberry bark, oak bark, or rhatany root make a good mouth wash.

Throat mullein, sage, Golden Seal, slippery elm.

Bronchioles: For steaming, use benzoin, eucalyptus, bay, or poppy seeds; to expel mucus, yerba santa, blood root, hyssop, or elecampine.

Lungs comfrey, mullein, lobelia, oat straw (for TB), pleurisy root (for pleurisy), lungwort, and garlic.

Heart three tbsp. wheat germ oil a day, hawthorne berry tea; tansy should be used for pounding of the heart.

Blood pressure European mistletoe, apple bark to lower, and asafoetida to increase.

Stomach raspberry leaf, dandelion root, angelica, centaury, agrimony, calamus, wormwood, and Oregon grape root.

Small intestines turkey rhubarb root, slippery elm.

Large intestines cascara sagrada bark, squaw vine for the transverse colon.

Liver Oregon grape root, dandelion, agrimony, maple bark, mandrake.

Gall bladder olive oil, bayberry bark, comfrey, and the above-mentioned liver herbs.

Spleen maple leaves and bark, hyssop tea taken with steamed figs, bayberry bark, angelica.

Pancreas cedar berries, yarrow, periwinkle, dandelion.

Kidneys dandelion root, uva ursi, white poplar bark, sandlewood, parsley.

Bladder: same as above, including juniper berries, buchu, wild carrot seed, gravel root, and hydrangea for stones anywhere in the kidneys or bladder.

Prostate pumpkin seeds, a combination of echinacea and saw palmetto berries, uva ursi, gravel root.

Fertility sarsaparilla, false unicorn, damiana, licorice.

Uterus and Vagina dong kwai, squaw vine, Golden Seal root, oak bark, white pond lily, trillium or beth root, uva ursi, angelica, myrrh, yarrow.

Muscles comfrey, alfalfa, saw palmetto berries to increase weight.

Bones comfrey, horsetail grass gathered in late summer.

Arteries remove salt from diet, kelp, hawthorne berries, wheat germ oil.

Skin chickweed, walnut husk tincture (see formulas).

Circulation system cayenne (most powerful, fast-acting, nonirritating if uncooked, antiinflammatory), ginger, bayberry bark, prickly ash (for the joints and extremities), myrrh.

Digestive system hops, papaya, mustard seeds (one-half tsp. of whole seeds in a cup of warm water 20 minutes before eating), apple cider vinegar and honey (a tsp. of each in a glass of warm water 20 mins. before eating), tonic bitters (should be taken unsweetened) including centaury, gentian, agrimony, Oregon grape root, wormwood.

Endocrine gland system ginseng, sarsaparilla, yarrow, licorice, false unicorn root, true unicorn root, pumpkin seeds, kelp.

Respiratory system cayenne, lobelia, hyssop, elecampine, oat straw, garlic (best carrier of oyxgen in the body).

Urinary system dandelion root, parsley root and herb, wild carrot seed, juniper berries, uva ursi.

Nervous system   skullcap, valerian, hops, lobelia, ladies slipper root, passion flowers, linden flowers.

Medicinal uses for culinary herbs are:[12]

Allspice   aromatic, carminative, stimulant. Added to a bath, allspice is said to have anesthetic effects.

Anise   antispasmodic, aromatic, carminative, digestive, expectorant, stimulant, stomachic, tonic. Anise promotes digestion, improves appetite, alleviates cramps and nausea and relieves flatulence, especially in infants. Promotes the flow of milk in nursing mothers. Promotes menstruation. For insomnia, steep a few seeds in warm milk before going to bed. It is said that a strong decoction applied to the head will kill lice.

Basil   antispasmodic, carminative, stomachic. Used for stomach cramps, gastric catarrh, and excessive vomiting. Hindus use this holy herb to disinfect their homes. Used externally, it draws out poisons from insect bites. Has been used for antidote for hemp overdose.

Bay laurel   astringent, carminative, digestive, stomachic. Stimulating to digestion. Poultice good for chest colds or insect stings.

Bean   (dry pods before fully matured) diuretic, useful in dropsy, kidney and bladder trouble, uric acid accumulations, and loss of albumin in urine during pregnancy. Bean meal applied directly to cases of eczema, eruptions, and itching is beneficial.

Caraway   antispasmodic, carminative, emmenagogue, expectorant. Use caraway for flatulent colic, particularly in infants and to relieve nausea. Promotes menstrual flow, relieves uterine cramps, promotes milk in mothers, and is mildly expectorant. Powdered seed used as a poultice for bruises.

Cardamom   carminative, stimulant, stomachic. Cardamom is rarely used alone but rather in combination with other herbs.

Cayenne   stimulant, digestive, irritant, sialagogue, tonic. Stimulating both internally and externally. Care should be taken when taking cayenne in capsules as it can cause catarrh when taken in large doses. Produces heat for cold feet when put into socks.

Celery   Plant: diuretic, emmenagogue. Seed: carminative, sedative. Celery promotes sleep. Should be taken in moderate amounts when pregnant as it will promote menstruation in larger doses. Very helpful in clearing skin problems. Good poultice for burns, etc. If crushed and applied to poison oak, celery will help take away the swelling.

222   herbs

Chervil   digestive, diuretic, expectorant, stimulant.

Chives   digestive—contain iron, thus may be helpful in anemia.

Cinnamon   stomachic, carminative, mildly astringent, emmenagogue. Useful in diarrhea, nausea, vomiting, and flatulence. The tincture is useful in uterine hemorrhage.

Clove   anodyne, antiemetic, antiseptic. Good for toothache and teething babies if dropped in cavity or rubbed on gums.

Coriander   antispasmodic, aromatic, carminative, stomachic. Good addition to herbal preparations to improve taste. Will stop griping caused by laxatives and will expel gas. Young plants make good salad greens. The greens are called cilantro.

Cucumber   aperient, diuretic. Important in heart and kidney problems because of its ability to eliminate water from the body. Also helps dissolve uric acid accumulations. Good for chronic constipation. Cucumber juice is beneficial for intestines, lungs, kidneys, skin. Good local application for burns. Cooling and soothing to skin.

Dill   antispasmodic, calmative, carminative, diuretic, stomachic. Increases mother's milk especially when combined with anise, coriander, fennel, and caraway. Chew the seeds for bad breath. Will expel gas.

Fennel   antispasmodic, aromatic, carminative, diuretic, expectorant, stimulant, stomachic. Increases mother's milk. Helps relieve abdominal cramps, flatulence, and will expel mucus. Will stop griping from laxatives. Similar in almost every respect to anise.

Fenugreek   expectorant, mucilagenous, restorative. Good for people recovering from illness. Use as a gargle for sore throat. Excellent poultice for wounds.

Flax   demulcent, emollient, purgative. A decoction of seeds is used for coughs, catarrh, lung and chest problems, digestive and urinary disorders. Excellent poultice for sores.

Garlic   antiseptic, anthelmintic, antispasmodic, carminative, digestive, diuretic, expectorant, febrifuge. To break a fever in a small child or baby, oil the bottom of the child's feet, rub garlic juice (from pressed garlic) on the soles of the feet, taking care to wipe off any chunks of garlic pulp. Put socks on the child, bundle him up, put him to bed. The garlic will be absorbed into his system and he will sweat. Garlic stimulates peristaltic action in the bowels. The tincture is good for coughs, sore throat, diarrhea. Good for treating worms when given with a laxative. Use a slide of garlic to relieve painful gums temporarily.

Ginger   adjuvant, carminative, diaphoretic, stimulant. Promotes cleansing of the system through perspiration. Good for suppressed menstruation, flatulent colic, and to stimulate flow of saliva.

Horseradish   diuretic, rubifacient, stomachic. Use in colic, bladder infections, use externally to stimulate circulation. Good for sinus conditions and at the first sign of a cold. Grate ½ teaspoon, add a drop of lemon juice, and hold in the mouth. Inhale up through back of nose. Don't overdo it, though.

Lettuce   anodyne, antispasmodic, expectorant, sedative. When lettuce has gone to seed it contains a milky substance which is sedative. Good for insomnia and nervous conditions. Useful in coughs, asthma, and cramps. Excellent green poultice for bruises and burns.

Marjoram   antispasmodic, calmative, diaphoretic, expectorant, stomachic, tonic. Good for colic in children.

Nutmeg   aromatic, carminative, stimulant. Small amount of the oil aids digestion and stops flatulence. Used in hot foot baths.

Oregano   antispasmodic, calmative, carminative, diaphoretic, expectorant, stomachic, tonic, antiseptic. Good for headaches, nervousness, upset stomach and indigestion. Oil dropped in cavity is good for toothache. Calming bath additive. Leaves makes good sleep pillow for insomnia. Mexicans use it as an antiseptic for cuts and wounds.

Parsley   antispasmodic, carminative, diuretic, emmenagogue, expectorant. Excellent for jaundice, fevers, stones in kidneys, difficult urination. Helps prevent illness. Good source of vitamins A and B. Seeds are a febrifuge.

Potato   Excellent poultice when grated and applied fresh to old sores and ulcers. Poultice must be changed often and a new one applied. Also useful for burns and scalds. Hot potato water is good for swellings and painful areas. Never peel a potato as most nutrients are in the peel. Mealy flour made from baked potatoes is a good application for frostbite. Raw potato juice is good for gout, rheumatism.

Rosemary   antispasmodic, emmenagogue, stimulant, stomachic. Old remedy for colds, colic, and nerves (good for headache). Good gargle for sore throat. Aids digestion. Good for female problems but should be avoided by pregnant women.

Sage   antispasmodic, astringent, carminative. Cold tea is used to dry up mother's milk. Good in lung troubles. Inhale vapors to treat asthma. Cleansing for old sores and ulcers. Soothing to nerves. Excellent hair rinse for dandruff. Given hot will produce sweat. When signs of cold begin, drink sage tea (2 cups), get into hot bath, and sweat. Good for baby's colic and strengthening digestive tract.

Salt   (crude sea salt, or earth salt). Use as a mouthwash for infections of the gums. Use hot salt pack for relief. A salt glow is good for low blood pressure and sluggishness. It is a vigorous rub with hot wet salt after a cold shower. Contains trace minerals.

Savory   astringent, carminative, expectorant, stimulant. Good remedy for stomach disorders. Good in diarrhea. Will stop bleeding of wounds.

Tarragon   diuretic, emmenagogue, stomachic.

Thyme   anthelmintic, antispasmodic, carminative, expectorant, sedative, emmenagogue. Will cause perspiration when taken hot. Taken cold, good for diarrhea, cramps in the stomach, gas and lung troubles. Should be taken in moderate amounts when pregnant as it will promote menstruation in larger doses.

In case you found some unfamiliar words used to describe the properties of herbs, some definitions follow, of herbal preparations and terminology.[13]

Decoction   Seeds, barks, roots, and other hard materials are prepared by decoction. Put 1 oz herb in 1½ pints cold water. Cover and simmer for ½ hour. Then cover and steep for 15–30 minutes. Honey or lemon can be added. Use porcelain or glass vessels.

Fomentation   Dip cloth in the infusion or decoction, wring it out, and apply locally.

Infusion   Leaves, flowers, and some roots are prepared as teas or as infusions. Take 1 tsp per cup or 1 oz per pint. Do not boil the herb. Bring water to boil and pour the water over the herb. Cover and steep for 10–15 minutes. Honey or lemon can be added. Use porcelain or glass vessels.

Oil   Mix 2 tablespoons minced or powdered herbs with ¼ pint of oil. Place in hot sun or heat daily in hot water. Shake daily. After three weeks, strain and use.

Ointment or salve   Take 4 parts Vaseline or like substance to 1 part herb. Stir and heat gently for 20 minutes. Cool slightly and strain. This works best if herb has been ground.

Poultice   Bruise the herb, add enough boiling water to moisten it, then apply it to the affected part of the body, covering it with a cloth wrung out in hot water.

Syrup   Boil tea for 20 minutes, add 1 oz glycerin, and seal up in bottles as you would fruit.

Tincture   Add 1 oz powdered herb to 8 oz alcohol and 4 oz water. Shake daily. Let stand for two weeks, then strain.

Alterative   Gradually altering or changing a condition, also a blood purifier.

Anodyne   Relieving pain.

Antiperiodic   Preventing the periodic return of certain diseases.

Antiseptic   Destroying infection-causing microorganisms.

Antispasmodic   Relieving or preventing involuntary muscle spasms or cramps.

Aperient   Mild and gently acting laxative.

Aromatic   Substance with a spicy scent and a pungent but pleasing taste. Useful for fragrance, and often added to medicines to improve their palatability.

Astringent   Temporarily tightening or contracting the skin or tissues. Checks the discharge of mucus and blood, etc.

Carminative   Checking formation of gas and helping to dispel whatever gas has already formed.

Cholagogue   Promoting the discharge of bile from the system.

Deobstruent   Clearing obstruction from the natural ducts of the body.

Depurative   Removing wastes from body, purifying blood.

Detergent   A cleansing action.

Diaphoretic   Promoting sweating. Commonly used as an aid for relief of the common cold.

Diuretic   Promoting flow of urine.

Emmenagogue   Promoting menstruation.

Emollient   Softening and soothing skin when applied externally.

Expectorant   Loosening phlegm in the mucous membrane of the bronchial and nasal passages, thus facilitating its expulsion.

Hemostatic   Checking internal bleeding.

Hepatic   Affecting the liver.

Laxative A gentle cathartic that helps to promote bowel movements.

Mucilaginous A soothing quality for inflamed parts.

Nervine Calming nervous irritation from excitement, strain, or fatigue.

Pectoral Relieving ailments of the chest and lungs.

Refrigerant Generally cooling in effect, also reduces fevers.

Rubefacient Causing redness of the skin due to increased blood supply; usually works by irritation.

Sedative Calming the nerves.

Sialogogue Used to excite salivary glands, provoke secretion, and increased flow of saliva.

Stimulant Increasing or quickening various functions of the body, such as digestion and appetite. It does this quickly, whereas a tonic stimulates general health over a period of time.

Stomachic Strengthening and toning the stomach and stimulating the appetite.

Tonic Invigorating or strengthening the system.

Vasodilator Widening blood vessels.

Vermifuge Destroying and helping to expel intestinal worms.

Vulnerary Application for external wounds.

Finally, there are herbs that may have toxic properties and effects.[14]

Diuretics
• *Juniper:* Gastrointestinal irritation

• *Shave grass and horsetail:* Nicotine, thiaminase (excitement, loss of appetite and muscular control, diarrhea, difficulty breathing, convulsions, coma, death—all of the before-mentioned effects were observed in animals)

Cathartics
• *Buckthorn and senna:* Severe diarrhea

• *Aloe:* Strong irritant used in veterinary medicine for constipated large animals

Anticholinergic or Psychotogenic Effects
• *Burdock:* Blurred vision, dilated pupils, dry mouth, inability to void, bizarre behavior and speech, hallucinations

- *Catnip, juniper, hydrangea, lobelia, jimson weed, wormwood:* Euphoria, stimulant, hallucinogen

- *Nutmeg:* Hallucinogen, liver damage, death, severe headaches, cramps, nausea

Allergenic Properties
- *Chamomile:* Contact dermatitis, anaphylaxis, other hypersensitivity reactions

- *St. John's wort:* Delayed hypersensitivity, sensitivity of the skin to light

Cardiovascular Toxicity
- *Licorice root* (in large quantities): Salt and water retention, decreased potassium in the bloodstream, high blood pressure, heart failure, cardiac arrest

Possible Abortifacients
- *Devil's claw root:* Oxytocic properties

- *Pennyroyal oil:* Induce menstruation, kidney and liver toxicity

Carcinogens
- *Sassafras:* Liver toxin

Hormones
- *Ginseng:* Estrogens, swollen and painful breasts, nervousness, sleeplessness, low blood pressure, tranquilizing effects, skin eruptions, edema, lack of menstrual periods, diarrhea, laxative effect, depression, euphoria

Poisons
- *Indian tobacco* (contains lobeline): Sweating, vomiting, paralysis, depressed temperature, coma, death

- *Mistletoe:* Gastroenteritis (in animals, the following has been observed: depolarization of skeletal muscles, contracture of smooth muscle, constriction of the blood vessels, shock, cardiac arrest)

- *Poke:* Gastroenteritis, diminished respiratory response, death (these results have been observed in persons who ingested uncooked poke plant)

- *Apricot, bitter almond, cassava, cherry, choke cherry, peach, pear, apple, plum (seeds, pits, bark, leaves):* Liberates cyanic acid which can cause cyanide poisoning

- *Cassava:* Goiter, *tropical ataxic neuropathy, tropical amblyopia*

• *Mate:* Liver damage, death (when mate is ingested in large quantities)

As time goes on, these herbal products are being tested. Some herbs are found to do the things that are claimed. The herb chamomile, for instance, not only has cosmetic properties but it has also recently been found to counteract the effects of the acid gastric juice, pepsin; it also has an anti-inflammatory action on the body (that is, it reduces inflammation).[15]

Yet others not only fail to do what they are said to do, but they are actually dangerous. Be very aware that many of the claims made about the medicinal properties of herbs have not been proven. Remember our caution: The information in this section is not intended to replace the services of a physician.

CAUTIONS

Since herbal teas and other products have increased in popularity with increasing consumer interest in natural or health products, the negative side to the herb question should also be examined. These products are presented more often as foods than as drugs that may cause dangerous effects with long-term or heavy use. The serious side effects that have been noted are: kidney irritation, pain, vomiting, diarrhea, slowed pulse, lowered blood pressure, tremors, respiratory problems, weakness in the limbs, and convulsions.

Many of these substances, which are readily available in health food stores or by mail order, contain large amounts of psychoactive (mind-altering) substances; sometimes their use has resulted in serious intoxication. Of the 396 herbs and spices on the market commercially, 43 contain psychoactive substances and have caused serious intoxications.[16] Many people cannot drink tea or coffee for health reasons, and so they resort to herbal teas because of their variety in flavor and aroma. Often, they consume the "safer" herbal teas in larger quantities, not knowing that they contain a mind-altering drug that is relatively safe in small quantities but that may produce allergies or dangerous side effects in large quantities. To confuse the question, some herbs are like a double-edged sword: They may cause side effects with some people while they do nothing to others. For example, an herb may be a diuretic for one person but cause kidney irritation in another.

To make matters worse, packagers of herb products are not allowed to state on labels what herb products can do, and they cannot make health claims of any kind on labels. So there is no control or warning on herbs for public use. "Just because herbs are for sale in a store does not mean that they are necessarily safe, or the right choice for you."[17]

Another problem with herbal products (especially teas) is that the mixtures are often not prepared in the same manner each time and are not tested for purity. In other words, their quality is not controlled. Sometimes the impurities can be in the form of fibers, irritants, pollen, insect parts, mold, or spores, which may cause allergies among susceptible people.

Many people do not realize that herbal products can cause dangerous reactions when taken at the same time prescription drugs are taken. Drug–plant interactions are for the most part unknown. Some herbs can slow down the absorption of drugs into the bloodstream so that a drug's effects may last longer than expected. Other herbs can alter medication to a point that it becomes useless to the body or that it becomes poisonous to the system. Still other herbs combine with medications so that the medication cannot work properly.

Some herbs are even too dangerous to be sold on the market. For example, horsetail has produced nervous system reactions in animals that have eaten it. Mistletoe is another example of a dangerous plant: It contains poisonous proteins that can cause anemia, bleeding in the liver and intestines, and glandular problems in laboratory animals.[18] Another controversial herb is sassafras, which contains safrole as its major ingredient. In 1960, the FDA showed that safrole caused liver cancer in rats. At one time, safrole was used in root beer and other soft drinks, but now, because of its supposed danger, the FDA requires safrole-free sassafras to be used. Ever since that time, sassafras has been under fire, and there has been a controversy as to what contains safrole and what does not.[19]

As consumers, you need to be cautious in your use of herbs. Before using any herb concoction, you should check with your doctor to make sure that the herb is safe. Some doctors are opposed to herbal medicine and refuse to recommend it; but you're not after a recommendation, only an assurance that you won't *hurt* yourself. You should use common sense during use of the herb, too: Find out if the herb agrees with you. If you start to develop adverse reactions, such as rash, dizziness, fainting, palpitations, blurred vision, diarrhea, or depression, stop using the herb! You should also realize that large quantities of herbs may not be good for you. Ara der Marderosian has said: " . . . Ninety percent of herbal teas are OK at least in moderation, but they are not perfectly safe. . . . You cannot assume that just because it is sold, because it is natural, it is safe. . . ." He further explained: ". . . Years ago, these herbals were available only through pharmacies and were used as medicines. The consumer had more respect for them and their effects because he bought them as drugs. Now that they are sold in the commercial market (as foods or beverages) . . . the consumer is frequently uninformed."[20]

Herbs should never be used to treat serious conditions, which should receive medical attention. Herbs may do nothing to treat such conditions, or they may aggravate a condition to a point where it becomes very serious.

19

vitamins and minerals

Most people agree that the basis of good health is a nutritionally balanced diet. But they may never realize that good nutrition and a sound diet may increase the body's resistance to disease, provide more control of metabolic disturbances, and promote more rapid healing. Some people go even further, claiming that nearly all foods have some medicinal effect in addition to their nutritional values. Henry David Thoreau indicated that "a man may esteem himself happy when that which is his food is also his medicine."[1]

However, caution is advised in thinking that all diseases of the body and mind can be therapeutically cured by good nutrition. "Good food goes a long way towards good health, but food is not medicine. It does not take the place of proper medical care, nor is it a treatment to be applied only when a health problem is present. A balanced diet will correct many nutritional deficiencies, but it is much more effective in preventing poor health than in curing illness."[2]

In this chapter you may become aware of some of the current trends in nutrition and its relation to illness and health. Many of the ideas presented are merely that—ideas, not final or completely proven solutions. As always, be cautious in accepting as gospel the principles discussed here. Many of the theories are still in the supposition stage, and, in fact, many have been discounted as having no worth. We remind you again that *this section is not intended to replace the services of a physician.*

"Vitamins are chemical substances essential for the health, growth, and survival of human beings. They insure growth of different types of tissues and are necessary for proper functioning of nerves and muscles."[3] Dr. Joseph DiPalma adds to this definition of vitamins by indicating that vitamins are, ". . . organic chemical substances that serve as precursors of certain cofactors essential to the vital metabolic processes of the body. Except for a limited amount of Vitamin D, they cannot be synthesized in the body but must be obtained from food. When one or more of them is lacking in the diet, a deficiency disease results."[4] Typically, vitamins, in conjunction with enzymes, promote the growth, maintenance, repair, and coordination of cell and tissue function.

Because of their importance in body function, we must be certain that we take in enough vitamins with our diets each day. So we may make sure that we do, the United States Food and Drug Administration has formulated a list of food sources for each vitamin. They have also established Recommended Daily Allowances (RDAs) for each of the vitamins so we know the amount of each vitamin needed daily. The RDA indicates the intake of essential nutrients considered adequate for the known nutritional needs of practically all healthy people to ensure optimal growth and body function. In effect, the RDAs are usually far above the actual nutrient requirements to meet these needs.

In addition, the RDAs do not account for special health problems that may require more vitamin intake: pregnancy, lactation, the taking of oral contraceptives, chronic disease, alcoholism, the taking of certain drugs that interfere with the body's ability to absorb certain nutrients, cigarette smoking, and stress conditions such as injury, fever, or infection. For example, smokers require more vitamin C. Heavy drinkers often have increased needs for vitamins B_1, B_6, and folic acid. Women taking oral contraceptives have lower levels of vitamins B_1, B_2, B_{12}, C, folic acid, and B_6; the need for B_6 can be two to ten times as great as that for women not on the Pill. Those who suffer from stressful conditions need extra portions of vitamins C, B_6, and pantothenic acid.

Most nutritionists agree that individuals can get all the vitamins they need to fulfill the RDAs from the foods they eat—provided they get the right kinds of foods. Eating the proper foods in the proper amounts from the Basic Four Food Groups (meat, milk and dairy products, fruits and vegetables, and breads and cereals) can ensure adequate intake of the vitamins and maintain a healthy body. Remember, though, that even if you are taking in the right foods in the proper amounts, those foods may not contain all the vitamins your body needs. Vitamins can be easily destroyed in several ways. Exposure to air, light, heat, and multiple handling can destroy the vitamin value of many of our foods. To ensure that you get the most vitamins from your food, you should:

- use fresh foods in your diet as much as possible,
- use a minimum of water in cooking foods,
- cook foods for the least possible time, and
- avoid storage of foods.

Although there are very few full-blown, clinical cases of vitamin deficiencies in the United States, nutritionists feel that, in many sub-clinical deficiencies, individuals do not manifest gross abnormalities or symptoms of the deficiency. The following table offers guidelines to discern less apparent vitamin deficiencies.

If you notice abnormalities in body tissues, it could mean a vitamin deficiency. Check with your doctor to be sure. Additionally, the following table has been designed specifically with you, the consumer, in mind. It gives you a brief but complete overview of the most common vitamins in your diet. It also helps you know what each vitamin does in your body to help it function and maintain its health. It lists the RDA for each vitamin, tells you the best food sources of the vitamin, indicates some of the problems that can result from not taking enough of the vitamin, states some of the claims and controversy surrounding megavitamin therapy for each vitamin, and suggests what to look for if you suspect that you are getting too much of the vitamin.

The existence of subclinical deficiencies is due to such things as personal likes and dislikes in food, ethnic preferences for certain foods, fixed incomes that limit the purchase of various kinds of foods, super-

SYMPTOMS AND POSSIBLE VITAMIN DEFICIENCIES

AFFECTED TISSUE	DEFICIENT VITAMIN
Skin	A, K, B_2, B_3, B_6, biotin, C
Mouth	B_2, B_3, B_6, B_{12}, biotin, C
Intestines	B_1, B_3, B_6,
Eye	A, D, K, B_1, B_2, B_3, C
Nervous system	B_1, B_3, B_6, B_{12}, folic acid
Blood (anemias)	E, B_2, B_{12}, biotin, folic acid
Heart and vessels	E, B_1, B_3, C
Skeleton	A, D, C

stition and fixed ideas about foods and nutrition, geographic and climatic differences that influence food and eating habits, and seasonal variations in food that make many foods unavailable at certain times.[5] Another recent factor is the rising popularity of eating convenience foods and eating away from home. Today, 36 percent of the total food dollar is spent on food away from home. In addition, soft drink consumption has increased 80 percent since World War II; pastry consumption has increased 70 percent in the same time period; and potato chip consumption has increased 85 percent. At the same time, dairy product consumption has decreased by 21 percent, the consumption of vegetables has decreased 23 percent, and fruit consumption has decreased by 25 percent.[6]

Some individuals do need vitamins supplements of some kind. Those who eat poorly, who are on fixed incomes, who have chronic disease, who are pregnant, who are experiencing growth and development spurts, and others may need extra vitamins. Before beginning a vitamin supplement program, though, you should keep the following items in mind:

1. Attempting to treat illness symptoms with vitamins is generally considered to be folly; vitamins are foods, not drugs.

2. Laypeople should not attempt to self-diagnose and/or treat vitamin deficiencies.

3. Do not begin vitamin supplementation without consulting your doctor who knows your specific needs.

4. Stop vitamin supplementation at the first sign of negative symptoms.

5. Avoid all nutritional fads and fetishes.

6. Vitamins alone do not promote good health; you should also follow other good health practices, such as getting enough exercise and rest, eating properly, abstaining from or limiting the use of alcohol and tobacco, and so on.[7]

Remember that "vitamin supplementation should not be used as an excuse for dietary slothfulness."[8] "The person who works on a supplement program and ignores the daily diet of whole food is like the runner who spends more time selecting a pair of track shoes than actually training."[9]

ORTHOMOLECULAR NUTRITION AND
MEGAVITAMIN THERAPY

Orthomolecular psychiatry deals with nutrition and the concentration of essential substances for optimum brain functioning. This approach may encompass several aspects of the nutrition area. So-called *orthomolecular nutrition* implies the absence of "junk foods" in the diet. Maintaining that the best foods are whole foods, it recommends the identification of food allergies so that the individual may stay away from those foods that cause allergic reactions. It also advocates a wide variety of foods, to be eaten more frequently and in smaller quantities. Probably the most well-known aspect of orthomolecular psychiatry is the megavitamin therapy approach, as advocated by Linus Pauling. Dr. Pauling indicates that the goal of megavitamin therapy is to "create the correct molecular environment for optimal health with certain elements."[10] To accomplish this, he endorses taking large amounts of vitamins (ten times or more above the RDA), moderate amounts of minerals, or eliminating certain harmful substances from the diet.

Megavitamin therapy—especially the B vitamins—is currently used in treatment of schizophrenia and other mental disorders. Take, for example, the case of Stephen Warner. While attending a college in New Jersey at the age of 19, Stephen began to act peculiarly. He played his stereo through the loudspeaker on the roof of his dormitory at 3:00 AM one morning, thus arousing the whole campus at that unearthly hour. Stephen, who was usually quiet, introspective, analytical, thoughtful, and a peacemaker, became argumentative and hysterical at times. His parents were extremely worried at the change that had come over their son, and their fears were not allayed when they called their son at the college, and his conversations with them were irrelevant and jumbled.

The Warners finally took their son to the family physician, and, after listening to the boy's symptoms and behavior, the doctor labeled the young man schizophrenic. The parents were heartsick over the diagnosis and quite unwilling to commit their son to an institution.

About this time, Stephen decided to leave college and go to the north woods to become a lumberjack. The college dean called Stephen's parents to tell them of this decision. Just as the parents decided to call the police for help, Stephen walked in looking disheveled, wild-eyed, and babbling.

After trying traditional approaches to the problem of Stephen's schizophrenia, the worried parents finally decided to try the orthomolecular psychiatry approach. Stephen was put on a no-junk food regimen with megavitamin and multimineral supplements. He also took minimal dosages of two tranquilizers.

In two weeks Stephen was responsive to conversations. He dressed more neatly, resumed eating with more enthusiasm, attempted to read, and called friends to report his progress. In four weeks, he had friends over to visit. He went to the library and the movies. Later, he began to go to college again—at first parttime and then fulltime. In time, Stephen Warner graduated magna cum laude with a BS in business, receiving some of the university's highest awards for scholarship and leadership. He also received scholarship awards for his outstanding achievement. He is now an executive with a noted business firm.[11]

With cases like Stephen's, enthusiasts support the claim that megavitamins enable individuals to function more efficiently, lose their anger and irritability, heighten perception and creativity, rid themselves of depression, and enjoy greater brain efficiency.[12] But schizophrenia and other mental disorders are not the only problems that are said to be relieved. Megavitamin therapy is currently used to treat a great variety of ailments—skin problems, reproductive disorders, gastrointestinal diseases, among others.

However they have a negative side. Note that the relief of these conditions is listed under the heading "Claims and Controversy" in the accompanying table. They are merely that—claims that are yet unproven and controversies that are as yet unresolved. The present knowledge about the safety or tolerance of massive doses of vitamins is still incomplete, and the evidence of potential hazards is still growing. The table shows that vitamin toxicities do occur, and some very serious and deadly symptoms can occur with overuse of vitamin compounds.

Apparently, part of the danger of megavitamin therapy and the possibility of toxicity relate to the fact that the concentration of vitamins necessary for tissue saturation is usually considerably lower than the megadose of the vitamin. In addition, some researchers have indicated recently that massive doses of vitamins may interfere with certain medications. If so, persons who need medication for medical problems may not derive all the benefits from the medicine they are taking. Other recent studies indicate that vitamin therapy for the treatment of diseases unrelated to vitamin deficiencies is effective in only a few instances. Besides, the prevention through megavitamin supplements of diseases not caused by a specific vitamin deficiency is extremely difficult to prove or disprove. These researchers conclude that there is no convincing evidence of unique health benefits occurring from the excessive consumption of any one vitamin or nutrient.[13]

We recommend extreme caution in using megavitamins as self-medication. They can be dangerous in that their claims may not be completely proven or justified.

OVERVIEW OF COMMON VITAMINS

VITAMIN	FUNCTION OF VITAMIN	RDA	FOOD SOURCES
Vitamin A	Important for normal growth and development of children. Necessary for good vision (visual purple, rod vision). Necessary for healthy skin, eyes, and hair; maintains the health of the skin and mucous membranes in general.	4,000 IU Women 5,000 IU Men	Beef liver, milk, butter, margarine, kidney, egg yolk, apricots, broccoli, cantaloupe, parsley, turnips.

Sources: Editors of *Consumer Guide*, *The Vitamin Book* (New York: Simon & Schuster, Inc., 1979), pp. 39–174; Nutrition Search, Inc., *Nutrition Almanac* (New York: McGraw-Hill Book Company, 1979), pp. 86–90; Morton Walker, "Vitamins: What They Can (and Can't) Do for You," *Consumers Digest* (January–February, 1979), p. 18; Robert J. Benowicz, *Vitamins and You* (New York: Grosset & Dunlap, Inc., 1979), pp. 73–87; Brent Q. Hafen *et al.*, *Food, Nutrition, and Weight Control* (Allyn & Bacon, Inc.: Longwood Division, 1980).

DEFICIENCY	CLAIMS AND CONTROVERSY OF MEGAVITAMIN THERAPY	TOXICITY
Xerophthalmia—night blindness, rough, dry, scaly skin, increased susceptibility to infections, frequent fatigue, loss of smell and appetite.	Arterial diseases: angina, arteriosclerosis, atherosclerosis, stroke, myocardial infarction, congestive heart failure, rheumatic fever. Glandular diseases: diabetes, hyperthyroidism, cystic fibrosis, prostatitis, goiter. Eye diseases: glaucoma, night blindness, cateracts, amblyopia, conjunctivitis. Nervous diseases: alcoholism, epilepsy, meningitis, schizophrenia. Gastrointestinal diseases: celiac disease, colitis, hemorrhoids, peptic ulcer, gastritis, gastroenteritis, gout. Kidney diseases: renal calculi, nephritis, cystitis. Liver diseases: cirrhosis, hepatitis, jaundice, gall stones. Lung diseases: allergies, asthma, bronchitis, emphysema, influenza, TB. Skin diseases: eczema, psoriasis, impetigo, shingles, acne, pyorrhea, boils, dandruff, warts, squamous metaplasia. Reproductive disorders: menopause, vaginitis. Miscellaneous: resistance to infection, aging, sore throat.	Retarded growth, increased skull pressure (severe headache), dizziness, diarrhea, cirrhosis-like symptoms, overabundance of calcium in the body, loss of appetite, blurred vision, loss of hair, dry flaky skin, enlargement of liver and spleen, rheumatic pain, menstrual cycle disturbance.

VITAMIN	FUNCTION OF VITAMIN	RDA	FOOD SOURCES
Vitamin E	Helps regulate lipid oxidation. Necessary for red blood cell functioning. Protects essential fatty acids.	12 IU Women 15 IU Men	Asparagus, broccoli, cabbage, chocolate, margarine, oils, peanuts, wheat germ, whole grains, yeast, lettuce.
Vitamin D	Aids absorption of calcium and phosphorous from the intestines so that strong bones and teeth are produced.	400 IU	Ultraviolet light, liver oils, margarine, egg yolk, lard, yeast, shrimp, salmon, tuna, fortified milk.

DEFICIENCY	CLAIMS AND CONTROVERSY OF MEGAVITAMIN THERAPY	TOXICITY
Rupture of red blood cells, muscular wasting, abnormal fat deposition in muscles.	Skin diseases: acne, baldness, boils, bruises, scarring, warts, liver spots, diaper rash, frostbite, sunburn. Lung disorders: allergies, lung damage caused by air pollution. Digestive disorders: gout, ulcers. Cardiovascular diseases: high blood pressure, heart disease, arteriosclerosis, angina. Blood diseases: decreases serum cholesterol, decreases clotting, hemolytic anemia in preemies. Skeleto-muscular disorders: pain from torn ligaments, bursitis, muscular dystrophy, calf pain when walking. Reproductive disorders: labor pains, miscarriage, sexual impotence, sterility, infertility. Miscellaneous: detoxification, aging, delays the process of oxidation.	Minimal toxicity.
Osteomalacia—soft bones in adults, rickets—poor bone and tooth formation, softening of bones and teeth, inadequate absorption of calcium, phosphorous retention in the kidneys.	Bone diseases: fractures, rickets, osteoporosis, osteomalacia, arthritis. Eye diseases: nearsightedness, bitot spots (spots on the conjunctive of the eye), glaucoma, cataracts. Lung disorders: colds, TB, allergies. Nerve disorders: sciatica, leg cramps, epilepsy, meningitis, backache. Reproductive disorders: menopause, premenstrual tension, menstrual problems. Gastrointestinal diseases: ulcers.	Calcification of the kidneys and other organs and soft tissues, weakness, lassitude, headache, nausea, vomiting, diarrhea, excessive urination, weight loss, absence of appetite, constipation.

VITAMIN	FUNCTION OF VITAMIN	RDA	FOOD SOURCES
Vitamin K	Essential for normal blood clotting.	60.0 mg	Intestinal bacteria, green leafy vegetables, beef, pork, cauliflower, tomatoes, peas, carrots.
Vitamin B₁ (thiamine)	Necessary for the normal metabolism of carbohydrates. Essential for normal heart and nervous system function.	1.00 mg Women 1.4 mg Men Based on 0.50 mg per 1000 calories	Brewer's yeast, beef kidney, ham, eggs, plums, prunes, raisins, wheat germ, whole grain flour, fish, poultry, lean meat, peanuts, legumes.
Vitamin B₂ (riboflavin)	Part of the body enzyme systems responsible for energy transfer. Necessary for building and maintaining body tissues. Promotes healthy skin. Helps prevent sensitivity of the eyes to light.	1.2 mg Women 1.6 mg Men Based on 0.60 mg per 1000 calories	Liver, heart, kidneys (beef, sheep, pork, veal); brewer's yeast; broccoli; eggs; enriched bread and cereals; lean meats; milk; leafy green vegetables.

DEFICIENCY	CLAIMS AND CONTROVERSY OF MEGAVITAMIN THERAPY	TOXICITY
Lack of prothrombin, increased blood clotting time—hemorrhagic disease of the newborn, hemorrhage in adults.	Digestive disorders: constipation, digestive disorders, liver toxicity. Cardiac diseases: high blood pressure. Reproductive disorders: menopause. Miscellaneous: fatigue.	Red blood cell destruction, antagonism of blood coagulants.
Beriberi—Gastrointestinal disorders, fatigue, loss of appetite, nerve disorders, heart disorders, constipation, labored breathing, nausea, tiredness of the calf, spastic colon, depression.	Stress diseases: mental illness, anemia, sciatica, alcoholism, neuritis, MS, Bell's palsy, toxic poisoning, diabetes, decreased adrenal gland function, anxiety neurosis. Heart diseases: coronary thrombosis, congestive heart failure. Eye and ear diseases: night blindness, lazy eye syndrome, Meniere's syndrome, infections. Skin diseases: shingles, dermatitis. Miscellaneous: increased energy.	No toxicity or undesirable side effects have followed use of large doses of thiamine.
Eye problems, cracks and sores in the mouth, dermatitis, retarded growth, digestive disturbances.	Nervous diseases: Parkinsonism, MS, migraines. Urinary disorders: nephritis. Reproductive disorders: inflammation of the vagina. Skeletal disorders: arthritis. Eye and ear diseases: Meniere's syndrome, glaucoma, conjunctivitis, xerophthalmia, cataracts. Digestive diseases: peptic ulcers, colon cancer.	No known oral toxicity.

VITAMIN	FUNCTION OF VITAMIN	RDA	FOOD SOURCES
Vitamin B₃ (niacin)	Used in conjunction with the enzymes involved in energy transfer and carbohydrate metabolism.	13 mg Women 18 mg Men Based on 6.6 mg per 1000 calories	Intestinal bacteria, liver, roasted peanuts, swordfish, tuna, halibut, yeast, lean meats, poultry, legumes, milk.
Vitamin B₆ (pyridoxine)	Part of the enzyme systems involved in protein metabolism and utilization of essential fatty acids.	2 mg	Liver, brewer's yeast, peanuts, herring, mackerel, salmon, soybeans, walnuts, lean meats, milk, legumes.

DEFICIENCY	CLAIMS AND CONTROVERSY OF MEGAVITAMIN THERAPY	TOXICITY
Pellagra—dermatitis, diarrhea, deterioration of mental function, loss of appetite, digestive disturbances, intestinal ulceration, swollen red tongue.	Mental illness: paranoia, schizophrenia, depression, anxiety neurosis, hyperactivity, mental retardation, alcoholism. Brain diseases: Parkinsonism, epilepsy, MS. Cardiovascular diseases: arteriosclerosis, atherosclerosis, elevated cholesterol, diabetes, high blood pressure, phlebitis, vessel dilator, heart attacks. Eye diseases. Gastrointestinal diseases: diarrhea, digestive disturbances. Lung diseases: asthma. Bone diseases: arthritis.	Flushing, pus formation, skin rash, heartburn, nausea, vomiting, diarrhea, activation of ulcer, low blood pressure, fainting, rapid heartbeat, jaundice, sensation of tingling or burning of the skin.
Anemia, mouth disorders, nervousness, muscular weakness, dermatitis, sensitivity to insulin, dizziness, nausea, weight loss, may reduce immunological protection.	Skin diseases: acne (premenstrual). Kidney disease: kidney stones. Arterial diseases: elevated cholesterol, pernicious anemia, low blood sugar, diabetes, anemia. Nervous diseases: epilepsy, mental illness, neuritis, Parkinsonism, MS, Bell's palsy, cerebral palsy, migraines, headaches, dizziness, insomnia, paralysis due to nerve damage. Bone and joint diseases: arthritis, muscle spasm. Gastrointestinal diseases: intestinal malabsorption disease, gastritis, colitis, vomiting, diarrhea, nausea due to morning sickness and anesthetics. Cardiovascular diseases: arteriosclerosis, atherosclerosis. Miscellaneous: sore throat, hemorrhoids, lack of energy, weak memory, breath holding in children, hangovers, suppression of lactation.	Convulsive disorders, may inhibit effect of levodopa (which is used to treat Parkinson's Disease), temporary dependency.

VITAMIN	FUNCTION OF VITAMIN	RDA	FOOD SOURCES
Vitamin B$_{12}$ (cyanoco-balamin)	Necessary for normal red blood cell synthesis. Contributes to the health of the nervous system. Necessary for proper growth in children.	3 mg	Intestinal bacteria, liver, egg yolk, crab, salmon, sardines, herring, oysters, lean meats, milk, kidney.
Pantothenic acid	Necessary for use of carbohydrates, fats, and proteins in the body.	No RDA established—5–20 mg usually meets daily requirements.	Almost universally present in plant and animal tissues, lean meats, egg yolk, peanuts, potatoes.
Biotin	Necessary for carbohydrate, fat, and protein metabolism. Utilization of other B vitamins.	100–300 mg usually meets daily requirements.	Egg yolk, green vegetables, milk, liver, kidney.
Folic acid	Necessary for red blood cell formation. Maintains the function of the intestinal tract.	400 mg	Leafy green vegetables, yeast, meats, fish, milk.

DEFICIENCY	CLAIMS AND CONTROVERSY OF MEGAVITAMIN THERAPY	TOXICITY
Pernicious anemia—brain damage, nervousness, neuritis, spinal cord degeneration.	Arterial diseases: anemia, angina, arteriosclerosis, atherosclerosis, diabetes, low blood sugar. Reproductive disorders: menstrual problems. Respiratory problems. Liver disease. Mental illness. Muscle and joint diseases: muscular dystrophy, osteoporosis, arthritis, bursitis. Gastrointestinal diseases: ulcers, abdominal cavity disease, gastritis. Miscellaneous: fatigue.	No toxic or adverse reactions have been known to occur following large doses.
Vomiting, restlessness, stomach stress, increased susceptibility to infection, sensitivity to insulin.	Gastrointestinal disorders: digestive disturbances, gout. Reproductive disorders: menopause. Bone and joint disorders: arthritis. Miscellaneous: restores color to gray hair, sore throat.	Essentially nontoxic.
Dermatitis, grayish skin color, depression, muscle pain, impairment of fat, metabolism, poor appetite.	Skin diseases: Leiner's disease (oily skin rash on infants who breast feed from malnourished mothers). Heart disease. Mental disorders.	No toxic or adverse reaction has yet been demonstrated.
Megaloblastic anemia—poor growth, gastrointestinal disorders, B_{12} deficiency, nutritional mecrocytic anemia.	Blood disorders: anemia. Mental disorders.	Decreased efficacy of phenytoin, increased size of kidney cells, may mask symptoms of pernicious anemia.

VITAMIN	FUNCTION OF VITAMIN	RDA	FOOD SOURCES
Vitamin C (ascorbic acid)	Necessary for healthy teeth, gums, and bones. Helps build strong body cells and vessels. Participates in many cellular metabolic functions.	45 mg	Green peppers, parsley, guava, broccoli, brussel, sprouts, strawberries, citrus fruits, melons, tomatoes, leafy green vegetables, cabbage, new potatoes.

DEFICIENCY	CLAIMS AND CONTROVERSY OF MEGAVITAMIN THERAPY	TOXICITY
Scurvy—bleeding gums, swollen or painful joints, slow-healing wounds, slow-healing fractures, bruising, nosebleeds, impaired digestion.	Stress diseases: lead poisoning, cancer, decreased adrenal gland function. Cardiovascular diseases: arteriosclerosis, atherosclerosis, anemia, pernicious anemia, angina (chest pains), elevated cholesterol, diabetes, hemophilia, high blood pressure, low blood sugar, leukemia, mononucleosis, phlebitis, stroke, varicose veins. Bone diseases; backache, osteoporosis, fractures, osteomalacia, rickets, arthritis, bursitis, gout. Gastrointestinal diseases; abdominal cavity disease, colitis, gastritis, gastroenteritis, peptic ulcer. Eye and ear disorders: glaucoma, focus disorders, cataracts, lazy eye syndrome. infections, corneal ulcers. Brain diseases: MS, Parkinsonism, mental illness, senility, meningitis, dizziness. Lung diseases: allergies, bronchitis, emphysema, influenza, pneumonia, TB, croup, colds. Glandular diseases; cystic fibrosis, goiter, prostatitis, swollen glands. Kidney diseases: nephritis, renal calculi. Liver diseases: hepatitis, jaundice cirrhosis. Muscle disorders: muscular dystrophy, rheumatism. Skin diseases; boils, bruises, pressure sores. Reproductive disorders: menstrual disorders. Miscellaneous: increased resistance to disease, fatigue, nosebleeds, sore throat, facilitation of electron transfer, inhibition of histamine action, bee stings.	Relatively safe, most doses are not toxic. The following toxic reactions may occur in only a few people when taking *large* doses: some people may experience abdominal discomfort, cramps, and diarrhea; a few people are prone to developing kidney stones faster; megadoses may interfere with urine and blood tests used for diagnosis of disease; may also affect drugs being used to dissolve blood clots; people who become conditioned to high levels may express symptoms of deficiency when they return to normal levels (this can also affect a baby in utero).

VITAMINS B$_{15}$ AND B$_{17}$

Recently, chemical substances have been discovered that have been labeled as "vitamins." Little is known or proven about the value of these substances in disease treatment or prevention. Two of the more popular "new" vitamins are vitamin B$_{15}$ and vitamin B$_{17}$.

Vitamin B$_{15}$. Pangamic acid, although commonly referred to as a vitamin, in reality has not been fully identified as a vitamin, since its need in human nutrition has not been established completely. B$_{15}$, discovered by American biochemist Dr. E. T. Krebs, apparently functions as a coenzyme in respiration, protein formation, and the regulation of steroid hormones.

Many benefits have been assigned to B$_{15}$, such as possible detoxification of environmental pollutants, protection of the liver, reducing the susceptibility to infection, promoting the activity of white blood cells, treating old age symptoms, prevention of premature aging, relieving emotional and mental problems, treating chronic alcoholism, treating gangrene, improvement of physical energy, lessening of fatique, increasing strength (especially in athletic events), causing injuries to heal faster, and treating diabetes.

As yet, these claims have not been totally substantiated. Food sources of B$_{15}$ are as follows: brewer's yeast, organ meats, whole grains, apricot kernels, rice bran, seeds, sunflower seeds, and pumpkin seeds.

Vitamin B$_{17}$. Better known as laetrile, this vitamin-like compound comes from the pits of apricots. It has been claimed to relieve the suffering of terminal cancer patients, and it has been further supposed to aid in the prevention of cancer as well.

Like B$_{15}$, B$_{17}$ has not been fully identified as a vitamin because the FDA also asserts that laetrile does not promote any physiological process vital to the existence of living organisms. So, no disease state is either produced or alleviated by the absence or presence of laetrile.[14] Even though laetrile is recognized as legitimate cancer therapy in more than twenty nations in the world, its questionable value has caused laetrile use in this country to be strongly opposed by the FDA and the medical profession.[15]

Not only is the therapeutic value of laetrile doubtful, then, but using the compound entails other dangers. Laetrile contains cyanide, a deadly poison; large amounts of laetrile would present a definite danger of cyanide poisoning. Also, laetrile is not subject to the FDA control for quality and purity, so often other toxic substances may appear in the drug, which might cause adverse or allergic reactions.

MINERALS

Besides nutrient materials such as proteins, carbohydrates, fats, water, and vitamins, one other category of nutrients is essential for a healthy body: minerals. Like vitamins, minerals are required for the maintenance of proper body function, and they are not synthesized or made by the human body. Also like vitamins, minerals are obtained through food intake. Generally, milk products, meats, grains, and vegetables, when consumed in varieties, have been shown to meet the basic RDAs. However, one other thing influences the mineral content of some foods to a certain extent, and that is the chemical composition of the water used for the preparation and cooking of the food. Foods cooked in soft waters (that is, waters low in mineral content) lose minerals, and foods cooked in hard waters (waters high in mineral content) may gain mineral content. Foods cooked or otherwise prepared in hard water, then, may contain the following minerals: iodine, calcium, chromium, lithium, silicon, magnesium, and fluorine.

The role of the minerals as they relate to the body and disease is unclear at this time. Yet this much can be said: Playing a subtle but crucial role in bodily functions, minerals have both building and regulatory functions. In building, the minerals promote the healthy formation of the skeleton and soft tissues of the body. And their regulatory function lies in the areas of heartbeat, blood clotting, internal pressures of body fluids, nerve response, oxygen transport to the tissues, hormone activation, and the activation of other biochemical molecules. Several degenerative diseases have been shown to be influenced by the minerals: atherosclerosis, muscular dystrophy, rheumatoid arthritis, and multiple sclerosis. Further research in these areas will undoubtedly reveal more substantial evidence as as time goes on. For now, this area remains basically a mystery.

The table that follows provides you with more information concerning minerals that appear in your diet. The minerals listed are those macroelements and microelements (trace elements) that are essential or are believed to be essential to your health, how these minerals function in your body, how much of each mineral is required for adults, the best food sources for each, and what happens to your body if there is a deficiency of a mineral.

MINERALS (INORGANIC ELEMENTS)

MINERAL	RDA	FOOD SOURCES	DEFICIENCY
Macroelements			
Calcium: Almost all of the body's calcium is in bones and teeth; only one percent is in body fluids; essential for blood clotting, muscle contraction, and transmission of nerve impulses.	RDA: 800 mg	Milk and dairy products are the best food sources. Green, leafy vegetables are good sources (except spinach and chard), citrus fruits, dried peas, and beans.	Caused only by low intakes, deficiency is extremely rare. It may occur secondary to vitamin D deficiency, adversely affecting bones and teeth.
Chloride: Components of stomach acid; with other elements helps to maintain acid-base balance in body fluids.	RDA not established	Chloride supplied by salt (sodium chloride) present in or added to foods.	Dietary deficiency does not occur in humans unless salt intake is severely restricted.
Magnesium: Most of the body's magnesium is in bones; the remainder is inside body cells taking part in many enzyme reactions. Important for nerve and muscle function.	RDA: Men: 350 mg; Women: 300 mg	Dried peas and beans, nuts, whole-grain cereals, cocoa, and chocolate are the best food sources. Green leafy vegetables are good sources.	Deficiency causes muscle tremors, convulsions, hyperexcitability, weakness, behavioral disturbances. Usually seen only in disease conditions, e.g., alcoholism, kidney disease, malabsorption syndromes.

Source: editors of *Consumer Guide, The Vitamin Book* (New York: Simon & Schuster, Inc., 1979), pp. 212–218.

MINERAL	RDA	FOOD SOURCES	DEFICIENCY
Phosphorus: Eighty percent of the body's phosphorus is in bones and teeth. Present in all cells as part of compounds vital for many reactions of metabolism; essential for energy production.	RDA: 800 mg	Milk, dairy products, meats, dried peas and beans, and whole-grain cereals are good sources. Fruits and vegetables have small amounts. Poultry, fish, eggs.	Dietary deficiency does not occur in humans. Deficiency may occur secondary to prolonged and excessive use of some antacids.
Potassium: Most of the body's potassium is present inside cells; very little is in body fluids. Helps to regulate acid-base and fluid balance; important for regulating muscle action and transmission of nerve impulses.	RDA not established; healthy adults need about 2.5 g per day.	Bananas, citrus fruits, carrots, green, leafy vegetables, potatoes, and tomatoes are rich sources. Whole-grain cereals, meats, and seafoods are good sources.	Deficiency usually seen only in disease conditions which cause excessive loss of body potassium.
Sodium: Sodium is present in fluids outside of cells; only small amounts are found within cells. Sodium functions with chloride and potassium to regulate water and acid-base balance and to regulate muscle and nerve action.	RDA not established; intakes probably range from about 2.5 g to 7 g per day.	Sodium content of animal foods (meats, dairy products, eggs) higher than that of fruits, vegetables, and cereals. Main source is salt used in processing, preservation, and seasoning. Some medications, such as laxatives, sedatives, cough medicines, also contain salt.	Dietary deficiency does not occur in humans. Excessive losses of body sodium in certain disease conditions may cause evidence of deficiency.

Microelements

MINERAL	RDA	FOOD SOURCES	DEFICIENCY
Chromium: Necessary for maintaining normal blood concentration of sugar (glucose).	RDA not established; the World Health Organization suggests 20 to 50 μg per day is needed to replace urinary losses.	Meats, especially liver, whole-grain cereals, and brewer's yeast are good sources. Availability from food varies widely. Beef, bread, mushrooms, green leafy vegetables.	Deficiency apparently causes disturbances in blood sugar metabolism. Marginal deficiency may exist during pregnancy, in diabetics, and in the elderly.
Cobalt: Functions only as integral part of vitamin B_{12}.	RDA not established; no need except as B_{12}.	Vitamin B_{12} present only in animal foods (meats, seafood, and dairy products).	No known symptoms due to cobalt deficiency.
Copper: Component of enzymes that function in energy production, amino acid metabolism, and iron metabolism. Necessary for making hemoglobin.	RDA not established; estimated need is about 2 mg per day.	Nuts, dried legumes, liver, oysters, other seafood, and green vegetables are good sources. Dairy foods, meats, cereals are relatively poor sources.	Not seen in human adults. In infants and children with poor diets, copper deficiency may contribute to anemia and poor bone development.
Fluorine: Necessary in teeth to provide maximum protection against decay. May contribute to maintenance of bone structure.	RDA not established; recommend addition to drinking water to provide about 1 mg per quart.	Most foods contain only small amounts. Seafoods are fair sources. Tea and small fish eaten with bones (sardines) are good sources.	In infants and children deficiency may have adverse effects on bone structure and strength.

MINERAL	RDA	FOOD SOURCES	DEFICIENCY
Iodine: Component of hormones produced by the thyroid gland. These regulate energy metabolism.	RDA: Men: 130 μg; Women: 100 μg.	Iodized salt and seafoods are excellent sources. Bread made by continuous-mix process has high content.	Deficiency affects function of thyroid gland and produces goiter. Severe deficiency causes impairment of physical and mental development.
Iron: Component of hemoglobin, which transports oxygen from the lungs to the cells of the body. Also part of many enzymes involved in energy production.	RDA: Men: 10 mg; Women: 18 mg.	Red meats and cereal foods enriched with iron are best sources. Liver is especially high in iron. Eggs, whole grains, dried fruits, legumes, spinach, peas, beans, fish.	Deficiency causes anemia or low hemoglobin concentrations. Especially prevalent in infants, pregnant women, menstruating women, individuals with some type of internal hemorrhage, and those with diseases that cause malabsorption of iron.
Manganese: Needed for normal bone structure, reproduction, and nerve function. Component of enzymes.	RDA not established; intakes of 2.5 to 7 mg per day meet requirements.	Peas, beans, nuts and whole-grain cereals are best sources. Tea is high in manganese. Fruits and vegetables are good sources; meats and seafood are not.	No evidence of manganese deficiency in humans.
Molybdenum: Component of several enzymes; possibly involved in iron metabolism.	RDA not established; tentative estimate is about 150 μg per day.	Content in foods varies widely. Good sources include legumes, whole grain cereal products, milk, leafy vegetables, and organ meats.	No evidence of molybdenum deficiency in humans.

MINERAL	RDA	FOOD SOURCES	DEFICIENCY
Nickel: Apparently functions in liver oxidation reactions in rats and chicks.	Believed but not proved essential for humans.	More research is necessary to determine food content	No evidence of deficiency in humans.
Selenium: Component of enzyme involved in maintaining integrity of cell membranes; may be important for protein synthesis; has antioxidant properties; may protect against toxicity of heavy metals (e.g., mercury).	RDA not established; actual human need not known.	Seafoods and meat have relatively high amounts. Fruits and vegetables are poor sources. Selenium content of foods varies widely depending on the soil in which they are grown. Organ meats, muscle meats.	No identification in humans of any symptoms resulting from selenium deficiency.
Silicon: Important for normal development of bones and connective tissues in rats and chicks.	Believed but not proved essential for humans.	No information available. (Silicon is one of the elements in sand and glass.)	No evidence of deficiency in humans
Tin: Appears necessary for normal growth and tooth development in rats.	Not proved essential for humans; assume daily intake of 3.5 mg meets any nutritional requirement.	No solid information available; may be incorporated into foods from tinfoil and cans, although practice of lacquering cans reduces tin content of canned foods.	No evidence of deficiency in humans.
Vanadium: Promotes normal growth and reproductive ability in chicks and rats.	Probably essential for humans, but requirement is not known.	Little available information; food content appears to vary widely.	No evidence of deficiency in humans.

MINERAL	RDA	FOOD SOURCES	DEFICIENCY
Zinc: Constituent of many important enzymes; necessary for normal growth and sexual maturity; appears to be involved in wound healing.	RDA: 15 mg.	Seafoods, especially oysters, are rich in zinc. Red meats and some cheeses are good sources. Whole-grain foods, nuts, dried peas and beans furnish good amounts. Chicken, vegetables.	Conditions in humans related to zinc deficiency include: growth failure, sexual immaturity, impaired wound healing, and reduced taste sensation, poor appetite.

The danger with the minerals is that they can become highly toxic. The information presently available on toxicity follows.[16]

Calcium   Very high intake of calcium may reduce the absorption of other important minerals, such as manganese, zinc, and iron. Excessive intakes of calcium may have side effects in certain persons such as hypercalcemia. This condition may result in excessive calcium deposits occurring in the bones and some of the soft tissues (especially the kidneys). Generally, however, there is no known oral toxicity of calcium.

Chloride   A daily intake of salt of 14–28 g is considered to be excessive. Large doses of sodium chloride (salt) may cause increases in heart disease (especially high blood pressure), stroke, and kidney failure.

Magnesium   Evidence suggests that there must be a balance in the body between magnesium and calcium; if the intake of one of these minerals is high, the intake of the other must be high also. If calcium intake is low and magnesium intake is high, there is the danger of a toxic reaction. However, this is a rare occurrence. Usually, even in large amounts, magnesium is not toxic for persons with normal kidney functions.

Sodium   See toxicity for chlorine.

Cobalt   Enlarged thyroid gland, diarrhea, vomiting, nerve disease, myxedema, increased red blood cell count, congestive heart failure.

Copper   Toxicity is rare, since only a small amount of copper is absorbed and stored. Toxicity usually occurs with Wilson's Disease, which causes abnormal copper metabolism. With Wilson's Disease, copper is retained in the liver, brain, kidneys, and corneas of the eyes; insomnia; insanity.

Fluorine Depression of growth, calcification of the liver and tendons; degenerative changes in the kidneys, liver, adrenal glands, heart, central nervous system, and reproductive organs; mottled tooth enamel; possible mongolism.

Iodine Impaired formation of thyroid hormones. There is little chance of iodine toxicity occurring from ingesting iodine in food and/or water. However, toxicities do occur when thyroid is taken as a drug.

Iron Iron deposits in the liver and spleen, which may result in cirrhosis, diabetes, and other pancreas disorders.

Manganese Reduced storage and utilization of iron, weakness, psychological and motor difficulties (in industrial contamination). Actually, manganese toxicity is quite rare except for industrial contamination.

Molybdenum Diarrhea, anemia, depressed growth rate; high intake may result in copper deficiency.

Selenium Selenium can be toxic in its pure form, so care should be taken in using supplements. Even so, selenium toxicity is quite rare.

Zinc High zinc intake interferes with copper utilization, thus producing incomplete iron metabolism; kidney damage.

The minerals presently believed to have no known toxicity are: phosphorous, potassium, chromium, nickel, silicon, tin, and vanadium.

In the case of many minerals, the margin between the beneficial dose and the toxic dose is extremely small. Sometimes we are not even entirely sure where that line lies. So, the consumer is advised not to take multiple doses of any mineral without the knowledge and consent of a doctor.

20

other nutritional treatments

The controversy has raged for years as to the role of fiber in the diet and its relationship to various disease conditions. The major advocate of high-fiber intake as a disease-prevention technique is Dr. Denis P. Burkitt. Dr. Burkitt indicated recently that the most common cause of death in North America is coronary heart disease; the most common intestinal disease is diverticular disease; the most common emergency abdominal surgery is the appendectomy; the most common venous disorders are hemorrhoids and varicose veins; the second most common cause of death is cancer of the colon and rectum; the most common nutritional disorder is obesity; and the most common endocrine disorder is diabetes.[1] Dr. Burkitt maintains that these disease conditions could be decreased among the general population by increasing the fiber content of the diet.

What is fiber? It consists of cell walls of plants that resist the digestive enzymes in the gastrointestinal tract. Some common types of fiber that you might recognize are cellulose, hemicellulose, mucilages, pectin, gums, and lignin. Certain food types contain varying degrees of fiber. Some foods that are high in fiber are whole grains and cereals, fresh fruits (don't forget that the peelings are a good source of fiber!), berries, legumes and nuts, tuberous root vegetables (such as potatoes, carrots, turnips, and parsnips), and other fresh vegetables (such as cabbage). The following table indicates the dietary fiber content of some foods, expressed as a percentage of the total weight of the food.

259

BREAD AND CEREAL GROUP

All-bran cereal	26.70%
Bran	44.00%
Cornflakes	11.00%
Puffed Wheat	15.41%
Shredded Wheat	12.26%
Wholemeal bread	8.50%
Wholemeal flour	9.51%
White bread	2.72%
White flour	3.51%

VEGETABLES

Beans, baked	7.27%
Broccoli tops, boiled	4.10%
Brussel sprouts, boiled	2.86%
Cabbage, boiled	2.83%
Carrots, boiled	3.70%
Cauliflower, boiled	1.80%
Lettuce, raw	1.53%
Peas, canned, drained	7.85%
Potato, raw	3.51%
Turnips, raw	2.20%

FRUITS

Apples, flesh only	1.42%
peel only	3.71%
Bananas	1.75%
Cherries, flesh and skin	1.24%
Peaches, flesh and skin	2.28%
Pears, flesh only	2.44%
skin only	8.59%
Plums, flesh and skin	1.52%

Source: D. A. T. Southgate et al., "A Guide to Calculating Intakes of Dietary Fibre," *Journal of Human Nutrition*, 30:303, 1976.

Dr. Burkitt, wanting to prove the benefits of a high-fiber diet, studied groups of people from different degrees of industrialized societies. He found that among less industrialized societies, with an unrefined high-fiber diet (primarily African tribal groups), "400 gm. of soft feces were voided without straining with an average transit time of 3-5 hours." By contrast, groups from more highly industrialized societies, who ate more refined, lower-fiber foods, "produced less than 150 gm. of stools daily after remaining in the gut 3-5 days."[2] Incidentally, refining does more than remove fiber. It also removes nutrient materials. For example, modern wheat refining means a 28-percent loss of the bulk of the wheat. Polishing rice means removing the outer bran layer—and with it essential nutrients. Flour, in fact, is refined to such a point that it has to be enriched.

So how does this all relate to disease conditions? Fiber affects the intestinal tract in several ways. Fiber collects and holds water as it passes through the intestinal tract, which makes for softer, bulkier stools. These bulkier stools pass through the intestinal tract much more rapidly than harder, smaller stools, which are characteristic of low-fiber diets. As these larger, softer stools pass more rapidly from the body, they decrease the internal pressure in the large intestine. High fiber in the diet also influences the bacterial environment of the intestinal tract. In addition, bile salts (which emulsify fats and oils so that they are absorbed from the intestinal tract into the bloodstream) and bile acids are not reabsorbed from the intestinal tract. So, more bile salts and bile acids are excreted from the body with the fats and oils that are bound to them.

Advocates of high fiber in the diet point to the fact that fiber promotes a lower blood level of cholesterol, which in turn decreases coronary heart disease. Because less bile salts and acids are reabsorbed into the body, and because these salts and acids carry bound fats and oils with them as they leave the body, there is less cholesterol formation in the body. Also, because the stools produced from a high-fiber diet pass more rapidly from the body, more cholesterol is likely to be excreted from the body. Simply stated, with less cholesterol in the bloodstream, atherosclerosis, arteriosclerosis, and in turn, heart disease are all less likely. The decreased reabsorption of bile acids and salts also plays a role in decreased gallstone formation.

Those who favor a high-fiber diet point also to the fact that softer, bulkier stools lessen the need to strain when having a bowel movement and decrease the pressure in the intestinal tract. With less pressure and straining, there is a decrease in diseases such as diverticulitis (which occurs when the pressure in the intestines is so great that small pouches are formed from the intestinal wall), appendicitis, hemorrhoids, varicose veins, deep vein thromboses, and hiatal hernia.

Researchers claim that cancer of the colon and rectum can be caused by a number of related factors, of which a low-fiber diet is just one. When the diet is higher in fiber, fecal material passes more quickly through the intestinal tract and out of the body. The shorter transit time of the feces means that there is less contact between potential cancer-causing materials and the sensitive lining of the large intestine. It is also thought that fiber might bind to cancer-causing materials, thus aiding in their removal from the body.

Other researchers, though, have indicated that low fiber may not be the only dietary factor that could produce colon and rectum cancer.

There may be a relationship between high red meat and high animal fat intake and colorectal cancer. These factors also seemingly alter the large intestines in various ways that may contribute to cancer production. Possibly, the partial reason that fiber, red meat, and animal fat may be related to these common types of cancers is that, generally, diets that are high in fats and red meats tend to be low in fiber; so the situation is aggravated in many ways.

Many feel that obesity can be relieved to some degree by taking in more fiber. It is felt that fiber is a natural obstacle to overnutrition and obesity for several reasons: Fiber is largely indigestible. Chewier, it is more difficult to eat in large quantities. More saliva and digestive juices are produced in an attempt to digest fiber, so that you experience more satisfaction from eating high-fiber foods. The faster movement of the feces through the intestinal tract may mean less intestinal absorption of digested material and more excretion of fat. The harder-to-eat qualities of fiber also make for less emotional comfort in eating.[3] All these factors tend to increase weight loss to a greater or lesser degree when you are on a high-fiber diet.

Many investigators have seen a relationship between a low-fiber diet and diabetes production. Some now believe that starches, which are low in fiber, are more rapidly converted to glucose (a type of sugar) than some of the more high-fiber carbohydrates. The glucose enters the bloodstream quite quickly and causes increased demands on the pancreas to produce insulin. This condition may make a person more susceptible to diabetes. In addition, a team in Grand Forks, North Dakota, found that the slower conversion of glucose, which accompanies the eating of high-fiber carbohydrates, may also aid in the treatment of diabetes.[4]

There can be negative aspects to the fiber question. Some types of fiber bind certain minerals and vitamins so that these nutrients are excreted from the body along with the fiber. This extra excretion may produce vitamin and mineral deficiencies. Also, when some individuals decide to go on a high-fiber diet, they feel that if a little fiber is good, a lot of fiber is better. However, eating too much fiber too fast can cause gastrointestinal upsets such as gas and diarrhea. So, anyone increasing fiber in the diet should use moderation to ensure proper gastrointestinal functioning.

ORGANIC AND NATURAL FOODS

One of the most heated controversies in nutrition and health centers around organic and natural foods and nutrients.

Organic refers to carbon-based molecules, which also contain oxygen and hydrogen, that are characteristic of living protoplasm. Proponents of organic foods believe that foodstuffs grown in soil should be fertilized with decomposed plant material (called *humus*) rather than inorganic, chemically produced fertilizers, which contain materials such as potash, nitrates, and phosphates. Those advocating this type of nutrition feel that the active organic substances used in soil fertilization and the organic foods resulting from this fertilization are more in harmony with the components of our bodies.

This concept is interesting, but many refute it by saying that organically grown foods are not necessarily superior to synthetically fertilized foods. The reason: Plants cannot tell the difference between inorganic and organic fertilizers; they use the available chemicals regardless of the source. One other consideration is that organically grown foods cost more. This, and the fact that plants can't differentiate between organic and inorganic fertilizers, may help you to be a wiser consumer in the area of organic foods.

Natural foods are those derived from plant or animal sources, including foods that do not contain artificial colors, flavors, or synthetic ingredients such as chemical additives. Advocates of natural foods and of other nutrient materials consider the following concepts important:

• Whole foods are more nourishing than processed foods, because they contain more vitamins and minerals and less chemical additives.

• Americans eat too much sugar.

• Survival depends on the intake of complete proteins, which supply all the essential amino acids for growth, repair, and maintenance of body tissues.

• Individuals should take into account seasonal dietary changes and occasional cleansing (fasting) regimens to ensure health.

• There is no need to eat when hunger is not present; eating three meals a day is merely a cultural habit.

• Specific foods are medicines for specific conditions.[5]

Considering the characteristics of natural foods, however, finding foods that do not contain additives or artificial colors or flavors of some type is difficult. Today, agricultural productivity is enhanced by fertilizers, pesticides, and other substances. These substances are in turn taken into the plants that grow in the area and into the animals that ingest the plans. So, chemicals such as DDT, DES (diethylstilbesterol—a hormone-like substance), Dieldrin, Aldrin, and PCBs (polychlorinated biphenyls) get into our food sources. Then, other foreign substances are added when foods undergo chemical processing. Of the 10,000 items in your local grocery store, it has been established that 8,000 have undergone some type of major chemical processing.[6] Each year, 140 pounds of additives are consumed by every man, woman, and child in this country.[7] Our meats contain drugs, antibiotics, pesticides, and environmental pollutants. Our fruits and vegetables contain fumigants, retardants, preservatives, drugs, and antisprouting chemicals.

Although it is frightening to know that we are taking in so many harmful substances each time we eat, there is another side to the story. Most of our natural foods also contain these same harmful chemicals as a natural part of their makeup. For example, cranberry juice naturally contains sodium benzoate, a chemical preservative added to many foods. Nitrates and nitrites, the additives that help preserve cured meats, occur naturally in many green, leafy vegetables. The aroma that comes from the coffee you perk contains some 42 chemicals such as acetaldehyde, acetic acid, acetone, acetylmethylcarbinol, methylmercaptan, ammonia, cresols, diacetyldiethylketone, dimethylsulfide, 2- and 3-dioxyacetophenone, esters, ethyl alcohol, eugenol, formic acid, furance, furfural, furfuryl acetate, and many others. So not all of that food that is considered "natural" is natural.[8] Since many natural foods, like organically grown foods, cost the consumer more, you should take into account that you are getting some of the same harmful chemicals in natural foods that you are in foods that are not considered to be natural. Make your purchases accordingly.

The natural-versus-synthetic vitamin controversy is somewhat like the organic-versus-inorganic fertilizer debate. Natural vitamins are considered to be superior to synthetic vitamins because they don't contain synthetic (or chemical) ingredients. However, let the consumer beware! Each vitamin has the same molecular structure whether natural or synthetic. The body (like the plants and their fertilizers) cannot tell the difference between the natural and synthetic vitamins because of their identical structure.

SUGAR

Do Americans consume too much sugar? Is sugar better for you than honey or vice versa? These questions continue through the years, and they remain unresolved.

True, sugar consumption in this country has increased drastically over the years. The consumption of sugar in 1815 was about 15 pounds per person per year, and this figure has increased to about 120 pounds per person per year at the present time. This means an eight-fold increase in about 150 years.[9] And it appears that this increased sugar consumption is producing detrimental health effects in the general population. First and foremost, dental decay and dental disease have increased from taking in too much sugar. Also, excessive sugar consumption causes increased stress on the pancreas. The pancreas produces a hormone called insulin, which enables the body to use the sugar that it takes in. When there is too much stress on the pancreas to produce insulin, an individual can be more susceptible to the development of diabetes.

Recently, another factor has come to light. It has been found that the metabolism of sugar is accomplished only in conjunction with other nutrients, such as vitamins and minerals. Too much sugar in the diet can cause a nutrient debt to occur, that is, the body uses so many nutrients to metabolize the sugar that it doesn't have enough to carry on the fundamental body processes. So an individual can be obese from too much sugar consumption, but malnourished because of nutrient deficiencies. Remember, sugar contains no nutrients—except calories.[10]

Sugar can also be indirectly related, it is thought, to heart disease. An increase in sugar intake causes increased levels of serum cholesterol and triglycerides (fatty acids). These elements, in turn, can cause an increase in athero- and arteriosclerosis, which may predispose an individual to increased heart disease.

Is honey better for the body than sugar? At present, there is no evidence that honey is easier to digest than other sugars. Table sugar (sucrose) is broken down into fructose and glucose, which are the same basic ingredients that make up honey. There is also the fact that some kinds of honey may be 40 percent sweeter than sugar.[11]

Even though sugar is an integral part of all living substances, and even though our bodies need some sugar to function efficiently, we as Americans need to cut down on our sugar consumption. Here are some concrete suggestions on how to cut sugar intake:

- Avoid or cut down on sugar-laden foods such as cakes, pies, candies, and the like.

- Read the labels on food packages and find out which products have the least sugar. Then purchase those products.

- Cut down on the sugar you add to coffee, tea, breakfast cereals, and so on.

- Cut down on between-meal snacks, especially those that contain sugar.

- Use moderation in your sugar intake. Your sugar intake should be kept to 5 percent of your total calorie intake.[12]

other nutritional treatments **265**

Of late, the cholesterol question has become closely related to heart disease. It has been found that saturated animal fats produce larger concentrations of cholesterol in the blood than unsaturated and polyunsaturated (vegetable) fats. Cholesterol is used beneficially in the body to form sex and adrenal hormones, produce bile acids, form cell membranes, and build brain tissue, However, when cholesterol from dietary sources (such as animal fats) combines with already existing sources of cholesterol in the body, a high cholesterol level results. Increased blood cholesterol can be deposited in blood vessel walls, forming placcques. These placcques may in turn contribute to heart and vessel problems by forming clots or by closing vessels.

Certain foods, high in animal fats, raise blood cholesterol levels in the body. Some of these foods are: red meats (especially those marbled with fat), butter, egg yolk, cheese, chocolate, whole milk, ice cream, and so on. It has been found that to protect the body from too much cholesterol in the blood, less than 10 percent of the fats found in the diet should be saturated. That fact means that you should eat less high-fats meats and more low-fat meats, such as fish and poultry. It also means that you should cut off all the fat on meat before cooking, and you should bake, broil, roast, and stew your meat rather than frying it. You should consider using margarine rather than butter—and fewer eggs. You should use polyunsaturated fats in cooking, such as vegetable oils; remember, polyunsaturated fats may in fact lower blood cholesterol levels. You should, lastly, achieve and maintain an ideal body weight by eating more fruit, vegetables, and whole grains and less sugar-sweetened foods and foods that contain saturated fats.[13]

One other consideration has recently come to light: It has been thought that lecithin should be taken to avert some of the danger of fats. Lecithin, a fat-like compound, appears to dissolve cholesterol and other fats. Beans and peas contain lecithin, and we may find, with more research and documention, that lecithin may well lower cholesterol in the body and prevent heart attacks.[14]

YOGURT

Several years ago, yogurt was introduced as a new health food. Actually, it is a food that has been eaten and enjoyed for thousands of years. As far back as ancient Persia, people were eating yogurt. In fact, ancient Persian tradition has it that the method of making yogurt was revealed to Abraham by an angel. The tradition also tells that the reason for Abraham's virility and long life was that he ate yogurt.[15]

Whereas yogurt is made with cow's milk in this country today, in ancient Asia, medieval Europe, and Africa, yogurt was made from a variety of milks, including sheep, buffalo, goat, mare, and llama. Regardless of the milk, though, the beneficial bacteria in yogurt is the same: *Streptococcus thermophilis* and *Lactobacillus bulgaris*.

Yogurt has been attributed with certain properties—some believable and some not so believable. Several of the benefits of yogurt-eating that have more scientific backing are as follows:

- The lactic acid bacteria, present in yogurt in the millions, hinder the growth of or kill several dangerous types of bacteria that can be responsible for illness or death. These harmful bacteria include typhoid, paratyphoid, diphtheria, and *Escherichia coli*.

- Milk that is made into yogurt is easily digestible by people of all ages, so most of the nutrients are readily available for use. Adults and children who may have trouble digesting cow's milk do not have digestive problems with yogurt.

- The biological value of fermented milk's protein increases during yogurt manufacture, and the formation of B vitamins takes place also.

- Eating yogurt while traveling in foreign countries can be a precaution against dysentery.

Other benefits have been attributed to yogurt that so far have not been proven. Can those multitudes of 120-year-old people who live in the secluded valleys and mountains of some of the remote parts of Russia actually attribute their health and long life to the eating of yogurt? This question is still under debate. However, most of the evidence points to factors other than yogurt, such as environment and different eating patterns as a whole. Yogurt has also been said to correct overweight, restore hair, tone up flaccid muscles, improve sexual prowess among the aging, and relieve some of the symptoms of arthritis. A UCLA research team found that eating three cups of ordinary yogurt per day can cut serum cholesterol almost 9 percent in a week. It seems that the calcium in yogurt may halt cholesterol absorption, but this is merely a supposition at present.[16]

Now for the bad news. There are some disadvantages to eating yogurt. After about seven days, many of yogurt's healthful benefits seemingly begin to decline. So, if you want to get the most from your yogurt, you should buy it from an establishment that sells it immediately after its manufacture. You should be aware that flavored yogurt is not a diet food. The fruit flavors in yogurt have sugar-laden preservatives that add calories. And if you eat specialty yogurts, such as Swiss yogurt, you may be getting even more calories than you bargained for. Frozen yogurt has come into vogue of late, but did you know that freezing kills the yogurt cultures? So, again, the healthful benefits of the yogurt may be destroyed. Interestingly enough, skim milk yogurt has been found to promote the formation of eye cataracts, whereas whole milk yogurt does not.[17]

So, you may continue to enjoy your yogurt, knowing that it may be bringing you certain health benefits, but be aware that there may be some disadvantages to certain types of yogurts.

MACROBIOTICS

Macrobiotics, as formulated by George Ohsawa, relates the ancient Oriental philosophy of yin and yang to diet. Macrobiotic philosophy maintains that the selection and preparation of food can relieve physical illness plus psychological, spiritual, and social malaise. This concept, then, emphasizes the therapeutic rather than the preventive aspects of diet.

In Oriental philosophy, the yin and yang are opposing forces that coexist harmoniously in the universe. The yin, signified by the color purple, represents centrifugal force and the tendency to expand. The yang, signified by the color red, represents the idea of centripetal force and the tendency to contract. These ideas of yin and yang are carried over into eating foods. Foods are categorized not only by their color, but also by other characteristics. For example, vegetables are assigned yin or yang characteristics by their season of growth, speed of growth, direction of growth, height, water content, cooking time, size, and so on. Animal foods, on the other hand, are assigned yin or yang properties by their growth, place of growth, action (how active they are), personality, food preference, water consumption, hibernation characteristics, and the like. By these criteria, meat, eggs, and most animal products are yang foods while sugar, fruits, and liquids are yin foods. Several yang elements, used in food preparation, can help to "yangize" yin foods. These are salt, pressure, heat, and dehydration. The object in assigning yin and yang values to foods helps individuals maintain a natural balance in their diets.

One more element enters into macrobiotics: Most advocates eat mainly vegetable foods. George Ohsawa maintains that, "we come from the food that we take in daily."[18] Further, he indicates that vegetation is the food origin of the whole animal kingdom. Also, only vegetation can assimilate inorganic matter and produce organic substances, so man's right foods are vegetation-type foods. Ohsawa feels that vegetation-eating produces a free man, while meat-eating produces an unfree man.[19]

Just as foods are yin or yang, so are illnesses categorized as yin and yang. Some examples of yin illnesses are introversion, worry, loneliness, alienation, melancholy, rheumatism, arthritis, hearing diseases, TB, epilepsy, polio, miscarriage, ulcer, high blood pressure, cancer, and mental sickness. Appendicitis, night walking, dancing sickness, elephantiasis, Addison's disease, liver disease and jaundice are examples of yang illnesses. The concepts of diet and disease interrelate. If a disease is yin-caused, for example, to cure the disease you should take in more yang foods (in other words, yangize your body) and take in less yin foods. If a disease is yang-caused, the opposite is the treatment. In this way, through yinnizing or yangizing the body, repair and restoration of the physical and mental self can take place.[20]

FASTING

The principle behind fasting is that a limited, but specific diet of foods, liquids, or broth, accomplishes elimination in and cleansing of the body. Advocates of fasting maintain that undigested residue and decomposed cells and tissues build up in the body. Illnesses begin with this buildup of toxic material in the body; when these poisons are eliminated, health returns. Fasting enables every system of the body to get physiological rest so that all systems are rejuvenated. In other words, fasting diverts body energy to healing, rather than to digesting.

What does fasting actually accomplish? Fasting halts the intake of what may be causing a disease condition. The storage organs of the body empty, and the eliminative organs, such as the kidneys, are able to deal with backlogs of accumulated toxic materials. These factors produce such effect as rapid weight loss, self-purification, euphoria, improved digestion and bowel action, clear eyes and complexion, reduced blood pressure, improved heart action, reduction of an enlarged prostate gland in males, increased sexual vigor, an improved sense of smell and taste, no shortness of breath, and improved capacity of the eliminative organs.[21]

How long should you fast? The answer to this query is quite simple. Hunger returns when the body has eliminated all of its accumulated waste and cleansed itself. When hunger returns—whether it is in two days, two weeks, or two months—you should resume eating.

What, then, is the difference between fasting and starvation? Fasting ends and starvation begins if the fast is continued after natural hunger returns. At this time body reserves are consumed.

Fasting, it should be noted, can be dangerous under certain conditions such as diabetes, pregnancy, lactation, and the like. So before beginning any type of fast, anyone with a disease condition or anyone under particular stress should consult with a physician to see if a fast endangers the existing problem. Never begin such a regimen without medical advice.

This chapter has been designed to inform you, as a consumer, about some of the background, benefits, dangers, and current trends in nutrition. Remember that you should never try to treat a serious illness or symptom with herbs, any other home remedy, or diet. One of the secrets to the sucessful use of medicine and drugs is the ability to know when you can safely treat yourself and when you should see a doctor, dentist, or some other medical professional.

part five

THE USE OF DRUGS

21

drug action and hazards

Drugs are like the famous two-edged sword. They are marvelous chemical mixtures that can relieve our symptoms, make us feel better, and even effect a cure for any number of illnesses. Drugs can soothe the pain of a sore throat or cool the most fiery fever. Vaccines can prevent diseases that claimed thousands of lives only decades ago. For all the good they do, however, drugs are still only chemicals that may react with each other or with chemicals in the body to produce serious—or fatal—side effects. In one three-year period, nearly 18 percent of all the patients admitted to an American hospital under study had problems related to OTC drug use—toxic or allergic reactions, overdoses, or interactions between a prescription and an OTC drug. The biggest mistake American consumers make is that they take too much of a drug.[1] It is therefore critical that we weigh the benefits against the disadvantages before starting on any program of drug therapy and before we prescribe over-the-counter drugs to cure our minor ailments.

DRUG ACTION

Drugs produce their effects in different ways inside your body, and they work in different areas of the body. Drugs can thus be categorized either according to the location of their action or according to how they work.

273

1. Drugs can be *local or topical* in action. This term means that the drug has its effect where it contacts the body. One of the best examples of a drug with local action is an external analgesic, such as Mentholatum Deep Heating Rub, which is an irritant that causes blood vessels to dilate where it is rubbed on. These effects are confined to just the area that the Mentholatum has contacted.

2. Other drugs are *systemic* in action. These drugs find their way into the bloodstream, and, from there, they are carried to the entire body. For example, penicillin can be taken orally or in injection form, but it eventually finds it way to the bloodstream where it is carried throughout the body.

3. Drug action may also be either *selective* or *general.* Selective drugs affect only a specific organ or organs. For example, antacids have a selective action; they work in a specific organ, the stomach, to help neutralize excess acid. Drugs are said to have a general action when the body as a whole is affected. Aspirin might be considered to have a general action when you take it to fight a cold. In this case, you are taking it to relieve symptoms that affect your entire body—aches, pain, and fever. And although aspirin cannot cure your cold, it can help relieve these symptoms.[2]

Now that you know *where* drugs work, you should also know *how* they work.

1. *Stimulants* cause an increase in activity, somewhere in the body or in the body as a whole. Nicotine is an example: The nicotine from cigarettes causes your heart to beat faster, your blood pressure to rise, and your breathing rate to increase.

2. *Depressants* cause certain functions in the body to decrease in activity. For example, you take barbiturates to combat insomnia because of their depressant effect; they slow your breathing and heart rate so you are not as active and find it easier to fall asleep and to stay asleep.

3. Other drugs *replace substances that are deficient* in the body. Probably the example you are most familiar with is insulin. For various reasons, the body cannot manufacture its own insulin so that sugar can be used. In such cases, insulin or insulin-like products must be given to replace the insulin that the body cannot make itself. When insulin is given, the body can again use sugar, and the diabetic condition is relieved.

4. Some drugs *kill* foreign organisms in the body, while others *weaken* the organisms so that the body can build up its resistance to kill them. For instance penicillin is effective in killing the bacteria that cause infections; remember—penicillin has no effect on invading viruses. On the other hand, tetracycline weakens foreign bacteria so that the body's own defenses can contain the infection.

5. Other drugs produce their effect by causing *irritation*. One of the best examples of an irritant is a liniment or other external analgesic. Such a drug causes irritation where it is applied so that blood vessels in that area dilate and bring added warmth to the painful area.

6. Many drugs produce a *demulcent* effect. In other words, they coat the tissues and thus protect them. Some liquid antacids claim to coat the stomach to protect the lining from excess stomach acid.[3]

FACTORS THAT MODIFY RESPONSE TO DRUGS
Age, weight, sex, heredity, the time of administration, your emotional state, your condition of health, and other drug use—all these factors may be responsible for different responses to drugs.[4] More specifically, certain processes in the body determine how the drug reacts and how much effect it has.

1. *Absorption* is the transfer of the drug from the site of administration to the bloodstream. Absorption is dependent on several factors:

• *How the drug is administered:* Administering a drug directly into a vessel causes faster absorption than giving a drug orally.

• *The physical and chemical characteristics of the drug:* It may be fat- or water-soluble, for example.

• *How much surface is available for the drug to penetrate:* The stomach provides more surface area, for example, than the mouth does.

2. The *distribution* of a drug throughout the body is another factor. Because a drug usually has to cross several membranes before it reaches its final site of action, not all the drug reaches its destination. How much reaches the destination determines how much effect the drug has.

3. *Metabolism* changes the drug from its original form into a form that the body can use more easily; or it changes the drug to a more water-soluble form so it can eventually be excreted from the body. This process generally takes place in the liver.

4. *Excretion* is accomplished primarily through the urine and feces, but some excretion also takes place from the respiratory system (exhalation), from saliva, from perspiration, and through the mother's milk.

DRUG HAZARDS

Along with all the good effects of drugs come the bad. When a drug reacts either with other drugs or with chemicals in the body to produce a mild poisoning effect, we say that it has become *toxic*. Any drug taken at a high enough dosage can be toxic. The most serious of the toxic effects, of course, leads to death,[5] which can occur as a result of an allergic reaction that is not treated, a massive overdose of a drug, or a drug used for the wrong purpose. Fortunately, death is not the most common effect of a toxic reaction from a drug.

You should suspect a toxic reaction if you develop suddenly any of the following symptoms after taking a drug:[6]

respiratory difficulties	vomiting
convulsions	cardiac arrhythmias
dizziness	skin irritations or rashes
diarrhea	loss of hearing
a fall or rise in blood pressure	loss of eyesight in one or both
fever	eyes
chills	

Any of these symptoms—especially if you experience two or more—can signal two things: (1) that you have absorbed either too much of the drug into your system or (2) that the drug is reacting with another chemical agent (possibly your body's own defenses, causing an allergic reaction). Call your doctor immediately. While some of the toxic reactions are mild and relatively noncritical (such as a skin rash or slight dizziness), others can be critical (such as respiratory problems that cause you to stop breathing)—and these require immediate medical attention.

If you begin to react severely to a drug, ask a family member or friend to drive you to the nearest hospital emergency room. Take the drug with you—making sure you include the drug's container—and be prepared to tell the physician at the emergency room how much of the drug you took and when. The drug in its original container gives the physician important information. If you have taken any other drugs within 24 hours, take them with you to the hospital too, and be prepared to relate the circumstances under which you took them.

Treating Overdoses
In case of an overdose, take the following steps:[7]

• Act fast to lessen the toxicity of the drug or to get it out of the body. To lessen the damage to the stomach lining and to add fluid to aid vomiting, have the victim drink water. A child should drink one cup of water, and an adult should drink two to three. Only in the case of a conscious person, use syrup of Ipecac to induce vomiting: one teaspoon for a child and one tablespoon for an adult. Follow the syrup of Ipecac with one to two glasses of water. To prevent further absorption of the drug into the bloodstream, put one to two ounces of activated charcoal in a glass of water. Repeat this procedure one to two times every thirty to sixty minutes.

• Take the patient to the hospital immediately.

• Help the patient remain calm.

• Keep accurate track of the progression of the symptoms, as well as of the times that water or other treatment was administered.

• Take a sample of the vomited material to the hospital for analysis.

• If you are in doubt as to what to do, call your nearest Poison Control Center.

Drug Allergies
An allergy—simply an exaggerated sensitivity to a substance or allergen—can develop whenever your body encounters a foreign substance and attempts to fight it with its own line of defense. When one of the weapons in that line of defense encounters a substance to which you are sensitive, and when enough of the antibodies rush to combat the allergen, you experience an allergic reaction.[8] Drug allergies develop in three stages:

• You have at least one prior exposure to the drug.

• You do not take the drug for quite some time. During that latent period, your body builds the antibodies that are sensitive to the drug. (This process requires at least one to two weeks.)

• You are exposed to the drug again, and the sensitized antibodies rush to fight the invasion.

A reaction can occur either shortly after you take the drug (within a few minutes or hours), or it may occur even days after your exposure. Don't disregard the possibility of an allergic reaction simply because the symptoms appear "too soon" or "too late."

A number of things can affect your development of an allergy to a drug. The route of application has a definite effect: Drugs that are applied to the skin carry a much greater risk of causing an allergic reaction than drugs that are injected. Both have a greater tendency to produce an allergic reaction than drugs that are taken orally. Your dosage schedule plays a part, too: If you use a drug off-and-on over a period of weeks or months, you have a greater chance of having an allergic reaction than if you use the drug continuously for the same period of time. The alternating usage and latent periods give your body a chance to build sensitive antibodies; continuous use does not.

Unfortunately, three of the most commonly used drugs cause almost 90 percent of all allergic reactions: penicillin, sulfa drugs, and aspirin. Other drugs that normally cause allergic reactions include antibiotics, anticonvulsants, barbiturates, local anesthetics, vaccines, tranquilizers, and antithyroid drugs. Iodides that are used as the contrast media for X-rays are also often the source of severe reactions.

How can you tell if your reaction to a drug is an allergic one? Look for these symptoms:

- general itching of the skin or some mucous membrane that came in contact with the drug;

- hives;

- massive swelling of body tissue, generally involving a large section of tissue;

- photosensitivity of the skin where a drug was applied;

- various widespread eruptions that include redness and scaling, especially on large body areas such as the trunk;

- eruptions where the drug was applied to the skin, usually of a fixed nature and occurring at the site of application only.

Sometimes it's difficult to decide whether you are having an allergic drug reaction or whether your symptoms are due to some other irritating agent or part of the disease you were treating with the drug. The only definite sign of an allergic drug reaction is a fixed eruption: The eruption is always found at the same site, and it is a well-outlined welt that is generally oval, swollen, and red.

Because drug agents are generally circulated throughout your body and absorbed by most of the organs and membranes, an allergic reaction can cause a symptom in any part of the body. The following are common symptoms of drug reaction:

a significant drop in blood pressure
weakness
a loss of consciousness
tightness in the chest
wheezing
inflammation of any glands in the body

development of shock (can lead to death)
difficulty in breathing
fever
general body rash
pain in the joints
development of asthma

Again, it is often difficult to determine whether the symptom is a sign of drug allergy or a symptom of the disease you were trying to treat. One of the most common symptoms of drug allergic reaction—fever—normally accompanies a number of diseases and is generally not suspected as a sign of an allergic reaction. If your symptom is severe, or if you suspect that you might be having an allergic reaction, it is best to check with your doctor, who can test you for an allergic reaction to a drug by giving you one of two kinds of skin tests. In one, a small amount of the allergen (the drug to which you are allergic) is placed in a small scratch on your skin, or a needle containing the allergen is used to prick the skin. If you are allergic to the drug, a raised red welt appears within fifteen minutes at the site where the allergen was applied. In the second test, a gauze patch soaked with the allergen is taped to the skin and left in place for 48 hours; if you are allergic to the substance, the skin beneath the patch becomes red and scaly.

Unfortunately, skin tests are pretty unreliable. You may be allergic to certain drugs only after they have broken down inside your body and have had a chance to mix with the unique chemicals in your body systems. Other tests that might be more reliable, but that are still in experimental stages, include those that use X-rays and blood reactions.

Knowing which drugs you are allergic to is important so that you can help prevent an allergic reaction. Of course, if you are conscious and a doctor asks you if you have any allergies, you can describe any sensitivities. If you are purchasing over-the-counter medications, you can read the labels and ask the pharmacist to help you if you are unsure about the ingredients of a specific brand. If you are unconscious, however, you must rely on someone else to relay the information—and you might not always be with a person who is aware of your allergy. You should carry a card in your wallet that explains your allergy; if you are allergic to a widely used drug, you might consider wearing a Medic Alert tag in case you are involved in an accident.

You should remember, too, that if you are allergic to one drug or substance, you might also be allergic to related drugs or substances. Ask your doctor to help you by listing all the related substances that might cause reaction; the allergy test might diagnose allergies to related substances also. Remember, the drug you are allergic to might be hidden in some other drug mixture; aspirin, for example, is found in many over-the-counter antacids, decongestants, cough remedies, and other medications. Become an expert at reading labels.

FOOD AND DRUGS

Drugs and food interact within your body in several ways. When you're taking drugs, certain foods can render the drugs ineffective or even cause an adverse reaction. Conversely, drugs can affect your body's ability to derive full nutrition from the food you eat.[9]

A single drug can cause any of the following problems, and if your drug therapy includes two or more drugs, your problems are compounded:

- Nausea and vomiting prevent you from absorbing food into your system.

- Diarrhea affects the way the intestinal tract works to absorb nutrients from the food.

- A drug can alter your body's ability to transport, use, or excrete the nutrients in your food.

- Antibiotics can destroy the bacteria in your intestinal tract that work to form the vitamins from the food you eat.

- A drug can cause you to lose your appetite, causing you to reduce the amount of food you take into your system.

If you are taking any drugs, you should take steps to correct deficiencies, either through diet (the preferred way) or through the use of synthetic vitamin and mineral supplements. It is important that you eat properly whenever you are taking medication of any kind, so that you can protect your body against nutritional deficiency.

The nutritional needs you should be especially aware of during drug treatment include the following:[10]

- *Oral contraceptives* increase the need for vitamin C2 and the B vitamins.

- *Mineral oil* hinders the passage of vitamins A, D, and K into the bloodstream.

- *Diuretics* cause the body to eliminate large amounts of potassium as waste products.

- *Antacids* cause the loss of thiamin (vitamin B1) through elimination as waste products.

- *Antibiotics* cause a general deficiency in all vitamins and reduces the intestinal tract's ability to absorb nutrients from the food (due to the destruction of normal bacteria that aid this process in the intestinal tract).

- *Aspirin*, taken over a long period of time or in large doses, causes deficiency in the B vitamins, vitamin C, and vitamins in general.

- *Cholesterol-lowering agents* cause deficiencies in the B vitamins along with vitamins A, D, E, and K; it also hinders the body's ability to utilize and store phosphorus, iron, calcium, sodium, magnesium, and potassium.

A drug may be rendered useless, or it may cause severe and sometimes fatal reactions when mixed with food.[11] If you are taking the following drugs, avoid foods specified, which cause a serious reaction:

- With *anticoagulants*, green leafy vegetables cause a cancellation of the blood's ability to thin.

- With *tetracycline*, dairy products cancel the effectiveness of the drug, neutralizing the chemical action.

- With *monoamine oxidase inhibitors* (such as Nardil or Marplan, taken to reduce depression), pickled herring, Chianti wine, chocolate, chicken livers, and ripened or aged cheese can cause death. They generally bring about a rapid rise in blood pressure, accompanied by violent headaches and vomiting.

- With *diuretics*, monosodium glutamate (frequently found in Chinese cooking) can cause the body to eliminate critical sodium from the body.

- With *penicillin*, *ampicillin*, or *erythromycin*, fruit juices neutralize the drug.

- With *any drug taken for heart disease or blood pressure*, licorice can cause high blood pressure, heart failure, severe headache, and a loss of potassium.

- With *antidiabetic drugs*, any food containing sugar blocks the action of the drug.

Timing of drugs in relation to your meals can affect the drug's effectiveness and its tendency to react with food in your body. Use the following guideline:

Take on an Empty Stomach:

benzathine

tetracyclines (except Declomycin, which can upset the stomach)

erythromycin

methacycline

Take 30 Minutes Before Meals:

belladonna

Donnatal

Ritalin

Preludin

Pro-banthine

Pyridium

Take With Your Meal or With Food:

antidiabetics

APC (pain reliever containing aspirin)

Artane

Dilantin

Dyrenium

Ponstel

prednisone

prednisolone

rauwolfia

reserpine

Flagyl

Do Not Take With Milk:

Dulcolax

potassium chloride

tetracyclines (except Vibramycin)

potassium iodide

Do Not Drink Alcohol While Taking:

antihistamines

Antivert

DBI

Diabinese

Dymelor

Flagyl

Librium

Lomotil

narcotics of any kind

Orinase

Quaalude

DRUGS AND DRUGS

Because of their incompatibility in chemical makeup and formula, some drugs interact with others to produce harmful and sometimes fatal effects.[12] Drugs taken together may act independently to either increase or decrease the effect of one or both drugs or to produce new and perhaps undesirable reactions. These drug interactions may achieve several different effects:

- *Idiosyncratic effect:* Some drugs, when taken together by certain people, may produce an effect that is totally unexpected.

- *Toxic effect:* Two drugs taken together in regular dosages may be poisonous.

- *Antagonistic effect:* One drug may counteract the action of another when the two are taken together.

- *Synergistic effect:* Taking two drugs together may increase the potency of both drugs. Here, the effects of both drugs are not merely added together; they are multiplied.[13]

You should not take the following drugs together:

- antibacterial drugs and barbiturates,
- tetracyclines and antacids,
- tetracyclines and iron supplements,
- lincomycin and products containing kaolin (Kaopectate, Donnagel),
- antidepressants and monoamine inhibitors,
- antidepressants and minor tranquilizers,
- oral anticoagulants and aspirin,
- oral anticoagulants and cholesterol-lowering drugs,
- oral anticoagulants and thyroid preparations,
- oral anticoagulants and barbiturates,
- oral anticoagulants and birth control pills,
- aspirin and arthritis medications,
- aspirin and oral antidiabetic drugs,
- nose drops and digitalis,
- cold medications and sleeping pills,
- cold medications and minor tranquilizers
- cold medicines and codeine,

- cough medicines and sleeping pills,
- cough medicines and minor tranquilizers,
- birth control pills and anticoagulants,
- birth control pills and antidiabetics,
- stimulants (diet pills) and antidepressants, or
- stimulants (diet pills) and Darvon.

Because listing a comprehensive group of drugs that cause serious interactions is impossible, you should always be cautious when you are taking two or more drugs at the same time. Follow the common-sense rules already explained and discussed. Make sure that a physician who prescribes a drug for you is aware of any other drug (prescription or over-the-counter) that you might be taking. If you are taking a prescription drug, call your doctor before you take an over-the-counter medication for the same or another illness. And call your doctor before you mix two over-the-counter drugs; it's better to be safe than sorry. Also, to avoid adverse drug interactions, make sure you know how drugs are to be taken—on an empty stomach, with water instead of milk, an hour after meals, and so on. Thoroughly read all labels so that you know which ingredients are in the medication you are taking; many preparations contain more than one ingredient. Also, inform yourself of warnings, if any, of adverse effects. You should know the chemical, generic, and brand names of all the drugs you are taking so that you will not unknowingly take the same medication twice by two different names. Don't take a drug prescribed for someone else, especially if you are taking other drugs at the same time. You don't know what someone else's medication may do to you by itself; when you are taking other medication, the danger is much greater. If possible, buy all your medications at the same pharmacy. Your pharmacist, who knows you and the medications you take, may even keep a written record of which drugs you are taking. At any rate, he or she can advise you when drugs should not be taken together. Finally, report any adverse reactions to your doctor immediately. You may need a change in the combination of drugs you take.[14]

DRUG-INDUCED DISEASES AND DISORDERS

A drug can cause a disorder or an actual disease.[15] As many as 5 percent of all hospital admissions are for diseases or disorders caused by drugs; 35 percent of all hospital patients suffer from some kind of drug-related disorder before they are discharged. This, of course, depends on the person's age, sex, rate of metabolism, blood group, and general state of health. For example, newborn infants are unable to metabolize certain drugs, and elderly people suffer from diminished kidney function, which causes drugs and other elements to remain in the system for longer periods of time. Females seem to have more adverse reactions to narcotics than males, and they develop a larger number of drug-induced disorders because of those reactions.

While a comprehensive list is difficult to compile, the following diseases and disorders can be induced by the following drugs:

- *Changes in hair color:* haloperidol.

- *Hair loss:* cyclophosphamide.

- *Increase in body hair:* steroids.

- *Rash:* allopurinal, barbiturates, diuretics, penicillin, salicylates (including aspirin), sulfonamides.

- *Change in skin color:* oral contraceptives.

- *Asthma:* aspirin (the most common cause), penicillin, oral contraceptives, iron dextran, indomethacin.

- *Gastrointestinal disorders* (including ulcers and hemorrhage): corticosteroids, salicylates, phenylbutazone, oxyphenbutazone, indomethacin, anticoagulants, reserpine, ethacrybuc acid.

- *Liver disease* (primarily hepatitis and jaundice): halothane, oral contraceptives, erythromycin, phenothiazines, and MAO inhibitors.

- *Diabetes out of control:* corticosteroids, furosemide, oral contraceptives, phenytoin, thiazide diuretics.

- *Kidney disease:* analgesics (including aspirin), anti-inflammatory agents, anticoagulants, anticonvulsants, and antimigraine preparations. Certain antibiotics have also been implicated in kidney disease.

- *Blood problems* (different types of anemia and clotting abnormalities): antimalarials, sulfonamides, methyldopa, penicillin, chloramphenicol, phenylbutazone, trimethidione, phenytoin, primidine, phenobarbital, corticosteroids, oral contraceptives.

- *Neurological dysfunctions* (such as shuffling gait or tremors): isoniazid, some antibiotics, phenothiazide, reserpine, oral contraceptives, corticosteroids.

- *Eye disorders:* thioridazine, thloroquine, some steroids.
- *Ear disturbances:* streptomycin, neomycin, kanamycin, salicylates.

Other diseases, such as systemic lupus erythematosis and gout, can be initiated or unmasked by taking certain drugs.

22
oral
contraceptives

Besides sterilization, oral contraceptives constitute the most effective way of preventing pregnancy.[1] "The Pill," as it is called in America, is in fact considered to be 99.5 percent effective.[2] It isn't messy, like diaphragms and jelly. It can't cause uterine infections, like an IUD. And it doesn't interrupt lovemaking, like condoms or foams. As a result, the Pill is extremely popular, used by approximately 10 million women in America and by 50 million throughout the world. Yet how much do we know about the Pill?

Before we can understand how the Pill works to prevent conception, we need to understand a few of the basics about human reproduction.[3] First the woman's body prepares itself for pregnancy once each month. This marvelous process begins with the *ovaries*—small organs about the size of walnuts that contain thousands of spherical arrangements called follicles. Each follicle contains an immature egg (or *ovum*). In a woman of child-bearing age, follicles release a hormone called *estrogen* about once every 28 days. A maturing process in the ovary starts moving the eggs towards the ovary's surface, until a follicle finally ruptures about midway through the cycle, releasing an egg and sending it into the fallopian tube. The release of a mature egg is called *ovulation*.

A second hormone enters the scene at this point. Working with estrogen, *progesterone* helps the body create an environment favorable for the fertilization of the egg and the nurturing of the fetus. The uterine lining, while building up, becomes enriched with thousands of

287

blood vessels that serve as the place where the fertilized egg can implant itself and begin to grow.

Fertilization can take place anywhere from four to seven days from the time the egg is released from the ovary. If fertilization does not take place, the egg disintegrates, and the uterine lining—now rich with blood—is shed, leaving the body through the vagina. This natural bleeding, which occurs once each month, is known as menstrual bleeding, or *menstruation*.

But what happens if a sperm enters the fallopian tube and fertilizes the egg? Instead of disintegrating, the fertilized egg travels the length of the fallopian tube, enters the uterus, and becomes implanted in the thick, blood-rich lining. There, nourished, it grows until it becomes a full-sized baby nine months later. Upon implantation, an increase in hormone production signals the woman's body not to release any more eggs until the baby has been delivered and the uterus is prepared to accept another fertilized egg.

Oral contraceptives, taken for 20 or 21 days of the menstrual cycle, somehow prevent fertilization of the egg. Yet we're not quite sure *how* they do so. All we can say for certain is that their active ingredients— estrogen and a man-made version of progesterone, called *progestogen*—prevent conception. At first the Pill contained high levels of both, but researchers eventually modified the drug and came up with less potent combinations that still do the job. But precisely how these ingredients affect the process of conception is still guesswork. Some doctors think that they have some effect on the fertilized egg that prevents it from implanting itself in the uterine lining. Others think the Pill actually suppresses ovulation: Where there is no egg, there can be no pregnancy. Others think that the Pill creates a false pregnancy that tricks the body into not releasing any more eggs. Still others think that the Pill makes the cervix secrete a thick mucous layer that the sperm cannot penetrate. However it works, one thing is clear: It works. Most users of the Pill succeed in preventing conception and enjoy a 99-percent success rate.[4]

CAUTIONS AND SIDE EFFECTS

If the Pill is so effective, then why doesn't everyone use it? The answer probably lies in the fact that the Pill has a number of unpleasant—even dangerous—side effects. In fact, statistically, there is a chance that you might even die from the Pill.[5] Of course, a number of factors increase your risk: Obesity, cigarette smoking, and certain medical disorders all make taking the Pill more risky. Further, some women who react more severely to synthetic estrogen than others are at a greater risk of developing dangerous complications.

Before you decide to use the Pill, you should be aware of possible complications and side effects that are relatively common in women who use oral contraceptives:[6]

1. *Birth defects.* A fetus exposed to an oral contraceptive during the first three months of pregnancy runs a greater-than-normal risk of developing congenital heart disease. Evidence indicates that the Pill may also be responsible for multiple defects of the limbs (or even missing limbs) and of the central nervous system. If you are taking the Pill and think you have gotten pregnant anyway, stop taking the Pill immediately and see your doctor. If you stop taking the Pill in the hope of getting pregnant, wait at least three months before you conceive so that the chemicals have time to leave your system.

2. *Alteration in the quality of the mother's milk.* Oral contraceptives alter the fat and protein content of mother's milk, so you should not take the Pill while you are nursing a baby.

3. *Development of blood clots.* You run a greater-than-normal risk of developing venous clots, which may be surface or deep and which may develop into pulmonary embolisms, eventually leading to death. The likelihood of clotting diseases is 4 to 11 times greater if you take the Pill than if you don't.[7] This risk may be due to the blood platelets' increased responsiveness in clotting and to the decreased flow of venous blood in the legs, lungs, or brain. Your risk of developing a blood clot following surgery is also severe. If you are taking the Pill, stop taking it four to six weeks before surgery, and wait until two weeks after surgery to start taking it again.

4. *Heart attack.* The risk of myocardial infarction—both fatal and nonfatal—is serious among women who use the Pill. Women over 40 who smoke cigarettes run the greatest risk of all. A British study showed that in women 30 to 40 years of age, the risk of heart attack is two-and-a-half times greater among those who take the Pill than among those who don't. And in women ages 40 to 44, those who take the Pill have a five times greater risk of heart attack than those who don't. These figures do not mean that women who take the Pill have 2.5 to 5 times more heart attacks; they mean only that they have 2.5 to 5 times more risk of having heart attacks.[8] Other factors that increase your risk of myocardial infarction while you are taking the Pill include obesity, diabetes, hypertension, and high cholesterol levels.

Why does the Pill have such an adverse effect on a woman's chances? Beside its effect on blood clotting, the Pill may also cause increasing coronary atherosclerosis (that is, the narrowing of the vessels due to lipid, or fatty, deposits); it causes cholesterol and triglyceride levels in the blood to increase slightly, which may cause blocking of the coronary vessels.

5. *General diseases of the cardiovascular system.* Myocardial infarction is only one of the diseases commonly associated with the Pill. Deaths have been reported from a number of other cardiovascular diseases aggravated by oral contraceptives.

6. *Cerebrovascular disease.* Women who take oral contraceptives run a nine-fold increase in the risk of cerebral hemorrhage or stroke.[9] Stop taking the Pill immediately and call a doctor, if you develop any of the symptoms of cerebral hemorrhage or stroke: loss of vision, the periodic loss of the use of a limb, transient numbness at the side of the tongue, transient speech defect, or a migraine-like headache that changes character.

7. *High blood pressure (hypertension).* The dosage and the length of time you use oral contraceptives determine their effect on your blood pressure. Hypertension does not appear until you take the Pill for three to nine months. At that time, the great majority of women on the Pill have a slight increase in both systolic (pumping) pressure and diastolic (resting) pressure. This increase in blood pressure can increase your risk of having kidney disease or a stroke.

If you are taking the Pill, you should have regular blood pressure readings to ascertain any rise in blood pressure. Report to your doctor any sudden gain in weight, which is indicative of water and sodium retention that sometimes accompanies an increase in blood pressure. If you do experience an increase in blood pressure, you should stop taking the Pill immediately; in most cases, your blood pressure returns to normal in about three months.

8. *Benign breast disease.* Again, the dosage and the length of use determine the development of benign breast disease, characterized by fibrous growths in the tissues of the breast. Fibrocystic growths are usually not apparent until you have taken the Pill for two years. Although benign, these growths enhance a woman's risk of developing breast cancer later on.

9. *Breast cancer.* While there is no definite causal link between breast cancer and the Pill, studies indicate that there is some sort of connection. If you are taking the Pill, you should perform regular and thorough breast self-examinations and go for a careful examination by a doctor every six months. You should consider being examined more often if your mother or sister has had breast cancer.

10. *Endometrial cancer.* Oral contraceptives may cause uterine dysplasia (that is, an abnormal development of the cells of the uterus), which may develop into cancer. Like breast cancer, endometrial cancer has not been definitely linked to use of the Pill, but a connection is suspected by many.

11. *Liver disease.* Generally occurring in women who have used the Pill for at least five years, liver disease that results from the use of oral contraceptives can be either benign or malignant. There is also an increase in hepatitis among Pill users. If you develop abdominal pain while you are taking the Pill, you should stop taking it and see a doctor. A common complication is the rupture of the liver nodes and intra-abdominal hemorrhage.

12. *Cervical cancer.* Women who are sexually active and who are using oral contraceptives run a higher risk of developing cancer of the cervix. Pap smears every six months are critical if you are taking the Pill. If cervical dysplasia occurs while you are taking the Pill, you should have a pap smear three months from that time and then every six months after that.[10]

13. *Abnormal lactation.* During or after the time you are taking the Pill, you may develop abnormal lactation—that is, a leakage of lactose from the breasts, not associated with childbirth or nursing. Since you will probably not notice the problem if the amount of lactic juice is minimal, you should be aware of the possibility and watch for leakage during your regular self-examination.

14. *Amenorrhea (cessation of the menstrual periods).* In some women, the use of oral contraceptives reduces the amount of menstrual bleeding that accompanies each menstrual period. In a few, the suppression of menstrual flow becomes so severe that the menstrual bleeding stops altogether. If either side effect happens, you should be tested for pregnancy immediately. If pregnant, you should immediately stop taking the Pill; if not pregnant, your doctor should determine how to treat you. For women who find the lack of menstrual bleeding emotionally upsetting, the physician may prescribe a brand of oral contraceptive that contains a higher amount of estrogen and a lower amount of progestogen, a combination that usually reestablishes the monthly bleeding.

15. *Oversuppression syndrome.* In less than 1 percent of the women who take the Pill, the amenorrhea continues for some time after they have discontinued the use of oral contraceptives. If your period does not return within six months (and you are definitely not pregnant), inform your doctor. He or she may want to consider testing your pituitary function to make sure the oral contraceptives did not permanently affect it.

16. *Eye problems.* You may experience a change in visual acuity, burning of the eyes, or intolerance to your contact lenses if you are taking the Pill. Eye problems will be more severe and more frequent if you also suffer from migraine headaches. If you develop an intolerance to your contact lenses, you should quit wearing them and see your eye doctor for a complete reassessment.

17. *Gallbladder disease.* You double your chances of developing gallstones (hard deposits of cholesterol in the gallbladder), which require surgery before the age of 60 if you are taking oral contraceptives.

In addition to these complications, you should know about other possible side effects that you can expect from the use of oral contraceptives:[11]

- nausea,
- vomiting,
- breakthrough bleeding from the vagina or menstrual blood spotting,
- tenderness or enlargement of the breasts,
- jaundice,
- rash (generally caused by allergy),
- inability to tolerate carbohydrates,
- cataracts,
- either an increase or decrease in appetite,
- headaches or worsened migraine headaches,
- dizziness,
- growth of body hair,
- loss of scalp hair,
- impaired kidney function,
- weight gain and bloating,
- complexion problems or darkening of the skin,

- mood changes,
- cramps,
- more tubal pregnancy,
- more severe epilepsy,
- decreased quantities of breast milk,
- temporary infertility after discontinuance,
- mental depression,
- vaginal infection,
- changes in libido,
- nervousness,
- changes in the surface of the cornea.

WHO SHOULDN'T USE THE PILL?

Keeping in mind the side effects and possible complications, certain women should not use the pill. Don't plan on a program of oral contraception if you have had:[12]

- thrombophlebitis,
- thromboembolic disorders,
- active liver disease (benign or malignant),
- classical migraine,
- any eye disorder (including the loss of vision),
- myocardial infarction,
- jaundice,
- known or suspected breast cancer,
- cerebrovascular disorders (including stroke),
- known or suspected cancer of the endometrium,
- undiagnosed vaginal bleeding,
- diabetes,
- hypercholesterolemia,
- chronic illness leading to immobility,
- a family history of vascular diseases,
- a family history of breast cancer,
- breast nodules or fibrocystic disease,

- abnormal mammograms,

- exposure to DES (diethylstilbesterol) or estrogen during your mother's pregnancy,

- depressive reactions, or

- varicosities (such as varicose veins).

Of course, you should never use oral contraceptives if you are pregnant or if you are nursing a baby.

It is recommended that women over 40 years of age not take oral contraceptives. It is strongly suggested that women who smoke not take oral contraceptives because it increases the risk of myocardial infarctions. This factor is so important that a warning now appears on oral contraceptive packages: "Caution: Cigarette smoking increases the risk of serious adverse effects on the heart and blood vessels from oral contraceptive use. The risk increases with age and with heavy smoking (15 or more cigarettes per day) and is quite marked in women over 35 years of age. Women who use oral contraceptives should not smoke."[13]

Young women who have not achieved their full growth should not take the Pill either.

THE PILL AND DIET

Women who are on the Pill have nutritional needs different from those who aren't.[14] The Pill seems to lower blood levels of several of the B vitamins, vitamin C, and some important minerals. Lowering of vitamin B12, vitamin B6, vitamin C, and folate seem to be a result of the oral contraceptive's effect on the body's ability to metabolize the vitamins. Other vitamin levels are increased in women who use the Pill: Women who take oral contraceptives have a higher concentration of vitamin A, vitamin K, and iron than those who do not. If you are using the Pill, then, you need to take active measures to increase your intake of vitamins C, B6, B12, and folic acid. Because your body can utilize vitamins and minerals found in natural foods better than those obtained from vitamin supplements, make an effort to eat some of the following:

- *Vitamin C sources:* Broccoli, horseradish, turnip greens, rose hips, brussels sprouts, kale, parsley, sweet peppers, collards, acerola, black currants, guava, cauliflower, kohlrabi, strawberries, lemons, oranges, beet greens, cabbage, chives, watercress, spinach, papayas, and mustard.

• *Vitamin B6 sources:* Eggs, butter, yeast, bananas, beef, lamb, pork, veal, cod, flounder, halibut, tuna, liver, herring, salmon, mackerel, sardines, blackstrap molasses, avocados, pears, barley, grapes, carrots, cabbage, corn, oats, tomatoes, turnips, yams, cauliflower, brussels sprouts, wheat, soybeans, spinach, potatoes, kale, peas, rye, peanuts, wheat germ, walnuts, and brown rice.

• *Vitamin B12 sources:* Egg yolk, clams, sardines, herring, oysters, crabs, salmon, heart, brain, liver, and kidney.

• *Folic acid sources:* Lima beans, snap beans, barley, oats, rye, wheat, liver, asparagus, spinach, wheat, bran, yeast, dry beans, kidney, corn, beet greens, broccoli, chicory, kale, parsley, endive, chard, turnip greens, watercress, almonds, peanuts, walnuts, filberts.

REDUCING RISK AND MANAGING SIDE EFFECTS

Is there a way to reduce risk and manage side effects of the pill? Yes, there is. The key is to have a complete and thorough physical examination before you make the decision to use an oral contraceptive.[15] If you are normal and healthy and young, you will probably not suffer such a great risk from oral contraceptives. Make sure:

• that your circulatory system is in good working order,

• that your blood pressure is normal and stable,

• that you are not pregnant,

• that your menstrual cycles have been normal and regular,

• that you are not diabetic,

• that you are not overweight,

• that you have not had a history of breast cancer and that your mother or sisters have not had breast cancer,

• that you are not over the age of 40,

• that you have not had a cerebrovascular disorder, and

• that you have not seen a doctor for severe depression.

If you decide to use oral contraceptives, you can do several things to manage the most common of the side effects and make your course of medication more comfortable:[16]

1. *Take the Pill after you have eaten a full meal.* Nausea is usually severe if you take the medication on an empty stomach.

2. *If you suffer from breakthrough bleeding, consult your doctor.* If a medical cause is ruled out, ask for a change to a pill containing a higher level of estrogen. The breakthrough bleeding will be controlled.

3. *If you are worried by the scanty appearance of your menstrual bleeding, have your doctor examine you to make sure nothing is wrong.* If the scanty bleeding is simply an effect of the oral contraceptives, ask for a Pill that is higher in estrogen.

4. *If you suffer from heavy menstrual bleeding while on the Pill, ask your doctor for a pill that contains more progestin and less estrogen.*

5. *Modify your medication if you put on weight for no apparent reason.* If you gain weight that is not related to a decrease in physical exercise or to an increase in caloric intake, ask your doctor to change your pill. A pill lower in estrogen helps control cyclic weight gain; a continuous weight gain can be controlled by lowering the progestin level.

CHOOSING THE RIGHT PILL

Oral contraceptives are manufactured with a variety of estrogen and progestin levels, and the one that your doctor chooses for you depends on your needs and on the hormonal balance that works best for you.[17] A doctor will probably advise you to use a compound that is the most effective and that has the widest safety margin in terms of side effects. Most women find that a pill containing 50 micrograms of estrogen works well with the least side effects. Brands in this category include Demulen, Norinyl 1 + 50, Ortho-Novum 1/50, Ovcon-50, Norlestrin 1/50, Zorane 1/50, and Ovral. Pills containing 100 milligrams of estrogen have more side effects and are used only in cases where a lower estrogen dosage doesn't work. If you need more estrogen than is contained in the standard pill, your doctor will probably prescribe Norinyl 1 + 80, Ortho-Novum 1/80, or Ovulen.

Sometimes the Pill is used for purposes other than contraception—such as the treatment of menopause—and is used for its estrogen. In these cases, when the woman requires a high estrogen content, the doctor may choose Enovid 5 mg, Enovid 10 mg, Enovid-E, Norinyl 2 mg, Ortho-Novum 2 mg, Ortho-Novum 10 mg, or Norlestrin 2.5/50. Women who need a reduced estrogen level will probably be given

Loestrin 1/20, Zorane 1/20, Loestrin 1.5/30, Zorane 1.5/30, Lo/Ovral, Brevicon, Modicon, or Ovcon-35. In some rare cases, some women may need a pill containing progestin only; Micronor, Nor-Q.D., and Ovrette fall in that category.

If you decide not to use the Pill, ask your doctor to explain the other options open to you for birth control. Safe and reliable methods are available for both men and women. Make sure that you understand how each method works, its possible side effects, and its reliability rate before you make a decision concerning the method of contraception to use.

23

drugs
and pregnancy

Good prenatal care is critical to the health of both the mother and the baby. A sound program of exercise, proper nutrition, regular medical care, and avoiding exposure to harmful chemicals and agents can help ensure the best health for the baby and the safest, most problem-free pregnancy for the mother.

The thalidomide tragedy of 1962, which left thousands of children without arms and with other serious birth defects, focused the nation's attention on the safety of drugs taken during pregnancy. Knowing which drugs are safe and which are not safe to take while you are pregnant or nursing a baby can help you avoid those that may result in serious defects or death.

An expectant mother should realize that birth defects can result from taking drugs during pregnancy. The extent of damage depends on the nature of the drug, the amount and frequency of dosage, and the stage of pregnancy when the drug is taken. The most precarious time for the fetus is the first trimester (three months) of pregnancy. The first trimester is especially important in the development of the unborn child because many important and vital organ systems are being formed. During this period, the fetus is most susceptible to the effects of drugs. The stretch of time between day 13 and day 56 of the pregnancy is particularly dangerous because a woman may not realize she is pregnant until the organ formation is nearly complete. She may not be under the care of a physician, and worse, she may be taking some kind of medication. Some of the critical times for organ damage are 15 to 25

298

days for the central nervous system, 24 to 30 days for the eyes, 24 to 36 days for the legs, and 20 to 40 days for the heart. Most damage to body structures and organs occurs up until the eleventh week of pregnancy, but, after that time, behavioral damage can occur, which might produce hyperactivity or learning disabilities. Besides timing, large and frequent doses make exposure of the fetus to the drug all the more likely, and greater exposure, of course, makes damage to the fetus ever more probable.[1]

There are times during pregnancy when drugs must be taken. When a mother has an infection, heart disease, thyroid disease, high blood pressure, diabetes, or seizures, drugs must be taken. But care must be used in taking only the medication that is needed—not medication just to relieve symptoms. Medications should not be taken unless the illness or condition might pose a risk to the health and welfare of the mother or fetus. Even then, it must be considered whether the risk outweighs the benefit. When a pregnant female takes any substance into her body, she has to remember that she is no longer affecting just one human being, but two—her unborn child and herself.

THE TRANSFER PROCESS

One thing pregnant women should remember, and bear in mind continually during their pregnancy, is that the mother and the fetal child are inseparable, one and the same thing; but it does not necessarily follow that medication that helps the mother will not harm the unborn child.[2]

The average pregnant woman ingests ten different drugs during her pregnancy, four of them prescription. These ten drugs do not include vitamins, iron supplements, cigarettes, intravenous fluids, or anesthesia. Some of these drugs and substances are taken orally; others are injected intravenously.

What happens if you take a drug while you are pregnant? How does a drug transfer from your body to that of your baby? Until recently, doctors thought that the placenta served as an effective barrier between the mother and the growing fetus, blocking the passage of drugs and other harmful substances while permitting an exchange of life-giving elements, like food and oxygen. We know now, however, that the placenta is like all other human membranes—capable of being penetrated by chemical substances, including drugs.[3]

What happens to a drug when it enters your body? If you take the drug orally (such as a tablet or capsule), you swallow it, generally with some kind of fluid that speeds its dissolving in your stomach. As the drug dissolves, it is absorbed directly into the tissues of the stomach, where blood vessels absorb it and carry it to the liver. In the liver, the drug undergoes certain changes before it reenters the bloodstream and is circulated throughout the body. Drugs that are injected directly into the bloodstream travel throughout the body in the plasma. As they pass through the liver, they also undergo transformation before reentering the bloodstream and general circulation.

At this point, the placenta comes in. Your blood circulates through arteries, which take it to the uterine wall and the placenta, and returns through veins, which lead from the placenta back to the uterine wall and eventually back to the heart. The fetus, on the other hand, has arteries that flow from its body through the umbilical cord and into tiny capillaries laced throughout the placenta, the *placental villi*. In the walls of the villi—those tiny capillaries—the exchange takes place; the thin membranes of the villi permit the exchange of food, oxygen, and other substances from the mother's blood to the fetus's blood. The fetal blood then flows back through veins in the umbilical cord to its body.

How do chemicals, molecules of oxygen, and other elements pass through the membranes of the villi?

The most important—and major—way is by simple diffusion. The blood (bearing all its chemicals and elements) simply diffuses from an area of greater concentration (the mother's arteries) to an area of lesser concentration (the baby's arteries). The process is quite a simple one; it requires no real energy, and there is no competition among molecules. The rate of diffusion is determined by how concentrated the blood is, how many lipids (fats or fat-like substances) are in it, and how large the molecules are. Blood with a high lipid content passes through easily; most drugs have a high lipid content, have small molecular structure, and have little trouble passing through the membrane.

Diffusion isn't the only way drugs can pass through the membrane. Drugs with extremely small molecules can pass directly through the pores in the membrane. Even smaller molecules of drug chemicals can be picked up by another molecule, which then penetrates through a pore in the membrane and is discharged on the other side.

Of course, not all the drug taken by a mother ends up in the fetus, but almost every drug that a pregnant woman takes reaches her fetus in some concentration. Many factors influence the degree of concentration and the amount of penetration through the placenta:

- how the drug is administered,
- what time the drug is administered,
- how the drug is distributed through the mother's body,

- whether the drug binds to protein or body fat,

- how the mother's body works to metabolize the drug,

- how the mother's liver functions,

- whether the mother suffers from any inherited enzyme deficiencies,

- how large the molecules are when the drug is dissolved,

- how the drug reacts to water (is it soluble?),

- how the fetus's liver responds,

- the presence of disease (such as diabetes or toxemia),

- the size and thickness of the placenta,

- which enzymes are present in the placenta,

- how fast blood flows through the placenta, and

- how old the placental tissue is.

One other characteristic of the unborn child makes it especially susceptible to the effects of drugs. Because the fetus's circulation is different from an adult's, there may be a lower blood plasma concentration of the drug in the child. As an effect, the drug may stay in the bloodstream longer and affect the child for a longer period of time. So, because the fetus and its body function are different from an adult's, the child may react in the same or a different way from the way an adult would react to the very same drug.

WHICH DRUGS ARE UNSAFE

Too many women think that the only drugs that hurt their babies are those brightly colored prescription pills, and they wrongly think that their doctor protects them from harm by not prescribing harmful medication during pregnancy. Both assumptions, of course, are partially true: Many of the prescription drugs that are otherwise safe should not be taken during pregnancy, and doctors do protect you against harmful medication as much as possible. But even the common drugs—the things we don't usually think of as drugs—can hurt a developing fetus, sometimes more severely than many drugs a doctor might prescribe. In this section, we will see how a number of drugs and categories of drugs adversely affect mothers and their babies.[4]

Alcohol

Used during pregnancy, alcohol stunts the growth of the baby both before and after birth, as well as causing psychomotor retardation and small eye fissures and joint abnormalities in the infant. It has been cited as a major cause of mental retardation at birth.

In 1973, researchers at the University of Washington in Seattle, identified a condition that resulted from mothers' drinking large quantities of alcohol during pregnancy. This condition has been given the name "fetal alcohol syndrome (FAS)."[5] Full-blown symptoms of FAS appear in children born to alcoholic mothers, but partial symptoms show up in children of mothers who have been moderate drinkers, social drinkers, or binge drinkers. Generally, it is thought that as the mother consumes more alcohol, she runs an increasingly greater risk of having an FAS baby. The National Institute of Alcohol Abuse and Alcoholism states that pregnant women who consume 3 ounces of absolute alcohol (or six average drinks) per day face a definite risk of having an FAS baby. The NIAAA even cautions that drinking 1 to 3 ounces of absolute alcohol (or two to six average drinks) per day may be risky.[6] Actually, no one has determined a safe level of drinking. Recent studies indicate that one or two births per one thousand produce an FAS baby; partial symptoms occur in three to five births per one thousand.[7]

Children with FAS show characteristic symptoms that can be classified by five catagories:

1. *Central nervous system defects.* FAS is the third leading cause of mental retardation in infants. The retardation may range from borderline to severe, and accompanying physical deformities may or may not be present. In one group of FAS patients from 10 months to 21 years old, the average I.Q. was 65,[8] and apparently the retardation was roughly as severe as the physical deformities. FAS babies may also be hyperactive or extremely nervous, have poor attention spans, and experience tremors.

2. *Growth deficiencies.* Babies with FAS tend to have low birthweights and continue to be underweight long after birth. They are also slow to grow and don't catch up in growth even later in life.

3. *Abnormalities of the face, head, and palms.* Most FAS children are slightly microcephalic and have small eyes with epicanthic folds, a "fish" mouth (with a convex upper lip), a short upturned nose with a sunken nasal bridge, a protruding forehead, a small mouth with a retracted upper lip, a receding chin, and deformed ears. These children also have abnormal creases of their palms.

4. *Heart defects.* Most often the heart problems of FAS babies show up as heart murmurs and septal defects, but there may also be a few cases of tetraology of Fallot (a condition with four defects) and coarctation (narrowing) of the aorta.

5. *Joint and limb deformities, such as a small jaw.* In moderate, social, and binge drinkers, these symptoms may not be as pronounced. Babies born to these mothers may have symptoms very like a baby in narcotic withdrawal. They may yawn, sneeze a lot, and have tremors and dazed eyes.

To curb the growing numbers of FAS babies born each year, doctors have suggested that alcoholics of child-bearing age should stop drinking prior to conception and should not drink while they are pregnant and nursing. Concerned legislators have suggested that warning labels be put on the bottles of alcoholic beverages, to read: "Caution—Consumption of alcoholic beverages may be hazardous to your health, may be habit-forming, and may cause serious birth defects when consumed during pregnancy."[9]

Amphetamines
Amphetamines, used during early pregnancy as an appetite suppressant, can cause congenital heart defects. Withdrawal symptoms are usually not present in the newborn.

Anticonvulsants
The anticonvulsants, such as dilantin, can produce deformity if they are taken in early pregnancy. Women taking anticonvulsant drugs have a two to three times higher incidence of malformed babies than women with seizures who are taking antiepileptic drugs. The defects may show up as: cleft lip and palate, congenital hip dislocation, microcephaly, eyes with epicanthic folds, low nasal bridge, wide mouth, undescended testes, and congenital heart disease (mostly septal defects). Affected children may also show slow growth and a lowered I.Q. Pregnant women with seizures should *not* stop taking anticonvulsants; they should have their doctors prescribe alternate drugs to control seizures.

Antiemetics
Antiemetics should not be used during pregnancy because of their possible toxic effect on the fetal liver.

Antihistamines
Antihistamines can cause bleeding problems in babies. It is also thought that these drugs can cause skeletal deformities, liver and brain damage, low blood pressure, and respiratory depression in the fetus.

Aspirin
Since a fetus does not have the capability to metabolize aspirin (salicylate), a large concentration of unaltered salicylate is usually found in the umbilical cord of mothers who take aspirin during their pregnancy. Even so, the effects of aspirin on a child are usually not significant unless the aspirin is taken within several weeks of delivery.

Even common aspirin, however, can take its toll. Aspirin, taken several weeks before delivery, can cause impaired platelet function, in both mothers and infants. Mothers who take aspirin throughout their pregnancies run a risk of anemia, excess hemorrhage at or following birth, prolonged pregnancy, complicated deliveries, and the loss of babies through stillbirth. The platelet dysfunction is more severe (and critical) in babies. Because the newborn is unable to respond to the usual stimuli that initiate the clotting response (due to the aspirin's effects), the blood is unable to clot normally; hemorrhage at birth may result.[10]

Additionally, aspirin, taken early in pregnancy, may cause babies to be lower in birth weight and have a lack of subcutaneous ("under-the-skin") fat. The skin may also be cracked at birth. Some evidence now indicates that deformities of the hands, feet, and heart may also result from taking aspirin in the early stages of pregnancy.

Doctors generally warn mothers against taking aspirin any time during pregnancy but especially during the last trimester. The warning extends to any product that contains aspirin, including many decongestants, cold medications, antacids, and pain relievers.[11]

Barbiturates
The barbiturates, including those in sleeping pills, readily cross the placental barrier and store up in toxic amounts in the fetal brain, fetal liver, and the placenta. The concentration in the fetus is greater than in the mother. Pregnant women should remember not to take barbiturates during the last trimester of pregnancy, or the infant will demonstrate withdrawal symptoms and respiratory depression shortly after birth.

Birth Control Pills
If taken during the first three or four months of pregnancy, hormones contained in most kinds of oral contraceptives—estrogen and progestin—can cause birth defects: specifically, vertebral, anal, car-

diac, esophageal, renal, and limb abnormalities. In addition, female children born to mothers who took estrogen during pregnancy have a high risk of developing a normally rare form of vaginal or cervical cancer.

Current medical knowledge concerning the effect of estrogen and progestin on unborn children has changed former methods of treatment using both drugs. Estrogen was once used to prevent miscarriages, and progestins were used in solutions as a test for pregnancy. Both uses have been discontinued, and the FDA now requires that all women who use estrogens be given a brochure explaining the possible effect of the drug on an unborn child.[12]

If you think you might have gotten pregnant while using an oral contraceptive, stop taking the contraceptive immediately and contact your doctor. If you stop taking oral contraceptives in the hope of getting pregnant, wait at least three months after you have stopped to conceive your child. You should consider using another form of birth control until the three-month period has passed.

Bromides
Bromides, including those found in some major antacids (as discussed in Chapter 1), cause retarded growth of the child, dilated pupils in the newborn, and lethargy following birth. Some children may suffer from dermatitis if their mothers use bromide salts during pregnancy.

Caffeine
That cup of coffee in the morning might really perk you up. Yet if you drink a lot of it during the first five months of your pregnancy, it does just the opposite to your baby; he or she will be less active at birth and suffer from poor muscle tone. Excessive coffee intake also increases your chances of having a breech delivery, a miscarriage, or a still-birth.[13]

The culprit is caffeine, a substance that occurs naturally in coffee, tea, cocoa, chocolate, and the kola nut used to make soft drinks. In an overdose, caffeine causes difficulty in falling asleep, disturbances in the heart rate, anxiety, irritability, and nervousness. Used heavily, it can also cause birth defects.[14] Most seriously, it may result in miscarriage, spontaneous abortion, and stillbirth—dangers that also result from cigarette smoking and the use of alcoholic beverages.

As a contrast study, researchers studied birth rates in Utah, whose population is predominantly Mormon—a religion that prohibits the use of coffee, tea, alcohol, and tobacco among its members. Utah, with the highest birth rate in the nation, also enjoys the lowest fetal, neonatal, and infant death rates.[15] While other factors undoubtedly play a part, researchers are convinced that the low consumption rate of tobacco, caffeine, and alcohol plays a major part in the normal and healthy deliveries among Utah's population.

Cancer-Treating Drugs
Drugs used to treat cancer should not be used during pregnancy, including procarbazine and triethylene melamine. Infants whose mothers undergo chemotherapy during pregnancy suffer kidney malformation and serious physical malformations.

Cigarettes
"A mother who smokes a pack a day runs twice the risk of the baby's dying as do mothers in the general population."[16] Yet 15 million women of child-bearing age (between the ages 15 and 44) are smokers. Cigarette smoking during pregnancy increases a woman's chance of having a miscarriage, premature birth, or a stillborn child.[17] Further, while cigarette smoking has not yet been definitely linked to birth defects, it is suspected as a cause of abnormalities, some of which are not detected immediately at birth.

Three substances in cigarette smoke are rapidly transferred across the placental barrier:

• *Carbon monoxide:* This gas decreases oxygen in the placenta and in the baby's tissues, thus affecting the baby's breathing. Special monitoring has recently revealed that fetal breathing movements are diminished when a mother smokes two cigarettes in succession. The regularity of the fetal breathing movements is generally regarded as a sign of fetal well-being.

• *Nicotine:* Transferred directly to the fetus, nicotine causes the fetal heart rate to increase, and it may cause fluctuations in the baby's blood pressure.

• *Carcinogens (or agents that may produce cancer):* Unborn children who are exposed to cancer-producing agents may have cancer at birth and may have a higher incidence of cancer after birth through the childhood years.

In addition to these problems, babies born to mothers who smoked during pregnancy tend to be smaller, weaker, and less developed at birth than children born to mothers who do not smoke. The low birthweight, with all its risks, is twice as common in mothers who smoke as in mothers who don't. If a mother stops smoking four months before her delivery, her chances of having a baby of low birthweight are greatly diminished. Babies born to smoking mothers weigh on the average 150 to 250 grams less than nonsmokers' babies.

Cytotoxic Drugs
Cytotoxic drugs, such as methotrexate, cause birth defects, notably hydrocephalus, limb abnormalities, and prenatal growth deficits. Neonatal death is frequent among those who use cytotoxic drugs during pregnancy.

Diazepam (Valium)
While diazepam is generally safe in low doses, increased doses can cause a slight depression of vital signs in infants and shorten the duration of normal labor. If a woman has had massive doses, the infant may experience withdrawal symptoms shortly after birth.

Hypoglycemic Drugs
Hypoglycemic drugs, taken orally, are extremely dangerous during pregnancy. Pregnant women should instead use insulin intravenously, which has been used safely with no side effects for years. Hypoglycemic oral drugs, on the other hand, cause prolonged hypoglycemia in infants and contribute to a high infant mortality rate.

Hormones
Besides those contained in oral contraceptives, certain hormones, especially testosterone, can cause hormonal changes in the fetus, leading to extreme masculinization of a female.

Librium
Librium is dangerous only if used during the first 42 days of pregnancy. If the drug is taken during this time, there is an increased risk of having a baby with a cleft lip or palate. You should avoid this drug if you suspect you might be pregnant.

Lidocaine
Lidocaine and other local anesthetics used during delivery can cause depression of vital signs among the newborn, especially respiration. Newborns who have high blood lidocaine levels usually require resuscitation at birth. Local anesthetics used during delivery can also cause heart abnormalities among the newborn.

Lithium
Lithium causes altered heartbeat and cardiac rhythm, goiter, altered thyroid function and jaundice in the child.

LSD
Lysergic acid diethylamide (LSD) causes chromosomal damage, birth defects involving the limbs, and malformations of the skeleton in children whose mothers used the drug during pregnancy. An increased

rate of spontaneous abortion among pregnant women who take LSD has also been noticed.

Mercury
Contained in organic salts, mercury causes mental deficiencies in the newborn and is a major factor in the development of hypertonicity and seizures. Infants born to mothers who used mercury during pregnancy often develop cerebral palsy-like symptoms similar to those seen in Minamata disease in Japan. Mercury may also be cause of chromosomal breakage, which can lead to birth defects.

Narcotics
When, after large doses of narcotics (particularly heroin), a mother is addicted and narcotics pass the placental barrier, the child also becomes addicted and subject to withdrawal. Between 50 and 90 percent of infants born to addicted mothers have withdrawal.[18] Withdrawal may occur any time between birth and two weeks after birth, with the average onset taking place 72 hours after birth.

Narcotic withdrawal has very distinct symptoms in the newborn. Withdrawing babies usually have a fragile appearance. They have increased muscle tone, moving with jerks or tremors. They are irritable and cry with an unmistakably shrill cry. They may be restless and hyperactive, but they are less mature in motor development. Withdrawal babies sweat, whereas normal newborns do not perspire for awhile. These children may also fail to cuddle, have sleep disturbances, suck excessively, and have vomiting and diarrhea. Unfortunately, however, withdrawal may not appear or be diagnosed before the baby leaves the hospital. Many babies are therefore not diagnosed and treated.

Treatment for addiction is easy. Many of these babies need only to be held, fed, and cared for to relieve the symptoms, but others must have drug therapy to overcome withdrawal. Usually, the drug of choice is chlorpromazine, but other drugs (such as valium, phenobarbital, or methadone) may be given.

In addition to causing physical dependence in the fetus, the narcotics, especially heroin, can cause damage to the chromosomes in the infant.

OTC Drugs
Another area of concern is the over-the-counter drugs that women often use to self-medicate. In today's society, self-medication seems to be a medical and social institution. Sixty-five percent of pregnant women self-medicate with OTC drugs, and 25 percent are chronic OTC drug users during pregnancy, because many of the complaints and discom-

forts of pregnancy can be relieved with them.[19] The safety of OTC drug use during pregnancy has not been completely proven, so pregnant women should steer clear of them.

Phenacetin
Phenacetin has been shown to cause blood disorders in newborns. It seems that this drug causes excessive breakdown of red blood cells, so it should not be used during pregnancy. Your doctor can substitute another, safer pain-killer in case of severe pain.

Quinine
This drug leads to congenital defects, including abnormal ear and eye formation, deafness, and abnormal development of the central vital signs, including a depression of respiration. The depressed symptoms usually last about thirty days.

Streptomycin and Dihydrostreptomycin
Streptomycin and dihydrostreptomycin, used to treat tuberculosis, cause some hearing loss in children and a greater percentage of hearing loss among mothers treated during pregnancy. The drug also causes toxicity among newborns. Despite possible side effects, steptomycin is the safest drug that can be used against tuberculosis. It should be used in tuberculosis therapy, but not to treat other infections.

Tetracycline
Tetracycline causes discoloration of the teeth and corrosion of the enamel in children whose mothers take the drug (or one similar to it) during pregnancy. Children whose mothers take the drug also experience a temporary stunting of long bone growth. Large doses of tetracycline, administered intraveneously, have caued death due to hepatic failure among women who have been given the drug while pregnant.

Thorazine
Thorazine can cause pigmentary abnormalities, jaundice, and chromosomal damage in infants. Typically prescribed for nausea, thorazine should not be used during pregnancy. Check with your doctor for a safe nausea treatment if you suspect that you might be pregnant.

Warfarin
Warfarin is sometimes used during pregnancy to treat phlebitis—vein inflammations, usually found in the legs. It can cause severe hemorrhage, and possibly death, of the fetus, in utero and during birth. Warfarin can also produce numerous birth defects, such as the malformation of the nasal bridge.

Environmental Agents

In addition to certain drugs, a number of environmental factors can contribute to birth defects and to problems of toxicity during pregnancy. While you take care to avoid the drugs that may harm you or your baby, you should also be careful to avoid the following harmful agents:[20]

1. *Radiation.* Exposure to X-rays can cause leukemia, as well as the destruction of the thyroid gland, in the child. Usually these drastic effects result only from massive does of X-ray, but it is difficult to ascertain which levels of radiation are safe. It is therefore wise to avoid any kind of exposure to X-rays. X-ray technicians generally ask you if you are pregnant before they begin X-ray treatment or tests; if you suspect that you might be pregnant but you are not sure, tell the technician so that protective measures can be taken.

2. *Diabetes* in the mother can increase the size of the infant and lead to a difficult pregnancy and birth.

3. *Herpes simplex,* a virus that causes cold sores and certain strains of venereal disease, causes damage to the child's central nervous system and results in skin lesions in the newborn.

4. *Rubella (German measles)* during the first trimester of pregnancy results in damage to the fetus, including deafness, cataracts and blindness, mental retardation, and congenital heart disease.

5. *Syphilis* in the mother can cause blindness, a low nasal bridge, and skeletal abnormalities in the infant.

6. *Injections, vaccinations* or *immunizations* present a danger of birth defects and other abnormalities. Live vaccines (such as those for measles, mumps, rubella, yellow fever, smallpox, and oral polio) are not recommended for pregnant women. The Rubella vaccine in particular can cause birth defects like those caused by the actual disease. To prevent birth defects, women should visit their doctors a few months prior to marriage and request an antibody titre for rubella. If the titre is low, the women should have a rubella vaccination which protects her and any children from rubella and its effects.[21] Killed or inactivated vaccines (such as those for *influenza, rabies, cholera, tetenus, diphtheria,* and *Salk polio*) should be given only when absolutely necessary.

Additional agents that are suspected of causing birth defects and neonatal abnormalities—but which are not confirmed—include: blighted potatoes, corticosteroids, hepatitis, influenza (flu), and the mumps.

DRUGS AND BREAST FEEDING

Many of the same drugs that should not be taken in pregnancy should also not be taken while breast feeding your baby. Many drugs can easily be transmitted from mother to child through the milk and in this way cause toxicities and overdoses in the baby.[22]

Whether or not the drug is transported via the milk depends on the lipid (fat) solubility of the drug, the pH of the milk, and whether the drug binds to protein. Drugs pass into the milk most often by diffusion (explained earlier in connection with the placental barrier). Just as with the placental barrier and transfer, the concentration of a drug in the mother's milk depends on how the mother metabolizes the drug and how her body handles the distribution and absorption of the drug. Infants may or may not be affected by the drug, depending on how much milk they consume, whether they take the same amount of milk at each feeding, how often they feed, how completely they absorb the drug, and how sensitive they are to the drug.

If you are nursing a baby, you need to exercise just as much caution about taking drugs as you do when you are pregnant. If you are in doubt as to what you should or shouldn't take, ask your doctor. A physician can advise you as to what is best for both you and your baby.

WHICH DRUGS ARE SAFE

All drugs should be used cautiously during the last trimester of pregnancy. Yet some drugs, when taken in therapeutic amounts as prescribed by your doctor, are generally safe to use during pregnancy:[23]

1. *Penicillin (G and V)* can be used to treat bacterial infections during pregnancy with no adverse effect on the developing fetus. Penicillin crosses the placenta easily, and it has been used for many years to treat infections among pregnant women.

2. *Ampicillin*, especially effective against urinary tract infections, can be used both orally and intravenously safely during pregnancy. Ampicillin does alter the chemical makeup of urine, detectable in laboratory testing, but it does not have any adverse effect on the fetus.

3. *Erythromycin* can be used to treat infection in women who are allergic to penicillin. It crosses the placenta in much lower concentrations than does penicillin, and it has no adverse effect on the fetus.

4. *Narcotic pain-killers* (such as morphine and meperidine) can be used safely in *some* pregnant women, and they are safer when used in small doses. Large doses can result in depression, hypothermia, bradycardia, and atonia in newborn infants.

Some expectant mothers should avoid them. Women who have an abnormal pregnancy history—including retardation of fetal growth, prematurity, or insufficiency of the placenta—should not be given narcotics, because those abnormalities restrict placental blood flow and cause the narcotics to concentrate more highly in the fetus. Narcotics have traditionally been used as pain-killers during delivery, but their risks should be carefully weighed, and patients should be carefully monitored.

5. *Salicylates* (including aspirin) are safe in low doses in otherwise healthy women who have not experienced abnormal pregnancies in the past. They should not be used during the last trimester of pregnancy, due to their tendency to thin the blood and to interfere with the body's platelet-forming mechanisms.

6. *Other drugs* that are generally safe during pregnancy include:

- skeletal muscle relaxants (such as diazepam),
- local anesthetic drugs (such as lidocaine and procaine),
- anticoagulants of some kinds (including heparin),
- thiazide derivatives used as diuretics,
- hormones extracted from thyroid,
- digitalis and other heart medications, and
- insulin.

In general you should take an active role in protecting both yourself and your baby by making intelligent decisions concerning drug use during pregnancy:

1. *If you suspect you are pregnant, visit your doctor as soon as possible.* Do *not* take any medication from the time you suspect pregnancy until you can ask a doctor's advice on safe medications.

2. *Make sure that any doctor who prescribes medication for you knows you are pregnant.* Don't forget that you may have to tell some doctors what is obvious to you. An orthopedic specialist who is treating you for a sprained hand, for instance, would have no reason to know that you are three months pregnant. A specialist may unwittingly expose you to harmful X-rays or prescribe an unsafe pain-killer unless you explain that you are pregnant.

3. *Be especially careful with over-the-counter drugs.* If you're in doubt about a drug, call your doctor and ask whether it is safe for you to take during pregnancy.

4. *Always consider your baby's health before you self-medicate.* Never take medications prescribed for or recommended by others unless you have asked your doctor.

5. *Take general precautions to protect yourself against disease, and limit your consumption of caffeine, tobacco, and alcohol.*

24

drugs and children

In this country, 90,000 harmful substances are ingested yearly by children under 5 years of age.[1] Newspapers and television news reports are dotted with tragic stories of children who die because they get into the medicine cabinet and, quite accidentally, eat all the pink capsules in the prescription bottle. They think the pills are candy. We hear grizzly accounts of the child next door who is rushed to the hospital to have his stomach pumped after taking a bottle of aspirin. He and a friend were practicing to be doctors. Perhaps your niece suffers severe acid burns around her mouth when she drinks a cleaning solution found in a bottle under the kitchen sink.

These stories are tragic—the more so because the heartbreak they bring seems avoidable if only people safeguard their medicines, keep them in cupboards that lock or that are too high for a child to reach, or store dangerous drugs and chemicals in child-proof packages.

Yet there are other stories, just as tragic, that we rarely hear about on television and that we rarely read about in the newspaper. Parents, in a well-meaning attempt to relieve a child's stuffy nose, may give a decongestant designed only for adults or a dose that is incorrect and unsafe for a child. When adults are insensitive to a child's special drug tolerance level, the results can be just as disastrous as the child's fumbling attempts at self-treatment (and subsequent poisoning). As a parent (or a responsible adult who is charged with the care of a child), you should be aware of special dosages and medications suited for

314

children, and you should make sure that you protect the child from unsuitable drugs.

DOSAGE GUIDELINES

A substantial number of those who take over-the-counter drug remedies are children. Yet many of these remedies fail to list dosage information for children on the labels.[2] If you have any question at all about the safety of the drug you intend to administer to a child, call your doctor or pharmacist. Either one will be happy to instruct you as to the safety, the possible side effects, and the correct dosage.

Generally, you can estimate proper dosages using the following guidelines:[3]

1. *Children under 2 years of age:* Never give a child under 2 years of age any kind of drug unless it is prescribed or recommended by the child's physician. Make sure that you understand the exact dosage of the drug and the proper method of administration. Ask the doctor to write any extra instructions (such as giving the medicine only at bedtime, with a light meal, or on an empty stomach). Don't feel foolish about asking the doctor to write down the instructions; it might save you from making a foolish mistake.

2. *Children 2 to 5 years old:* Generally, a child between 2 and 5 should be given one-quarter of the adult dose for cold or flu medication. A child between the ages of 2 and 5 should never be given a cough medicine unless it is prescribed by the child's doctor. Again, make absolutely sure that you understand the directions and that you administer the proper dosage. Never give a child who is under the age of 6 a cough or cold medication that contains over 10 percent alcohol.

3. *Children 6 to 11 years of age:* In general, administer half the adult dose of cold and cough medications to children between these ages.

ALTERNATIVES TO DRUGS

We have become a drug-happy society, with a tendency to use that magic bottle of pills to cure all kinds of ills and discomforts. In certain cases, however, children are better off when they undergo a treatment program that excludes—not includes—drugs. Let's examine two examples, bedwetting and hyperactivity.

BEDWETTING

Imipramine (sold under the brand names Tofranil and Presamine) was originally prescribed for severely depressed adults who suffered bouts of suicidal psychological depression. One of the side effects it consistently produced was difficulty in urination. Because it tended to make urination difficult, physicians started prescribing it for children who had a problem with wetting the bed.[4] But Imipramine brought along with its seemingly simple cure of bedwetting a host of other, more serious side effects: restlessness, difficulty in sleeping, nausea, tearfulness, nervousness, inability to concentrate, and irritability. Some children suffered from symptoms like constipation, anxiety, and weight loss.

Before you allow a doctor to prescribe *this or any drug* for your child, you should be aware of certain facts associated with its use:

1. *The long-range effects are unknown.* Doctors have not yet been able to determine the long-term effects of the drug on a child's growth and development.

2. *Serious side effects result in children under 6.* Since many bedwetters are five or younger, the drug really shouldn't be considered as a part of their therapy.

3. *No drug should be used when bedwetting is only an occasional problem or when the bedwetting episode is clearly related to emotional stress* (such as a death in the family). A child who is undergoing emotional stress or who has experienced a crisis that has caused the bedwetting should not be given any kind of drug. Young children especially do not understand drugs, and they may become even more distraught and upset at the prospect of taking the medication.

4. *Drugs don't really cure the problem.* They simply make it difficult for the child to urinate. When the drug is discontinued, most children resume wetting the bed.

5. *A drug can hide the real problem.* A drug, administered to a child to curb bedwetting, might keep a doctor from carefully examining the child to determine whether the bedwetting is caused by a serious disease of some kind. Some children who wet the bed do so because they have a serious urinary infection; others have a small bladder capacity, an abnormally formed bladder, or some other physical defect. Any child who experiences consistent or even occasional bedwetting should be given a complete physical examination, and the doctor should try to get to the source of the problem instead of simply treating the symptom.

316 drugs and children

Nonmedicinal Treatment

What are the alternatives to drug therapy for children who wet the bed? First of all, have the child examined completely by a competent doctor who is willing to spend the time to search out a possible physical cause. Then, as a parent, you can do the following:

1. *Don't lose your cool.* Children need to be accepted and to know that they are loved during times of sadness.

2. *Don't punish them.* Since many cases of bedwetting are caused by emotional stress (such as the arrival of a new baby or the fear of beginning school), punishment only makes matters worse. You should adopt a positive attitude and work to reinforce good behavior instead of punishing bad behavior.

3. *Don't ridicule children in front of their brothers and sisters or in front of friends.* This is a personal problem that should be kept personal between you and the young person with the problem.

4. *Make a chart, and let children keep track of wet and dry nights.* Don't punish them for the wet nights, but reward them for the dry ones. Praise them freely for the times that they stay dry. By asking them to mark the chart, you help them understand that they are responsible for their own actions.

5. *When children wet the bed, help them clean up.* Assist them in removing the wet sheets and other bedding and in putting them into a place appropriate for dirty linens, The first few times you can help, but then make them do it themselves. Again, this kind of assignment helps children understand that they are responsible for their own actions. Before you make such an assignment, though, you should make sure that they know how to remove the soiled bedding, how to place fresh bedding on the bed, and where to put the wet sheets. If they do not know the proper procedure, their frustration serves only to increase their emotional stress.

6. *Restrict children's fluid intake a few hours prior to bedtime.* Don't make a big deal out of denying the drink. If they ask for a glass of milk, calmly say that you don't think it's a good idea because it's so close to bedtime and that they would have to wake up in the middle of the night to go to the bathroom. If they insist on having the milk (or water or juice), let them have it, but give them only a portion of what they normally drink.

7. *Help bed-wetting children wake up to use the bathroom.* If children seem unable to overcome the problem at first, you and your spouse might take turns waking them up and taking them to the bathroom at night. It may be difficult to judge exactly when children should be awakened, but the fact that someone comes to help may be reassuring and may help them overcome the problem.

8. *If you can't help in any other way, consider buying a battery-operated device that sounds an alarm when your child starts to urinate.* Two that are sold widely are Wee Alarm and Wee-Alert. This sort of device is placed under the child's sheet; when a drop or two of urine contacts two electrodes, a circuit is closed and the alarm sounds, waking the child. If you decide to use such a device, you should follow some specific guidelines:

> • Make sure that you completely explain the apparatus to the bedwetter (what it is for), and make sure he or she understands that it will not hurt in any way.

> • Make sure your child understands how the device works. You might want to put it in place, set the alarm, and spill a few drops of water on it to let the child see and hear what happens.

> • Teach the child how to set the alarm.

> • Tell the child what is expected. Explain that when the alarm goes off, it is time to get up and go to the bathroom. Explain also that when he or she comes back from the bathroom, the alarm must be reset. You might have to wake up and take the child to the bathroom for the first week or two until he or she gets used to the device and the alarm.

> • Provide a great deal of assurance. Make sure the child understands that the alarm is not a punishment, but a help. Describe the alarm as a friend that will help to stop the bedwetting problem.

> • Have the child sleep without pajama bottoms. The alarm is more efficient and works quicker if the urine doesn't have to penetrate pajamas or a nightgown before activating the buzzer.

> • Continue the treatment for about a month after the child has stopped wetting the bed.

HYPERACTIVITY (HYPERKINESIS)
About 10 percent of all children—about 5 million children in the United States—suffer from *hyperkinesis,* a disease that causes strenuous physical activity, distractibility, impatience, impulsiveness, and an inability to concentrate.[5] Of course, all children manifest one or more of

these symptoms sometimes; hyperkinetic children are ones whose symptoms disrupt their normal lifestyles and negatively affect their ability to make and keep friends, to get along with members of their families, or to perform normally in school. Hyperkinetic children may have normal I.Q.s yet do poorly in school because they can't seem to sit still for even five minutes at a time. Disruptive behavior often results in temper tantrums, and these children are often the victims of wide swings in mood.

Researchers attempting to find a cause and a cure for hyperkinesis found a startling irony: *Amphetamines,* which are used by adults to keep them awake and stimulate them, actually work to calm down hyperkinetic children. Benzedrine, Dexedrine, Ritalin, and Cylert—all powerful amphetamines—began to be prescribed widely in the treatment of children who seemed to be hyperkinetic.

Do these drugs really work? Or do they just work against symptoms? Amphetamines can combat the nervousness, the irritability, the tearfulness, the spurts of physical activity, and the inability to concentrate. But amphetamines do not cure hyperkinesis. Results of in-depth studies show that children who were treated with amphetamines are the same as children who were not treated, once the amphetamines are no longer administered.

What about side effects? Even though the drugs seem to work in calming the children down, they involve some real concerns. A major side effect that should keep doctors from prescribing amphetamines is their stunting of growth. A number of others also result in physical damage and emotional stress.

Nonmedicinal Treatment

What are the alternatives? Recent research reveals that hyperkinesis may actually be an allergic reaction—the child's way of reacting to certain foods and chemicals, most notably artificial flavors and colors found in many processed foods. San Francisco allergy specialist Dr. Ben Feingold has come up with a diet that includes the following restrictions:

1. *Eliminate any foods that contain artificial colors or flavors from your child's diet.* These include foods such as candy bars, powdered drink mixes, soft drinks, hot dogs, luncheon meats, and ready-to-eat cereals. Even some of the flavored toothpastes especially designed for children contain harmful color and flavor additives.

2. *Never give your child medicine or vitamins that are colored or flavored.*

3. *Don't let your child take aspirin.* The salicylate promotes hyperactivity.

4. *Eliminate from your child's diet all fruits and vegetables that contain the natural chemical salicylate.* These include prunes, peaches, raspberries, strawberries, apples, apricots, currants, grapes, oranges, cherries, and cucumbers. You might try reintroducing some of these, one at a time, to your child's diet after you have eliminated them for a period of six weeks. If you introduce them one at a time, you can discern whether any of them cause a reaction and can then consider permanent elimination from the diet.

GENERAL GUIDELINES

To best protect your children from becoming poisoned by drugs (either through their own clumsy attempts at taking the drugs or through your unknowledgeable administration of them), consider these guidelines:

1. *Keep all drugs out of the reach of children.* You read this caution on labels constantly, but it's probably the most important piece of advice you receive on preventing the misuse of drugs. If you have a locked cabinet, use it to store drugs. Keep your cleaning solutions, furniture polish, and cleansers there, too. Think twice before you carelessly leave a bottle of medicine on a nightstand, next to the bathroom sink, or in the cabinet where the child goes every morning for toothpaste. Keep hazardous substances in their original containers. Do not change or combine medication in a different container. And don't change medications to containers that are normally not used for medications. Children may not know that the change has occurred and inadvertently try the contents of the new container. Dispose of unused, old, or unwanted medications by flushing them down the toilet. Then, wash the container out so no residue of the medicine remains.

2. *Ask your pharmacist to put all your prescriptions into child-proof packaging.* Bottles with lids that are difficult to open are widely available in pharmacies everywhere, and your pharmacist will be happy to put your medicine into such a container.

3. *Never tell your children that medicine is candy in an effort to get them to take it.*

4. *Ask your pharmacist to fill a child's prescription with an unflavored pill or liquid if one is available.* A child is much less likely to seek a nasty-tasting solution in the bathroom cabinet than one that tastes like cherries.

5. *Ask your doctor to write down any instructions when prescribing a medicine for your child.*

6. *Never give any medicine to a child under the age of 2 unless your doctor prescribes it.*

7. *Read the labels when you buy over-the-counter remedies for a child's cold or cough.* Many major manufacturers make medicines for children; if one is available, choose it. Call your doctor or pharmacist if the label is unclear or if it gives no precise instructions regarding dosages for children.

8. *Never give your children medicine in the dark.* You should administer medicine in a well-lighted room and double-check the label on the medicine to make sure that you have the right one. Don't stagger into the bathroom in the dark, reach into the cluttered medicine cabinet, pull out the bottle that you think contains your child's cough syrup, and fumble down the hall to give him a spoonful in the dark—so you don't wake him up too much—only to find that you have administered a potent formula prescribed for your husband, who is suffering from bronchitis.

9. *Don't let your children see you taking medicine.* Children are great imitators, and they'll mimic anything they see you do.

10. *Don't use medicine as a threat.* For instance, don't tell children that if they don't pick up their toys, they'll have to gag down a spoonful of castor oil. Children should understand that a drug is not a method of punishment.

11. *Help children understand the purpose of medicine.* Tell them that medicine is used to make sick people better, and that people who are already well have no need to take medicine. Help them understand that medicine is neither a reward nor a punishment, but that it has a definite purpose and that it should be used only for that purpose.

12. *Be prepared for accidental poisoning.* Have Syrup of Ipecac or Activated Charcoal on hand to help induce vomiting when that is indicated. Keep the number of the nearest poison control center next to your telephone, and call for help if your child accidentally poisons himself.

13. *Watch children carefully after you have given them medication of any kind.* Call your doctor if children begin to act in an unusual way or if they manifest any out-of-the-ordinary symptoms. Call your doctor if in doubt.

By following these guidelines, you can take an active part in protecting your children against the kinds of tragedies that result from the misuse and abuse of drugs, both prescription and over-the-counter. Your patience and consideration in helping them understand the nature of drugs give them a lifelong gift of good experiences with drugs, as well as a lifetime free of the harm that can result from ignorance and the careless use of medication.

chapter notes

Chapter 1

[1]Editors of *Consumer Guide*, "Nonprescription Drugs" (Skokie, Ill.: Publications International, Ltd., Fall, 1979), p. 5.

[2]*Consumer Guide*, p. 7.

[3]The Food and Drug Administration, the United States Department of Health, Education, and Welfare, *We Want You To Know What We Know About Medicines Without Prescriptions* (Washington, D.C.: Government Printing Office, 1973).

[4]Richard Bauman, " 'Harmless' Drugs and Driving," *Life and Health* (March 1978), pp. 16–17.

[5]Morton K. Rubinstein, *A Doctor's Guide to Non-Prescription Drugs* (New York: Signet Books, 1977), p. 25.

[6]"Drugs Can Skew Clinical Tests," *FDA Consumer* (July/August 1979), pp. 27–28.

[7]Keith W. Sehnert, *How to be Your Own Doctor—Sometimes* (New York: Grossett & Dunlap, Inc., 1975), p. 19.

[8]DeWitt F. Helm, Jr., "Self-Medication: Its Present and Future As a Vital Part of Total Health Care," *American Druggist* (April 1977), pp. 38, 43, 62.

Chapter 2

[1]Editors of *Consumer Guide*, *Nonprescription Drugs* (Skokie, Ill.: Publications International, Ltd., Fall, 1979), pp. 21–23.

[2]Rubinstein, p. 5.

[3]Consumer Reports, *The Medicine Show* (New York: Pantheon Books, 1977), p. 27.

[4]Rubinstein, pp. 1–4.

[5]Robert J. Benowicz, *Non-Prescription Drugs and Their Side Effects* (New York: Grosset & Dunlap, 1977), p. 24.

[6]Erwin DiCyan and Lawrence Hessman, *A Guide to the Selection and Use of Medicines You Can Get Over-the-Counter for Safe Self-Medication* (New York: Simon and Schuster, 1972), p. 25; Consumer Reports, p. 29.

[7]DiCyan and Hessman, pp. 25–26.

[8]DiCyan and Hessman, pp. 27–30.

[9]Richard Harkness, *OTC Handbook: What to Recommend and Why* (Oradell, N.J.: Medical Economics, Inc., 1977), pp. 4–6.

[10]DiCyan and Hessman, pp. 31–33.

[11]DiCyan and Hessman, pp. 31–33.

[12]Harkness, p. 1.

[13]Harkness, p. 2.

[14]Harkness, pp. 2–4.

[15]Harkness, p. 2.

[16]Harkness, p. 5.

[17]Harkness, pp. 2–4.

[18]Ibid.

[19]Benowicz, pp. 25–27.

[20]Rubinstein, pp. 10–11.

[21]Consumer Reports, p. 42.

[22]Rubinstein, p. 26; DiCyan and Hessman, p. 36.

[23]Rubinstein, p. 25.

[24]Rubinstein, p. 25.

[25]Rubinstein, pp. 26–27.

[26]Rubinstein, pp. 26–30; Harkness, pp. 9–15.

[27]John E. Cormier and Bobby G. Bryant, "Cold and Allergy Products," *Handbook of Nonprescription Drugs*, 6th edition (Washington, D.C.: American Pharmaceutical Association, 1979), pp. 87–88.

[28]Harkness, p. 15.

[29]Consumer Reports, p. 45.

[30]Rubinstein, p. 30.

[31]Consumer Reports, p. 48.

[32]Michael Barletta, "What Every Pharmacist Should Know About Influenza," *American Druggist* (October 1978), pp. 68, 72–75.

Chapter 3

[1]Leon Gruberg, "What You Should Know About Laxatives," *American Druggist* (June 1976), p. 51.

[2]Roy C. Darlington, "Laxative Products," in *Handbook of Nonprescription Drugs* (Washington, D.C.: American Pharmaceutical Association, 1977), pp. 37–48.

[3]Rubinstein, p. 56.

[4]Rubinstein, pp. 57–59.

[5]Benowicz, pp. 66–67.

[6]Ghislain Devroede, "A Commonsense Approach to Overcoming Constipation," *Drug Therapy* (November 1978), pp. 114–115.

[7]Rubinstein, p. 59; Benowicz, pp. 65–66.

[8]Rubinstein, p. 59; Benowicz, pp. 65–66.

[9]Harkness, pp. 23–28. Lawrence W. Lamb, ed., *The Health Letter,* Vol. XII, No. 8 (October 27, 1978), San Antonio, Texas: Communications, Inc.

[10]Benowicz, p. 74.

[11]R. Leon Longe, "Antidiarrheal and Other Gastrointestinal Products," in *Handbook of Nonprescription Drugs,* 6th ed. (Washington, D.C.: American Pharmaceutical Association, 1979), p. 25.

[12]Rubinstein, pp. 48–54.

[13]Benowicz, pp. 77–78.

[14]Rubinstein, p. 52; Benowicz, p. 76–77.

[15]Rubinstein, pp. 52–53.

[16]Benowicz, pp. 77–78.

[17]Rubinstein, p. 67.

[18]Rubinstein, pp. 68–69.

[19]Rubinstein, pp. 67–68; Benowicz, p. 84.

[20]Rubinstein, pp. 70—71.

[21]Benowicz, p. 83.

[22]Benowicz, p. 83; Rubinstein, p. 70.

[23]Benowicz, p. 85.

[24]Harkness, pp. 57–59.

Chapter 4
[1]Benowicz, p. 24.

[2]W. Kent Van Tyle, "Internal Analgesic Products," in *Handbook of Nonprescription Drugs* (Washington, D.C.: American Pharmaceutical Association, 1977), p. 114.

[3]Benowicz, pp. 14–15.

[4]Benowicz, pp. 13–14.

[5]Harkness, pp. 37–39.

[6]Harkness, p. 38; Richard S. Farr, "Aspirin: Good News, Bad News," *Saturday Review* (November 1972), pp. 60–63.

[7]James F. Toole, "Can An Aspirin a Day Keep a Stroke Away?" *Executive Health* (January 1979), p. 3.

[8]DiCyan and Hessman, p. 110.

[9]Rubinstein, p. 114.

[10]Rubinstein, p. 124.

[11]Paul Shierkowski and Nancy Burdock, "External Analgesic Products," in *Handbook of Nonprescription Drugs* (Washington, D.C.: American Pharmaceutical Association, 1977), p. 289.

[12]Rubinstein, p. 136.

[13]Shierkowski and Burdock, p. 289.

[14]Shierkowski and Burdock, p. 290.

[15]Shierkowski and Burdock, p. 290.

[16]Shierkowski and Burdock, p. 292.

[17]Rubinstein, p. 155.

[18]Harkness, p. 98.

Chapter 5
[1]Consumer Reports, *The Medicine Show* (New York: Pantheon Books, 1977), p. 80.

[2]Rubinstein, pp. 25–36.

[3]Benowicz, p. 56.

[4]Benowicz, pp. 55–56; Rubinstein, p. 37.

⁵Rubinstein, p. 43.

⁶Harkness, p. 22.

⁷Rubinstein, p. 40.

⁸Benowicz, pp. 55–56.

⁹Harkness, pp. 17–18; Rubinstein, pp. 40–43.

¹⁰William R. Garnett, "Antacid Products," in *Handbook of Nonprescription Drugs* (Washington, D.C.: American Pharmaceutical Association, 1977), p. 7.

¹¹Harkness, pp. 18–20.

¹²Consumer Reports, pp. 83–84.

¹³Consumer Reports, pp. 89–90.

Chapter 6
¹Nathan A. Hall and James W. McFadden, "Burn and Sunburn Products," in *Handbook of Nonprescription Drugs* (Washington, D.C.: American Pharmaceutical Association, 1977), p. 271.

²Hall and McFadden, p. 271.

³John Henderson, *Emergency Medical Guide* (New York: McGraw-Hill Book Company, 1973), p. 240.

⁴Hall, p. 271.

⁵Henderson, p. 237.

⁶Hall, p. 271.

⁷Hall, pp. 272–274.

⁸Harkness, pp. 61–63.

⁹Henderson, p. 236.

¹⁰Henderson, p. 241.

¹¹"We've Been Asked How to Deal with the Sun," *U.S. News & World Report* (July 14, 1975), p. 62.

¹²"We've Been Asked How to Deal with the Sun," p. 62.

¹³"You and the Sun and Those Tanning Lotions," *Changing Times* (June 1977), p. 19.

¹⁴"Help For Your Sunburn-Prone Patients," *Patient Care* (June 1, 1976), pp. 41–42.

¹⁵"Help For Your Sunburn-Prone Patients," p. 43.

¹⁶Paula Siegel, "Convincing Patients About the Dangers of Excessive Solar Exposure," *Practical Psychology for Physicians* (July/August 1974), p. 68.

¹⁷"You and the Sun and Those Tanning Lotions," p. 20.

[18]Annabel Hecht, "Sunbathing Without Burning," *FDA Consumer* (June 1978), p. 22.

[19]Hecht, p. 22; "Help For Your Sunburn-Prone Patients," pp. 42–45.

Chapter 7
[1]Rubinstein, p. 107.

[2]Rubinstein, pp. 104–105.

[3]Harkness, pp. 53–55.

[4]Keith O. Miller, "Optic Products," in *Handbook of Nonprescription Drugs* (Washington, D.C.: American Pharmaceutical Association, 1977), p. 219.

[5]Miller, p. 223.

[6]Consumer's Guide, p. 153.

[7]Harkness, p. 124.

[8]Miller, p. 224.

[9]*Consumer Guide*, p. 153.

[10]Miller, p. 225.

[11]Rubinstein, p. 139.

[12]Glenn D. Appelt, "Weight Control Products," in *Handbook of Nonprescription Drugs* (Washington, D.C.: American Pharmaceutical Association, 1977), p. 177.

[13]Appelt, p. 177.

[14]Appelt, p. 179.

[15]Appelt, p. 181.

[16]Harkness, pp. 102–103.

[17]James P. Caro, "Sleep Aid and Sedative Products," in *Handbook of Nonprescription Drugs* (Washington, D.C.: American Pharmaceutical Association, 1977), p. 185.

[18]Benowicz, p. 49.

[19]Rubinstein, pp. 168–169.

[20]Benowicz, p. 48.

[21]Benowicz, pp. 48–49.

[22]Harkness, pp. 49–50.

[23]Judith Willis, "Biggest Recall of All Hits Sleep-Aid Products," *FDA Consumer* (July/August 1979), pp. 22–23.

[24]Harkness, pp. 50–51.

25Rubinstein, pp. 167–168.

26James P. Caro and Charles A. Walker. "Sleep Aid, Sedative, and Stimulant Products," in *Handbook of Nonprescription Drugs*, sixth edition (Washington, D.C.: American Pharmaceutical Association, 1979), p. 233.

27Caro and Walker.

28Benowicz, p. 53.

29Caro and Walker, p. 234.

30Benowicz, p. 51.

31Benowciz, p. 111.

32Benowicz, p. 112.

33Benowicz, p. 113.

34Benowicz, pp. 113, 115.

35Benowicz, p. 112.

36Benowicz, p. 100.

37Benowicz, pp. 101–102.

38Benowicz, p. 100; Nicholas G. Popovich, "Foot Care Products," in *Handbook of Nonprescription Drugs*, sixth edition (Washington, D.C.: American Pharmaceutical Association, 1979), p. 440.

Chapter 8
1Lynne Lamberg, "Your Doctor's Prescription: Is It Greek To You?" *Better Homes and Gardens* (February 1977), pp. 47–51.

2Anabel Hecht, "On Reading Prescriptions," *FDA Consumer* (December 1976–January 1977), pp. 17–18. Brent Q. Hafen and Brenda Peterson, *Medicines and Drugs*, 2nd ed. (Philadelphia: Lea and Febiger, 1978), pp. 38–44.

3Hecht, p. 18.

Chapter 10
1"Will PPI's Affect Your Patient's Attitudes?" *Patient Care* (February 15, 1979), p. 195.

2"Holding Down Prescription Drug Costs," *FDA Consumer* (December 1975–January 1976), pp. 9–10; "How to Pay Less for Prescription Drugs," *Consumer Reports* (January 1975), pp. 48–52; and "Prescription Drugs—the War Over Secret Prices," *The Kiplinger Magazine* (February 1973), pp. 13–16.

3Florence and Gerald Schumacher, "Rx for Choosing a Pharmacist," *Family Health/Today's Health* (June 1977), pp. 48–49.

4James W. Long, *The Essential Guide to Prescription Drugs* (New York: Harper and Row, 1977), pp. 14–16.

[5]Charlotte Isler, "Teaching the Elderly to Avoid Accidental Drug Abuse," *RN* (November 1977), pp. 39–42.

Chapter 11

[1]James W. Long, *The Essential Guide to Prescription Drugs* (New York: Harper and Row, 1977), pp. 711–717.

[2]Information for this section, except where otherwise noted, was taken from Brent Q. Hafen and Brenda Peterson, *Medicines and Drugs*, 2nd ed. (Philadelphia, Penn.: Lea and Febiger, 1978), pp. 29–35.

[3]Long, p. 703.

[4]Anabel Hecht, "Controls Urged on Top Rx Pain Drug," *FDA Consumer* (November 1976), p. 19.

[5]E. Stanton Shoemaker, *et al.*, "Estrogen Treatment of Postmenopausal Women," *JAMA* (October 3, 1977), p. 1529.

Chapter 12

[1]Margaret Morrison, "Cosmetics," *FDA Consumer* (April 1977), p. 18.

[2]Edwin Kiester, "Ugly Truths About Today's Beauty Aids," *Today's Health* (June 1971), p. 17.

[3]Kiester, p. 17.

[4]Morrison, p. 18.

[5]Deborah Chase, "Inside the Laboratories of the Beauty Makers," *Family Health/Today's Health* (June 1976), p. 54.

[6]Morrison, p. 18.

Chapter 13

[1]Joe Graedon, *The People's Pharmacy* (New York: St. Martin's Press, 1976), pp. 92–96.

[2]The information in the following section is taken from L. Kirk Benedict, "O-T-C Dental Drug Products: A Review," *U.S. Pharmacist* (May 1977), pp. 40–49; and "Toothpaste," *Consumer Reports* (April 1972), pp. 251–54.

[3]Robert L. Day, "Dental Products" in *Handbook of Nonprescription Drugs* (Washington, D.C.: American Pharmaceutical Association, 1977), p. 251.

Chapter 14

[1]This and the following information is taken from Adelaide P. Farah, "Soap," *Family Health* (November 1977), pp. 41, 60–61.

[2]"Toilet Soaps," *Consumer Reports* (March 1977), p. 128.

[3]"Soap," p. 60.

[4]"Soaps That Claim to Kill Germs and Odors," *Changing Times* (May 1975), pp. 13–15.

[5]"Soaps That Claim to Kill Germs and Odors," pp. 13–15.

[6]Margaret Morrison, " 'Hypoallergenic' Cosmetics," *FDA Consumer* (April 1978) p. 13.

[7]The following information is taken from Margaret Morrison, "Cosmetics: The Substances Beneath the Form," *FDA Consumer* (April 1977), pp. 19–20.

[8]Morrison, " 'Hypoallergenic' Cosmetics," p. 13; " 'Hypoallergenic' Cosmetics," *FDA Consumer* (June 1974), pp. 17–18.

[9]Graedon, p. 96.

[10]Adelaide P. Farah, "Be Armed Against Perspiration," *Family Health/Today's Health* (June 1976), p. 52.

[11]Farah, "Be Armed," p. 52.

[12]Morrison, "Cosmetics: The Substance Beneath the Form," p. 21.

[13]Graedon, pp. 97–98.

[14]Farah, "Be Armed," pp. 52, 58.

Chapter 15
[1]Laurence H. Miller and Angela A. Martin, "What You Should Know About Acne," *Pharmacy Times* (June 1977), p. 46.

[2]"Treatment and Management of Acne," *American Druggist* (December 1, 1974), pp. 46–48; Miller and Martin, pp. 47–48.

[3]"Treatment and Management of Acne," pp. 46–48.

[4]Robert G. Pietrusko, "Anti-Acne Aids," *The New Environment of Pharmacy* (November/December, 1976), p. 8.

[5]Graedon, pp. 337–39; "Treatment and Management of Acne," p. 49; Miller and Martin, p. 49; Melva Weber, "Acne Myths and Facts," *Family Health* (August 1975), p. 45.

[6]Graedon, pp. 335–37.

[7]Graedon, p. 339.

[8]Jonathan Zizmor and John Foreman, "For the New Year: Clearer, Cleaner Skin!" *Family Health/Today's Health* (January 1978), pp. 14–15; Weber, pp. 43–45; "Treatment and Management of Acne," p. 48.

Chapter 16

[1]"What You Should Know About Shampoos," *American Druggist* (August 15, 1974), p. 29.

[2]"Shampoos," *Consumer Reports* (November 1976), pp. 618–19.

[3]Charles F. Barfknecht, "Dandruff and Its Control," *U.S. Pharmacist* (March 1977), p. 48.

[4]Barfknecht, p. 49.

[5]Jane Heenan, "If You're Coloring Your Hair," *FDA Consumer* (November 1974), pp. 23–27.

[6]Joseph Hanlon, "Tint of Suspicion," *New Scientist* (May 11, 1978) pp. 352–56; Annabel Hecht, "Hair Dyes: A Look At Safety and Regulation," *FDA Consumer* (June 1978), pp. 16–19.

[7]"Bare Facts About Hair Removal," *Family Health* (September 1977), p. 11.

[8]Grace Lichtenstein, "Is Electrolysis For You?" *Family Health* (November 1977), pp. 33, 39.

Chapter 17

[1]Warren E. Schaller and Charles R. Carroll, *Health, Quackery, and the Consumer* (Philadelphia: W. B. Saunders Company, 1976), p. 33.

[2]Carol Bishop, *The Book of Home Remedies and Herbal Cures* (London: Octopus Books Limited, 1979), pp. 162, 170, 174.

[3]Schaller and Carroll, p. 33.

[4]Alex Comfort, "Folk Medicine Isn't All Bunk," *Medical Opinion* (November 1976), p. 47.

[5]Nelson Coon, *Using Plants for Healing* (Emmaus, Penn.: Rodale Press, 1979), p. 4.

[6]Graedon, pp. 53–56.

Chapter 18

[1]M. R. Stuart, "Herbalism," *Nursing Times,* (September 25, 1975), p. 1528.

[2]Carol Bishop, *The Book of Home Remedies and Herbal Cures* (London: Octopus Books Limited, 1979), p. 13.

[3]William H. Hylton, *The Rodale Herb Book* (Emmaus, Penn.: Rodale Press Book Division, 1974) pp. 41, 45, 47.

[4]"Back to Folk Medicine: The Pros and Cons," *Medical World News,* (December 1, 1973), p. 68.

[5]Siri Von Reis Altschul, "Exploring the Herbarium," *Scientific American* (May 1977), p. 99.

[6]Stuart, p. 1530. Von Reis Altschul, p. 99.

[7]Michael Tierra, *The Way of Herbs* (Santa Cruz, California: Unity Press, 1980).

[8]Edward Bauman, *et al.*, eds. *The Holistic Health Handbook*, Berkeley, Cal.; (And/Or Press, 1978), p. 135.

[9]Bishop, pp. 152–174.

[10]Bauman, *et al.*, pp. 124–125.

[11]Bauman, *et al.*, p. 133.

[12]Compiled by Ginny Clark, from *Well-Being*, edited by Barbara Salat and David Copperfield (Garden City, NY: Anchor Books/Doubleday, 1979), pp. 43–45.

[13]Nutrition Search, Inc., *Nutrition Almanac* (New York: McGraw-Hill, 1979), pp. 182–183.

[14]"Toxic Reactions to Plant Products Sold in Health Food Stores," *The Medical Letter* (April 6, 1979), pp. 29–31.

[15]Ara der Marderosian, "Medicinal Teas—Boon or Bane?" *Drug Therapy* (February 1977), p. 185.

[16]Ronald K. Siegel, "Herbal Intoxication: Psychoactive Effects from Herbal Cigarettes, Tea, and Capsules," *JAMA* (August 2, 1976).

[17]Linda Clark, *How to Improve Your Health: The Wholistic Approach* (New Canaan, Conn.: Keats Publishing, Inc., 1979), p. 52.

[18]der Marderosian, p. 185.

[19]"Herb Teas: How Safe?" *Consumers' Research Magazine* (March 1977), pp. 35–36.

[20]Ara der Marderosian, "It May Be Natural, But Is It Good for You?" *San Francisco Examiner* (June 8, 1977) p. 17.

Chapter 19

[1] Coon, p. 5.

[2]Linda Pelstring and Jo Ann Hauck, *Food to Improve Your Health* (Los Angeles: Pinnacle Books, 1975), p. 155.

[3]"Vitamins: Gear Their Intake to Your Special Needs," *Science Digest* (July 1979), p. 82.

[4]Joseph DiPalma, "Vitamins: Facts and Fancies," *RN* (July 1972), pp. 57–66.

[5]Erwin DiCyan, *Vitamins in Your Life* (New York: Simon & Schuster, Inc., 1974), p. 32.

[6]Rudolph Ballentine, *Diet and Nutrition: A Holistic Approach* (Honesdale, Penn.: The Himalayan International Institute, 1978), pp. 7–9.

[7]Robert J. Benowicz, *Vitamins and You* (New York: Grossett & Dunlap, Inc., 1979), pp. 125–126.

[8]The Editors of *Consumer Guide*, *The Vitamin Book* (New York: Simon & Schuster, Inc., 1979), p. 182.

[9]Mark Bricklin, *The Practical Encyclopedia of Natural Healing* (Emmaus, Penn.: Rodale Press, Inc., 1976), p. 182.

[10]Bricklin, p. 374.

[11]Morton Walker, *Total Health* (New York: Everest House, 1979), pp. 66–72.

[12]Lee R. Steiner, *Psychic Self-Healing for Psychological Problems* (Englewood Cliffs, N.J.: Prentice-Hall, Inc., 1977), p. 136.

[13]Brent Q. Hafen et al., *Food, Nutrition, and Weight Control* (Boston: Allyn and Bacon, 1980). The Editors of *Consumer Guide*, p. 179.

[14]Hafen et al.

[15]Benowicz, p. 124.

[16]*Consumer Guide*, *The Vitamin Book*, pp. 198–218; Nutrition Search, Inc., *Nutrition Almanac* (New York: McGraw-Hill Book Company, 1979), pp. 63–92.

Chapter 20

[1]Denis P. Burkitt, "The Link Between Low-Fiber Diets and Disease," p. 34.

[2]Joann J. Morris, et al., "Is Fiber the Answer to Constipation Problems in the Elderly? A Review of Literature," *International Journal of Nursing* (March 1978), pp. 107–113.

[3]"An Apple a Day . . ." *Nursing Times Community Outlook* (April 12, 1979), p. 93.

[4]Burkitt, p. 40.

[5]Bauman, et al., p. 121.

[6]Benowicz, p. 18.

[7]Benowicz, p. 20.

[8]Martha E. Rhodes, "Do You Believe This Food Myth?" *Science Digest* (October, 1979), p. 28.

[9]Ballentine, p. 59.

[10]Ballentine, p. 64.

[11]Hafen et al.

[12]J. A. Scharffenberg, "Diet and Heart Disease," *Life and Health*.

[13]Bauman, et al., p. 122. Scharffenberg, pp. 4–6. Lynne Scott et al., "The Help Your Heart Eating Plan," *Health Values: Achieving High Level Wellness*, 2:311 (November/December, 1978).

[14]Ballentine, pp. 102–103.

[15]Mort Walker, "Exploring the Yogurt Mistique," *Consumers Digest* (March/ April, 1978), p. 37.

[16]"Yogurt Cuts Lipids, Doctor Claims," *Medical World News* (March 19, 1979), p. 44.

[17]*Consumers Digest*, pp. 37–38.

[18]George Ohsawa, *Practical Guide to Far Eastern Macrobiotic Medicine* (Oroville, Ca: George Ohsawa Macrobiotics Foundation, 1976), p. 57.

[19]Ohsawa, p. 57.

[20]Ohsawa, p. 64.

[21]Norman D. Ford, *Good Health Without Drugs* (New York: St. Martin's Press, 1977), p. 86.

Chapter 21

[1]Editors of *Consumer Guide, Nonprescription Drugs* (Skokie, Ill.: Publications International, Ltd., Fall, 1979), p. 5.

[2]Mary W. Falconer, *et al.*, *The Drug, the Nurse, the Patient* (Philadelphia, Penn.: W. B. Saunders Company, 1968), pp. 31–32.

[3]Benjamin J. Kogan, *Health* (New York: Harcourt Brace Jovanovich, 1979), p. 389.

[4]Kogan, 370.

[5]Brent Q. Hafen and Brenda Peterson, *Medicines and Drugs*, 2nd ed. (Philadelphia, Penn.: Lea and Febiger, 1978), p. 66.

[6]Hafen and Peterson, p. 66.

[7]*Consumer Guide*, p. 11.

[8]United States Department of Health, Education, and Welfare, *Drug Allergy* [National Institute of Health, Washington, D. C.: Government Printing Office, 1974, DHEW Publication No. (NIH) 75–703].

[9]Cal Pierce, "Medicine on the Menu," *Life and Health* (July 1978), p. 11.

[10]Pierce, pp. 11–12.

[11]Martin L. Lambert, Jr., "Drug and Diet Interaction," *American Journal of Nursing*, Vol. 75, No. 3 (March 1975), pp. 402–406; Hafen and Peterson, pp. 75–76.

[12]Hafen and Peterson, pp. 76–79.

[13]Michael A. Barletta, "A Realistic Look at Drug Interactions," *American Druggist* (September 1978), p. 26.

[14]Midge Lashy Schildkraut, "Danger! Which Drugs Don't Mix with What," *Good Housekeeping* (November, 1976), p. 164.

[15]H. David Bergman, "Drug-Induced Diseases and Disorders," *The Apothecary* (July/August 1977), pp. 16–18, 56.

Chapter 22
[1]"What We Know About the Pill," *Changing Times* (July 1977), p. 21.

[2]"About New Report on 'The Pill,'" *U.S. News & World Report* (December 29, 1975), p. 46.

[3]*Changing Times*, p. 21.

[4]*Changing Times*, p. 21.

[5]*Changing Times*, p. 21.

[6]List compiled from Ron Gray, "How Safe Is the Pill?," World Health (August 1978), pp. 12–15; Patricia S. Coyne, "The Estrogen Controversy," *Private Practice* (February 1976), pp. 26–31; "The Pill: Weighing the Cancer Risk," *Emergency Medicine* (October 1977), p. 238; Social Welfare of Canada, *Report 1978: Oral Contraceptives*, 1978, pp. 1–15; and "What We Know About the Pill," pp. 22–23.

[7]*U.S. News & World Report*, p. 46.

[8]U.S. News & World Report, p. 46.

[9]Anita Johnson, "The Risks of Sex Hormones as Drugs," *Women and Health* (July/August, 1977), p. 9.

[10]Ronald M. Chez, "Taking Some Risk Out of the Pill," *Emergency Medicine* (October, 1977), p. 232.

[11]*Report 1978*, p. 14.

[12]*Report 1978*, p. 4.

[13]"Studies Show Smoking Raises 'Pill' Risk," *FDA Consumer* (November 1978), p. 3.

[14]Daphne A. Roe, "How the Pill Affects a Woman's Nutritional Status," *Medical Opinion* (September 1978), pp. 58–61; and Barbara Luke, "Think 'Nutrition' If She's On the Pill," *RN* (March 1976), pp. 33–37.

[15]Chez, pp. 231–237.

[16]Alvin Langer, Mona Devanesan, and Marco A. Pelosi, "Choosing the Appropriate Oral Contraceptive," *Drug Therapy* (June 1978), p. 120.

[17]Langer *et al.*, p. 119.

Chapter 23
[1]Molly J. Brog, "Is There a Relationship Between Birth Defects and Drugs We Commonly Use?" *Life and Health* (to be published).

[2]Leland Cooley and Lee Morrison Colley, *Pre-Medicated Murder* (Radnoe, Penn.: Chilton Book Company, 1974), p. 166.

[3]Thomas E. O'Brien and Carol E. McManus, "Drugs and the Human Fetus," *Grassroots* (March 1978 Supplement), p. 3. Information for the rest of the section on drug transferral from the mother to fetus is taken from this source.

[4]Information taken from Fehr, pp. 42–46; Jon M. Aase, "Environmental Causes of Birth Defects," *Continuing Education* (September 1975), pp. 39–46; O'Brien and McManus, pp. 9–13.

[5]Pat Horning, "Fetal Alcohol Syndrome—The Avoidable Tragedy," *Life and Health* (March 1979), p. 7.

[6]Horning, p. 6.

[7]Brog.

[8]Ann P. Streissguth, "Maternal Drinking and the Outcome of Pregnancy," *Grassroots* (September 1978), p. 30.

[9]Fritz Witti, "Alcohol and Birth Defects," *FDA Consumer* (May 1978), p. 23.

[10]Sumner J. Yaffe, "Drug Use During Pregnancy," *Drug Therapy* (June 1978), pp. 144–45.

[11]Laurel J. Stortz, "Unprescribed Drug Products and Pregnancy," *JOGN* (July/ August 1977), p. 11.

[12]Pauline Postotnik, "Drugs and Pregnancy," *FDA Consumer* (October 1978), p. 8.

[13]"Coffee May Perk Up Pregnant Mom, But Not Her Baby," *Medical World News* (April 17, 1978), p. 8.

[14]"Birth Defect Warning Asked for Caffeine," *FDA Consumer* (November 1978), p. 22.

[15]Paul. S. Weatherbee, Larry K. Olsen, and J. Robert Lodge, "Caffeine and Pregnancy," *Postgraduate Medicine*, Vol. 62. No. 3 (September 1977), pp. 64–69.

[16]Sidney S. Field, "What Smoking Does to Women," *Reader's Digest* (January 1976), p. 95.

[17]American Academy of Pediatrics, "Effects of Cigarette Smoking on the Fetus and Child," *Pediatrics*, Vol 57, No. 3 (March 1976), pp. 411–412.

[18]"Neonatal Narcotic Dependence," *National Clearinghouse for Drug Abuse Information* (February 1974), p. 2.

[19]B. Schenkel and H. Vorhers, "Nonprescription Drugs During Pregnancy: Potential Teratogenic and Toxic Effects Upon Embryo and Fetus," *Grassroots* (October 1974), pp. 1–2.

[20]Aase, pp. 44–45.

[21]Postotnik, p. 8.

[22]Lenor Rivera-Calimlim, "Drugs in Breast Milk," *Drug Therapy* (December 1977), p. 62.

[23]Peter E. Fehr, "Guidelines for Prescribing in Pregnancy," *Modern Medicine* (June 15, 1976), pp. 42–46.

Chapter 24

[1]Anabel Hecht, "Keeping Poisons and Children Apart," *FDA Consumer* (February 1979), p. 25.

[2]Brent Q. Hafen and Brenda Peterson, *Medicines and Drugs*, 2nd ed. (Philadelphia, Penn.: Lea and Febiger, 1978), p. 16.

[3]Hafen and Peterson, p. 16.

[4]Graedon, pp. 221–24.

[5]Graedon, pp. 224–28.

index

339